MICROCAPSULES AND OTHER CAPSULES

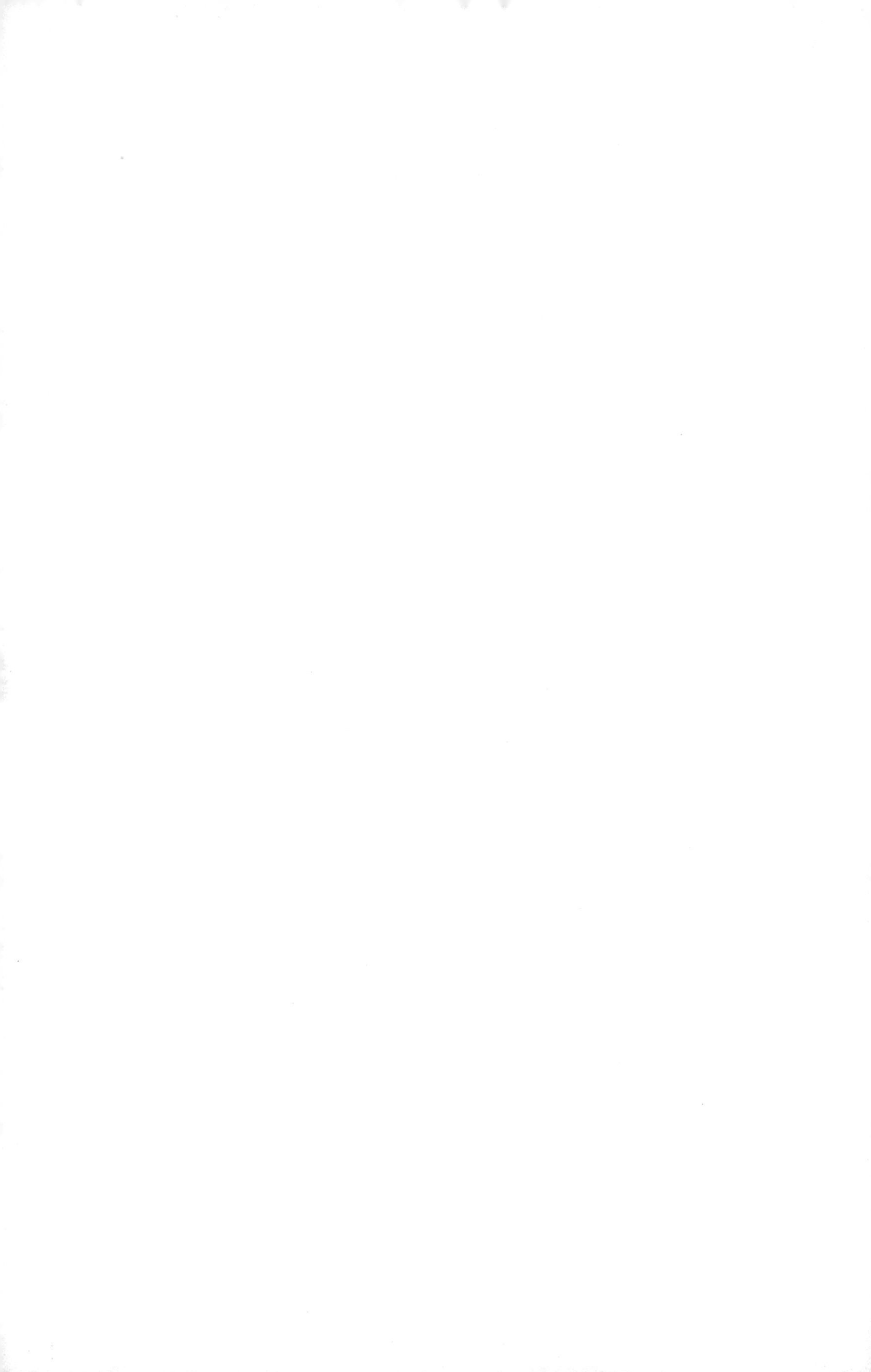

MICROCAPSULES AND OTHER CAPSULES

Advances Since 1975

M.H. Gutcho

NOYES DATA CORPORATION
Park Ridge, New Jersey, U.S.A.
1979

Library of Congress Catalog Card Number: 79-15917
ISBN: 0-8155-0766-6
Printed in the United States

Published in the United States of America by
Noyes Data Corporation
Noyes Building, Park Ridge, New Jersey 07656

Library of Congress Cataloging in Publication Data

Gutcho, M
Microcapsules and other capsules.

(Chemical technology review ; no. 135)
Includes indexes.
1. Microencapsulation--Patents. I. Title.
II. Series.
TS198.C33G89 621.7'57 79-15917
ISBN 0-8155-0766-6

FOREWORD

The detailed, descriptive information in this book is based on U.S. patents, issued since February 1976, that deal with microcapsules and other capsules. This title contains all recent advances since our previous titles *Microcapsules and Microencapsulation Techniques* published in 1976 and *Capsule Technology and Microencapsulation* published in 1972.

This book serves a double purpose in that it supplies detailed technical information and can be used as a guide to the U.S. patent literature in this field. By indicating all the information that is significant, and eliminating legal jargon and juristic phraseology, this book presents an advanced, commercially oriented review of recent advances in the manufacture and application of microcapsules and other capsules.

The U.S. patent literature is the largest and most comprehensive collection of technical information in the world. There is more practical, commercial, timely process information assembled here than is available from any other source. The technical information obtained from a patent is extremely reliable and comprehensive; sufficient information must be included to avoid rejection for "insufficient disclosure." These patents include practically all of those issued on the subject in the United States during the period under review; there has been no bias in the selection of patents for inclusion.

The patent literature covers a substantial amount of information not available in the journal literature. The patent literature is a prime source of basic commercially useful information. This information is overlooked by those who rely primarily on the periodical journal literature. It is realized that there is a lag between a patent application on a new process development and the granting of a patent, but it is felt that this may roughly parallel or even anticipate the lag in putting that development into commercial practice.

Many of these patents are being utilized commercially. Whether used or not, they offer opportunities for technological transfer. Also, a major purpose of this book is to describe the number of technical possibilities available, which may open up profitable areas of research and development. The information contained in this book will allow you to establish a sound background before launching into research in this field.

Advanced composition and production methods developed by Noyes Data are employed to bring these durably bound books to you in a minimum of time. Special techniques are used to close the gap between "manuscript" and "completed book." Industrial technology is progressing so rapidly that time-honored, conventional typesetting, binding and shipping methods are no longer suitable. We have by-passed the delays in the conventional book publishing cycle and provide the user with an effective and convenient means of reviewing up-to-date information in depth.

The table of contents is organized in such a way as to serve as a subject index. Other indexes by company, inventor and patent number help in providing easy access to the information contained in this book.

15 Reasons Why the U.S. Patent Office Literature Is Important to You –

1. The U.S. patent literature is the largest and most comprehensive collection of technical information in the world. There is more practical commercial process information assembled here than is available from any other source.

2. The technical information obtained from the patent literature is extremely comprehensive; sufficient information must be included to avoid rejection for "insufficient disclosure."

3. The patent literature is a prime source of basic commercially utilizable information. This information is overlooked by those who rely primarily on the periodical journal literature.

4. An important feature of the patent literature is that it can serve to avoid duplication of research and development.

5. Patents, unlike periodical literature, are bound by definition to contain new information, data and ideas.

6. It can serve as a source of new ideas in a different but related field, and may be outside the patent protection offered the original invention.

7. Since claims are narrowly defined, much valuable information is included that may be outside the legal protection afforded by the claims.

8. Patents discuss the difficulties associated with previous research, development or production techniques, and offer a specific method of overcoming problems. This gives clues to current process information that has not been published in periodicals or books.

9. Can aid in process design by providing a selection of alternate techniques. A powerful research and engineering tool.

10. Obtain licenses — many U.S. chemical patents have not been developed commercially.

11. Patents provide an excellent starting point for the next investigator.

12. Frequently, innovations derived from research are first disclosed in the patent literature, prior to coverage in the periodical literature.

13. Patents offer a most valuable method of keeping abreast of latest technologies, serving an individual's own "current awareness" program.

14. Copies of U.S. patents are easily obtained from the U.S. Patent Office at 50¢ a copy.

15. It is a creative source of ideas for those with imagination.

CONTENTS AND SUBJECT INDEX

INTRODUCTION

The techniques of microencapsulation, currently used successfully for a variety of commercial purposes, are expected to find other new and exciting applications. Microcapsules are composed of a polymeric skin or wall (shell) enclosing a core. The capsule wall is inert to the substance it contains, is strong enough to permit normal handling without rupture, and is relatively thin so as to permit a high core to wall ratio. The contents of the capsule are contained within the shell until released by means that serve to break, crush, melt, dissolve or rupture the capsule wall, or until the internal phase is caused to diffuse through the capsule wall.

Handling problems are facilitated when encapsulated compositions are used. Materials which would react with one another on contact can be individually encapsulated and then mixed without premature reaction. Liquid core microcapsules have low vapor pressure, therefore eliminating any toxicity hazard during handling. Microcapsules can be uniformly distributed on a coating or matrix body. They can be used to fill macrocapsules. Since the encapsulated fills are protected from air, moisture and contaminants, spoilage is reduced and shelf life increased.

Microcapsules are used advantageously in many fields. The encapsulation of volatile aromas and flavors protects them from physical oxidation and from thermal decomposition. For medicinals, encapsulation serves to mask unpleasant odor and taste, and to protect against oxidation and spoilage. In addition, encapsulation can be such that the medicament will be selectively absorbed in the intestine rather than the stomach, or released gradually to provide action over a long period of time.

Encapsulated perfumes can be coated on paper to make fragrance sheets. The polymeric capsule shell can be made susceptible to decomposition in certain environments, or be of a kind to permit diffusion through the capsule wall. This is particularly adapted to allow for the slow prolonged release of agricultural chemicals such as fungicides, herbicides and insecticides.

An important use of microcapsules is in pressure-sensitive, mark-forming, sheet material systems to replace carbon paper and typewriter ribbons. These systems may be autogenous, in which the encapsulated mark-forming components are all present on a single sheet. Or they may be of the transfer type, where the dye intermediate is encapsulated and coated on a transfer sheet, and "transferred" to a copy sheet which has an adsorbent coating containing material to coreact with the dye. When the dye-containing microcapsule is broken, colored marks appear.

The processes in this book are concerned with microcapsules having natural or synthetic materials as wall formers. The microencapsulation techniques encompass phase separation and polymerization as well as physical, interfacial and other methods. Many techniques are applicable to encapsulate a wide range of core materials. Others are particularly beneficial with a specific product in mind. The preparation and use of a large variety of microencapsulated products is described.

COMPLEX COACERVATION

SHOCK-PREVENTING AGENTS

Anionic High MW Polyelectrolyte plus Anionic Surface Active Agent

Conventionally known processes for preparing oil-containing microcapsules are described, for example, in the specification of U.S. Patent 2,800,457 and Japanese Patent 3875/62. The process of U.S. Patent 2,800,457 comprises the steps of:

(1) emulsifying a water-immiscible oil in an aqueous solution of a first hydrophilic colloid to be ionized in water (the first sol), (the emulsifying step);

(2) admixing an aqueous solution of a hydrophilic colloid in the emulsion of (1) forming the second sol, the first sol having an electric charge opposite to that of the second sol, and either adding water thereto or adjusting the pH thereof to cause coacervation, thus obtaining coacervates wherein the complex colloid is fixed to (i.e., surrounds) the individual oil drops (the coacervation step);

(3) cooling the coacervates to cause gelation thereof (the gelation step); and

(4) adjusting the pH to from 9 to 11 and adding a hardening agent (the hardening treatment).

The process of *H. Matsukawa, S. Katayama and M. Kiritani; U.S. Patent 3,970,585; July 20, 1976; assigned to Fuji Photo Film Co., Ltd., Japan* is an improvement of a well-known complex coacervation process for producing microcapsules. The preliminary steps of forming a coacervate dispersion of a complex gelatin-containing colloid (as the microcapsule wall material) deposited around individual oil droplets is well-known (U.S. Patent 2,800,457). To obtain the product microcapsules, the coacervate dispersion is cooled to gel the complex gelatin-containing colloid followed by hardening thereof by adding thereto a hardening agent and adjusting the pH to the alkaline region to promote hardening. The improvement in this process is in adding to the dispersion, after gelation but prior to hardening, a combination of the anionic high molecular weight electrolyte shock-preventing agent and an anionic surface active agent. The process is operable with any anionic high molecular weight electrolyte shock-preventing agent. Suitable surface active agents are: alkali metal naphthalene sulfonates such as methyl naphthalene potassium sulfonate, dodecyl naphthalene sodium sulfate, 2-butyl-3-ethoxy-naphthalene sodium sulfonate and their acid forms. The sodium or potassium salts of the naphthalene sulfonic acid-formalin condensates are suitable in addition to the free acid form of the condensate.

Suitable alkali metal polyoxyethylene sulfonates are ethyl polyoxyethylene sodium sulfonate, dodecyl polyoxyethylene sodium sulfonate, phenyl polyoxyethylene sodium sulfonate, etc. The potassium salts and the free acid forms are also suitable.

Suitable examples of the phenyl polyoxyethylene sulfuric acids are phenyl polyoxyethylene sulfuric acid, methyl phenyl polyoxyethylene sulfuric acid, and ethyl heptadecoxy phenyl polyoxyethylene sulfuric acid. The sodium and potassium salts of these acids are also suitable. Suitable sulfosuccinic acids are ethyl sulfosuccinic acid and octadecyl sulfosuccinic acid as well as their sodium and potassium salts. The complex coacervation process caused by water dilution or pH adjustment will suffice to prepare microcapsules containing an oily liquid according to the process.

Example 1: 10 parts of an acid-treated pigskin gelatin having an isoelectric point of 8.2 and 10 parts of gum arabic were dissolved in 50 parts of warm water at 40°C, and 0.15 part of Turkey red oil was added as an emulsifier. 50 parts of chlorinated diphenyl were added to the aqueous solution of the gelatin-gum arabic under vigorous stirring for emulsification to form an oil-in-water type emulsion. Stirring was discontinued when the size of the oil droplets became 6 to 10 μ. 310 parts of warm water at 40°C were added.

An aqueous solution of 5% acetic acid was added dropwise under mild stirring to adjust the pH to 4.35. The colloid accumulated around the oil droplets was gelled and solidified by cooling from the outside of the vessel while continuing the stirring. 4 parts of 37% aqueous formaldehyde solution were added when the liquid temperature reached 8°C.

Further, 25 parts of an aqueous solution (5%) of the sodium salt of carboxymethylcellulose (viscosity, 16 cp in 2% aqueous solution at 25°C; etherification degree, 0.75) as a shock-preventing agent and 6 parts of a 20% naphthalene sulfonic acid-formalin condensate (Lavelin S), as an anionic surface active agent, were added thereto.

Two minutes after the addition, while continuing the stirring, a 10% aqueous solution of sodium hydroxide was added dropwise over 20 minutes to adjust the pH of the liquid to 10.5. The viscosity of the capsule dispersion increased with pH and reached the maximum point at a pH of 7.5 to 8.0 and thereafter the pH decreased. The stirring was continued and the liquid temperature was raised to 40°C for 15 minutes to harden the wall film, and a mononuclear microcapsule containing chlorinated diphenyl as the nucleus having a heat resistance of above 125°C was obtained. The viscosity of the capsule dispersion system in individual steps is as follows.

	No Shock-Preventing Agent	Independent System Using Shock-Preventing Agent Only	Shock-Preventing Agent and Anionic Surface Active Agent
		.cp.	
After addition of formaldehyde	98	98	98
Shock-preventing agent	–	76	68
Anionic surface active agent	–	–	47
Maximum viscosity during pH conversion	coagulate	135	62

In the independent system 60 parts of a 5% aqueous solution of carboxymethylcellulose were used as a shock-preventing agent. The viscosity was measured by means of Brookfield type rotation viscometer. As is apparent from the above table, the system which does not contain a shock-preventing agent was coagulated in the pH conversion step. The independent system of shock-preventing agent gave multinuclear microcapsules without coagulation during the pH conversion step. Further, the system combining naphthalene sulfonic acid-formalin condensate, as the anionic surface active agent, was more remarkable in lowering viscosity and preventing an increase in viscosity both after addition and during the pH conversion step than that in the independent system.

Example 2: Example 1 was repeated except that combinations of shock-preventing agents and anionic surface active agents shown in the Tables 1 and 2 below were employed instead of the combination of the sodium salt of carboxymethylcellulose and naphthalene sulfonic acid-formalin condensate, respectively, used in Example 1. The viscosity values are shown in Table 3, and all of the combinations provided mononuclear (single emulsified droplet) microcapsules as compared to the use of the respective shock-preventing agents alone. In Table 1, DOEs represents degree of esterification and DOEt is degree of etherification.

Table 1

Compound No.	Shock-Preventing Agent	DOEs	DOEt
1	Sulfated cellulose*	0.75	–
2	Phosphated cellulose*	0.64	–
3	Carboxymethylhydroxyethylcellulose*	–	0.72
4	Sulfated hydroxyethylcellulose*	0.52	–
5	Phosphated hydroxyethylcellulose*	0.4	–
6	Carboxymethyl-starch*	–	0.65
7	Sulfated starch*	0.65	–
8	Phosphated starch*	0.45	–
9	Pectin	–	–
10	Pectic acid	–	–
11	Copolymer of acryloylmorpholine and vinylbenzenesulfonate**	–	–
12	Copolymer of acryloylmorpholine and acrylic acid***	–	–

*Sodium salt.
**Potassium salt, vinylbenezene sulfonate 53.7 mol %.
***Sodium salt, acrylic acid 50.6 mol %.

Table 2

Compound No.	Anionic Surface Active Agent (sodium salt)
I	Dodecyl naphthalene sulfonic acid
II	Naphthalene sulfonic acid-formalin condensate
III	Polyoxyethylene dodecyl sulfonic acid
IV	Methyl phenyl polyoxyethylene sulfuric acid
V	Diethyl ester of sulfosuccinic acid

Table 3

Shock-Preventing Agent	Anionic Surface Active Agent	Viscosity*	Maximum Viscosity**
1	–	74	143
1	III	52	68
2	–	86	167
2	II	46	48
3	–	65	120
3	V	50	82
4	–	73	135
4	I	56	74
5	–	94	170
5	IV	72	110
6	–	54	95
6	II	28	40
7	–	62	115
7	IV	41	63
8	–	71	130
8	V	48	74
9	–	85	170
9	I	65	120
10	–	90	175
10	III	67	115
11	–	78	164
11	II	45	77
12	–	85	158
12	V	70	115

*After adding shock-preventing agent.
**During pH conversion.

As is apparent from the above tables, particularly Table 3, the viscosity of the microcapsule dispersion system containing a combination of a shock-preventing agent and an anionic surface active agent, was more effective in lowering viscosity and preventing an increase in viscosity both after addition and during the pH conversion step than that of the microcapsule dispersion system containing only shock-preventing agents.

Polyelectrolytes Having Anionic Functional Groups

S. Katayama, H. Matsukawa, J. Matsuyama and M. Yamamoto; U.S. Patent Reissue 28,779; April 20, 1976; assigned to Fuji Photo Film Co., Ltd., Japan are concerned with producing mononuclear oil-containing microcapsules which are capable of being coated at higher speeds and which dry in a shorter period of time. This is accomplished by forming a film of polyvalent electrolyte colloid (second sol) around hydrophobic oil drops by the coacervation method to prepared coacervates, gelling the wall film of the coacervate and adding a shock-preventing agent.

Preparation of oil-containing microcapsules may be carried out by the complex coacervation method induced by water diluting or by pH control. That is, the formation of the complex coacervate from liquid-liquid phase separation is based upon an operation wherein two or more hydrophilic colloid sols are combined and one is separated in a colloid rich phase while the other is maintained in a colloid poor phase. At this time, the coacervated colloid must contain at least two hydrophilic colloids having opposite charges from each other, at least one of the colloids being gelled.

Examples of hydrophilic colloids are natural or synthetic high molecular weight compounds such as gelatin, casein, alginate, gum arabic, styrene-maleic anhydride copolymer and polyethylene-maleic anhydride copolymer.

The nucleus of the individual capsule may comprise natural mineral oils, animal oils, plant oils and synthetic oils. An anionic, cationic or nonionic surface active agent is used so as to emulsify or disperse an oily liquid into a nuclear material in water. It prevents reversing, i.e., the formation of a water-in-oil type emulsion.

An oil-in-water type emulsion can be obtained by emulsifying an oily liquid as the nuclear material in an aqueous colloid solution as the wall material. The emulsion is subjected to water diluting and pH control to accumulate coacervate around the emulsified oil drops. At the same time, the coacervation condition is preferably reduced in order to make mononuclear capsules.

The coacervate accumulated on the surface of the oil drop after the coacervation step is cooled from the outside to gel the wall film. For example, formaldehyde is added to harden the wall film and the pH of the system is controlled to alkalinity. This treatment for prehardening results in coagulation of the microcapsules under unstable coacervation conditions unless there is a shock-preventing agent. The hardening of the microcapsule wall is further advanced and the heat resistance of the formed capsule is increased by warming. Addition of the shock-preventing agent is carried out at a temperature lower than the setting point of the gelatin wall film, generally below 2°C, preferably below 15°C.

The capacity of the shock-preventing agent, depends upon the degree of polymerization of the cellulose and the degree of esterification or etherification. The higher the degree of polymerization, esterification and etherification, the better are the results in that the capacity of the shock-preventing agent is increased. However, in view of solubility and viscosity considerations, the degree of polymerization is preferably 50 to 500 and the degree of esterification or etherification is preferably 0.5 to 1.2. The shock-preventing agent may be present in an amount of about $\frac{1}{12}$ to $\frac{1}{2}$ the amount (by weight) of the two or more hydrophilic colloids having different charges.

The shock-preventing agent may simplify the hardening pretreatment of microcapsules under insufficient coacervation conditions to give a high concentration capsule liquid. Employing encapsulation by a combination of water dilution and pH control, as disclosed is U.S. Patent 2,800,457, the amount of water is 20.5 g per 1 g of the two or more colloids having different charges at a pH of

4.5. If the amount of water is reduced in that method, the capsules will be coagulated during the hardening pretreatment. However, by adding the shock-preventing liquid after the gelling operation, it is possible to reduce the amount of water to 15 g.

Shock-preventing agents which may be used are polyelectrolytes having an anionic functional group. Such polyelectrolytes include modified cellulose, an anionic starch derivative, an anionic acid polysaccharide, a condensate of naphthalene sulfonic acid and formalin, a hydroxyethylcellulose derivative, a copolymer of vinylbenzene sulfonate and a copolymer of sodium acrylate.

Example 1: Use of CMC Shock Preventer – 6 parts of an acid-treated gelatin having an isoelectric point of 7.8 and 6 parts of gum arabic were dissolved in 35 parts of water at 45°C. To the resulting solution were added 0.3 part of sodium alkylbenzenesulfonate as an emulsifier and then 35 parts of dichlorodiphenyl in which 2.0% of crystal violet lactone (CVL) had been dissolved to thus prepare an oil-in-water emulsion. The oil drop size was in a range of 8 to 12 microns. To 200 parts of an aqueous solution containing 0.08% of sodium sulfate at 45°C were added while stirring the foregoing emulsion, and 70% aqueous solution of acetic acid to adjust the pH to 4.3.

The system was cooled from the outside of a vessel to a liquid temperature of 8°C. Then, 3.0 parts of 37% formaldehyde and 25 parts of 7% aqueous solution of CMC (degree of etherification 0.95, degree of polymerization 250) were added. A 10% aqueous solution of caustic soda was added in 15 minutes to adjust the pH to 10.0. The viscosity at a pH of 7.5 was 110 cp (B_2 30 rpm). The solution was warmed to 50°C. The resulting capsules, 99% or more of which were mononuclear, had a heat resistance of 5 hours at 150°C.

Example 2: Use of Naphthalene Sulfonic Acid-Formalin Condensate – 10 parts of an acid-treated gelatin having an isoelectric point of 7.9 and 10 parts of gum arabic were dissolved in 50 parts of water at 40°C. To the solution, oil having 0.3 part of sodium alkylbenzene sulfonate was added thereto as an emulsifier. 60 parts of chlorinated paraffin having chlorination degree of 40% and molecular weight of 1,000 was added to the colloidal solution to form an oil-in-water emulsion. The average oil drop size reached 6 microns. 290 parts of 0.05% aqueous solution of sodium chloride at 45°C was added thereto.

While further stirring, 10% sulfuric acid was added in drops to adjust the pH to 4.3. The emulsion was cooled to 8°C from the outside to gel and fix the accumulated colloid walls. 3.5 parts of 37% formaldehyde solution was added, after which was added 25 parts of 20% aqueous solution of sodium salt of naphthalene sulfonic acid-formalin condensate. The pH of the capsule solution was adjusted to 6.5 over a period of 15 minutes.

Dropping of 10% caustic soda solution was then started. The viscosity of the microcapsule solution was 68 cp (B_1 60 rpm). The pH was adjusted to 8.0 after another 15 minutes, the viscosity being 440 cp (B_2 30 rpm). Alkali was further added in drops until the pH was 10.0. Thereafter, the liquid temperature was elevated to 50°C to harden the wall of the microcapsules, which were mononuclear microcapsules containing chlorinated paraffin and having excellent heat resistance.

Low Isoelectric Point Gelatin Derivatives

The process of *H. Matsukawa, K. Saeki and T. Shimada; U.S. Patent 3,944,502; March 16, 1976; assigned to Fuji Photo Film Co., Ltd., Japan* relates to microcapsules containing hydrophobic oil drops, characterized in that, in the preparation of microcapsules by a complex coacervation method using gelatin as at least one kind of the hydrophilic colloid, a gelatin derivative having an isoelectric point lower than the gelling point of the gelatin employed for the formation of the wall is added in order to prevent an increase of the viscosity due to the reaction of gelatin and aldehyde in the prehardening treatment and to carry out the prehardening treatment rapidly.

Examples of suitable gelatin derivatives for use as shock preventing agents are the reaction product of gelatin and an aromatic or aliphatic anhydride, the reaction product of gelatin and a compound having a reactive halogen atom, the reaction product of gelatin and isocyanate, and the reaction product of gelatin and N-arylvinylsulfonamide. Processes for preparing these materials are described in U.S. Patents 2,525,753, 2,614,928 and 2,614,930.

The preparation of microcapsules containing hydrophobic oil drops may be carried out by the method of complex coacervation caused by dilution with water and/or adjustment of the pH. The production of coacervates due to liquid-liquid phase separation is based on an operation of separating a phase richer in colloid from a phase poorer in colloid, each phase consisting of two or more sorts of hydrophilic colloid sols.

In this operation, it is necessary that at least two hydrophilic colloids having electric charges opposite to each other are contained in the colloid and at least one of the two colloids is gelable. Examples of natural or synthetic hydrophilic colloids are gelatin, casein, alginate, gum arabic, styrene-maleic anhydride copolymer, and polyethylene-maleic anhydride copolymer. Among those mentioned, gelatin is absolutely necessary for the formation of wall films.

The amount of the shock preventing agent added is more than 1/20, preferably 1/10 to 1/2 the total weight of the two or more hydrophilic colloids having different electric charges and capable of forming the wall. The addition of the shock preventing agent makes the prehardening treatment of capsules under the insufficient condition for coacervation easy whereby capsule liquid can be obtained in high concentration.

Example 1: Preparation of m-Carboxybenzenesulfochloride Derivative – 100 g of gelatin, isoelectric point 4.90, was dissolved in 625 ml of water and heated to 50°C, and then a 10% aqueous solution of caustic soda was added to the solution with stirring to adjust the pH of the solution to 10. The solution thus obtained was stirred for thirty minutes, and 10.5% of m-carboxybenzenesulfochloride dissolved in 50 ml isopropyl alcohol was added while the system is maintained at pH 10 by the addition of a 10% aqueous solution of caustic soda.

After stirring for 10 minutes at 50°C, dilute sulfuric acid was added to the mixture to reduce the pH to 7. The mixture was cooled, washed with water and dried with hot air. The gelatin thus obtained had an isoelectric point of 4.20.

Example 2: Control – 6 parts of acid-treated gelatin, isoelectric point 7.8, and

6 parts of gum arabic were dissolved in 30 parts of water, heated to 40°C. To the solution, 0.5 part of Turkey red oil as an emulsifier was added. Into the colloid solution, 30 parts of a 2.0% dichlorodiphenyl solution of CVL were emulsified with vigorous stirring to prepare an oil-in-water emulsion having a particle size of 6 to 10 microns. To the emulsion, 190 parts of water heated to 45°C were added.

While further stirring, a 50% aqueous acetic acid solution was added dropwise to adjust the pH of the system to 4.4. After maintaining the temperature for 15 minutes, the resulting mixture was cooled from the outside of the reaction vessel to gel the wall of the coacervates. When the temperature of the system was 15°C with stirring, 3.0 parts of a 37% formaldehyde solution were added.

When the temperature of the liquid was 10°C (the viscosity of the capsule liquid was determined at 10°C to be 35 cp by use of a B-type rotating viscosimeter, 30 rpm No. 1 rotor, hereinafter referred to as B_1 30 rpm), a 10% aqueous solution of caustic soda was added while adding the aqueous solution of caustic soda for 15 minutes, the pH of the capsule liquid was adjusted to 6.5, in which the viscosity of the liquid was 125 cp (B_1 30 rpm).

While adding the aqueous solution of caustic soda for a further 10 minutes, the pH of the liquid was 7.0, in which the viscosity of the liquid was 850 cp. When the pH of the liquid reached 7.3, the capsule liquid coagulated. The capsules had uneven form and the size of the larger capsules was 5 to 10 mm.

In this example, the addition of alkali and formalin for prehardening treatment was carried out by the following two methods: (1) formaldehyde was added after the pH of the capsule liquid was elevated to the alkaline side (pH 9.5); and (2) alkali and formaldehyde were added simultaneously from two nozzles, respectively. Capsules aggregated in both methods.

Example 3: *Process* – 6 parts of acid-treated gelatin, isoelectric point 7.8, and 6 parts of gum arabic were dissolved in 30 parts of water heated to 40°C. To the solution, 0.5 part of Turkey red oil as an emulsifier was added. Into the colloid solution, 30 parts of a 2.0% dichlorodiphenyl solution of CVL were emulsified with vigorous stirring to prepare an oil-in-water emulsion having a particle size of 6 to 10 microns. To the emulsion, 190 parts of water heated to 45°C were added. With further stirring, a 10% aqueous sulfuric acid solution was added dropwise to adjust the pH of the system to 4.2.

After maintaining the temperature for 15 minutes, the resulting mixture was cooled from the outside of the reaction vessel to gel the wall of the coacervates. When the temperature of the liquid was 10°C, 30 parts of a 5% aqueous solution of a m-carboxybenzenesulfochloride derivative of gelatin (isoelectric point 3.98) were added.

Afterwards, when the temperature of the liquid was 15°C with continued stirring, a 37% aqueous formaldehyde solution and a 10% aqueous solution of caustic soda were added simultaneously at the same addition speed from two nozzles, respectively. The other steps were the same as those in Example 2. The viscosity was 98 cp at pH 7.5. Thus obtained capsules were mononuclear and strong during the heat-resisting test.

HARDENING AGENTS

Slow Hardening Agent Followed by Rapid Hardening Agent

S. Egawa, M. Sakamoto and T. Matsushita; U.S. Patent 4,082,688; April 4, 1978; assigned to NCR Corporation are concerned with a process for producing oil-containing microcapsules consisting of coacervate capsule walls of colloidal material. These microcapsules are prepared by a coacervation process, using gelatin as at least one of the hydrophilic colloids and a negatively-electrically charged hydrophilic polymeric material as at least one of the hydrophilic colloids.

The process comprises using at least two kinds of hardening agents in a hardening step. Negatively-electrically-charged hydrophilic materials include gum arabic; maleic anhydride copolymers such as vinyl methyl ether, styrene, acrylic acid, vinyl acetate and ethylene; carboxymethylcellulose; and alginates such as sodium alginate and carrageenan.

The process is suitable to produce mononucleic microcapsules containing an oily liquid, which capsules afford less contamination in the pressure-sensitive paper due to less breakage of the capsules. The process comprises: forming films of colloid of multivalent electrolyte around hydrophobic oil droplets by a coacervation process to prepare coacervates; gelating wall films of coacervates at a pH less than 7.0; adding thereto, first, a relatively slow acting hardening agent thereby to effect gradual hardening; adding thereto, second, a relatively rapid acting hardening agent in the presence of a negatively-electrically-charged hydrophilic polymeric material; and converting the system to an alkaline condition greater than pH 8.0.

The relatively slow acting hardening agents include: formaldehyde; 2,3-dihydroxy-1,4-dioxane; glyoxal, and the relatively rapid acting hardening agents include: glutaraldehyde; 2-methylglutaraldehyde; and acrolein. The relatively slow acting hardening agents are used in an amount of preferably 5 to 10% by weight, based on the gelatin, and the relatively rapid acting hardening agents are used in the amount of preferably 5 to 10% by weight. Negatively-electrically-charged hydrophilic polymeric materials are used in an amount preferably 80 to 200% by weight, based on the gelatin.

Example 1: 22 g of acid-treated gelatin was dissolved in 216 g of water at 46°C, and 164 ml of a 3:1, by volume, solvent mixture of diallylethane and kerosene containing 2.0% of crystal violet lactone (CVL) in a solution state was added to the colloidal solution, and emulsified with vigorous agitation, whereby an oil-in-water emulsion was formed. The vigorous agitation was discontinued when the sizes of oil droplets reached 1 to 2 microns. 200 g of an 11% aqueous gum arabic solution at 55°C was added thereto, with moderate stirring which was continued. 680 g of warm water was added thereto, while continuing the stirring. Then, 50% aqueous acetic acid was added thereto, dropwise, to adjust the pH to 4.85.

The vessel was cooled from the outside, while the stirring was continued, and colloidal walls thus accumulated were fixed to the oil droplets. When the liquid temperature reached about 10°C, 4 ml of 37% aqueous formaldehyde was added. 33 ml of 5% aqueous solution of poly(methyl vinyl ether-comaleic anhydride) (hereinafter designated as PVM/MA) was added thereto. Viscosity of the system was temporarily increased by the addition of the PVM/MA, but decreased again to a lower viscosity after addition of a sufficient amount thereof. Then, 2.5 ml of 50% aqueous glutaraldehyde was added thereto, while keeping the solution temperature at about 10°C, and the system was converted from pH 5.5 to 11.0 with a 20% aqueous sodium hydroxide solution to complete the hardening. The time required for the dropwise sodium hydroxide addition was about 5 minutes.

Microscopic observation of the capsule system, thus obtained, revealed that more than 95%, by number, consisted of mononucleic capsules of single emulsified droplets. The capsules were coated upon test paper and subjected to a heat resistance test at 150°C for 3 hours, and then the dye-containing capsule paper, thus prepared, was used in copying with a sensitized receiving sheet, whereby clearly color-developed marks were obtained.

Example 2: Microcapsules were prepared in the same manner as in Example 1, using 3.5 ml of 40% aqueous glyoxal in place of the hardening agent formaldehyde and 6 ml of 25% aqueous 2-methylglutaraldehyde in place of glutaraldehyde of Example 1. It was found that more than 95%, by number, of the capsules were mononucleic, as in Example 1. The capsules were coated upon test paper and prepared into copying paper, which produced clearly color-developed marks.

Oxidation Product of a Polysaccharide

K. Saeki and H. Matsukawa; U.S. Patent 4,016,098; April 5, 1977; assigned to Fuji Photo Film Co., Ltd., Japan describe a hardening process which enables microcapsules which possess high impermeability, high strength and high resistance against influence of humidity to be produced. This is achieved by microencapsulating hydrophobic oil droplets by complex coacervation using at least two hydrophilic colloids having opposite electric charges and being ionizable in water with at least one of the colloids being gelable by using as a hardener an oxidation product of a polysaccharide in the hardening step of the coacervate wall conducted in the presence of hardener and the adjustment of pH to the alkali side (e.g., pH 7 to 13).

As the coacervate-forming hydrophilic colloid, natural or synthetic hydrophilic colloids can be used. For example, gelatin, saccharides, gums, maleic anhydride copolymers, e.g., with monomers having at least one addition polymerizable unsaturated bond, and olefins, can be used. Whether the hydrophilic colloid to be used possesses a positive or a negative charge is relative. For example, where gelatin is used, gelatin has a positive charge and the other hydrophilic colloid (as given above) has a negative charge.

The oxidation product of the polysaccharide is obtained by converting the secondary alcohol groups contained in the saccharide units forming the polysaccharide to aldehyde groups through oxidation using an aqueous solution of an oxidizing agent such as periodic acid, a salt of periodic acid (e.g., the alkali metal Na, K, etc., salts) or a like inorganic peroxide, preferably at room temperature (e.g., 20° to 30°C) for 2 or 3 days (the oxidation ratio being preferably not less than about 20%), followed by separation, washing and drying, e.g., as disclosed in U.S. Patent 3,057,723.

The oxidation product of the polysaccharide is added in an amount sufficient to harden the complex coacervate. A suitable amount of the oxidation product of the polysaccharide can range from 3 to 200% by weight, most preferably 10 to 80% by weight based on the weight of the gelable colloid, such as gelatin. As the examples of polysaccharides whose secondary alcohol groups can be oxidized to aldehyde groups, there are illustrated homoglycans such as glucans (e.g., cellulose, carboxymethylcellulose, starch, etc.), fructans (e.g., inulin, levan, etc.), mannans (e.g., *Phytelephas macrocarpa* mannan, etc.), xylans (e.g., xylan of straw, etc.), galacturonans (e.g., pectic acid, pectin, amylopectin, etc.), mannuronans (e.g., alginic acid, etc.), N-acetylglucosamine derivatives (e.g., chitin, etc.), heteroglycans such as diheteroglycans (e.g., chondroitin sulfuric acid, hyaluronic acid, heparin, etc.), triheteroglycans (e.g., mesquite gum, ghatti gum, tragacanth gum, etc.), and tetraheteroglycans (e.g., gum arabic, etc.).

Example 1: Synthesis – 500 ml of distilled water and 11.5 g of periodic acid were placed in a 1 liter three-necked flask equipped with a magnetic stirrer, a thermometer and a cooling bath (5°C). This mixture was stirred to form a uniform solution and cooled to 20°C. Then, 50 g of gum arabic was added thereto and stirred to form a uniform solution. After the reaction solution temperature increased to 35°C, the system was cooled externally to 20°C. The reaction was continued for 23 hours under stirring.

The resulting reaction mixture was poured into 5 liters of tert-butyl alcohol. The precipitate formed was filtered out using a Buchner funnel and repeatedly washed with ethanol until iodic acid was removed. The washed product was dried at 40°C for 18 hours under reduced pressure. 46 g of a white powder of aldehyde-gum arabic was obtained with the oxidation ratio of 57%.

Example 2: Encapsulation – 6 parts of acid-processed pigskin gelatin having an isoelectric point of 8.2 and 6 parts of gum arabic were dissolved in 30 parts of warm water at 40°C, and 0.2 part of sodium nonylbenzenesulfonate was added as an emulsifier.

Then, 30 parts of diisopropylnaphthalene containing dissolved therein 2.5% by weight of crystal violet lactone and 2.0% by weight of benzoyl leucomethylene blue was added to the above described colloid solution under vigorous stirring for emulsification to form an oil-in-water emulsion. The stirring was discontinued when the size of the oil droplets became 6 to 10 μ. 200 parts of warm water at 40°C was added thereto. A 20% aqueous acetic acid solution was added dropwise thereto, while continuing the stirring, to adjust the pH to 4.4. The colloid wall accumulated around the oil droplets was gelled by cooling from the outside of the vessel while continuing the stirring.

20 parts of a 5% aqueous solution of the hardener obtained in Example 1 was added under stirring when the liquid temperature reached 10°C. 20 parts of an aqueous solution, 7% by weight, of the sodium salt of carboxymethylcellulose (etherification degree 0.75) was added thereto as a shock-preventing agent. A 10% by weight sodium hydroxide aqueous solution was added dropwise thereto until the system reached a pH of 10, and the temperature of the system was increased from outside of the vessel and maintained for 1 hour at 40°C to obtain color-former-containing microcapsules.

The microcapsules obtained in this example are useful as microcapsules for pressure-sensitive copying papers. A coated paper was prepared by adding 10 parts of a 10% aqueous solution of PVA-210 (polyvinyl alcohol, Kuray) and 3 parts of cornstarch to 100 parts of the resulting capsule slurry and coating on a 50 g/m^2 paper in an amount of 5.5 g/m^2, followed by drying. On the other hand, a coated paper for comparison (Comparative Example) was prepared by adding 10 parts of a 10% solution of PVA-210 and 3 parts of corn starch to 100 parts of a capsule slurry (obtained in the same manner as described above except for using 2.0 parts of a 37% formaldehyde solution in place of the compound in Example 1 and coating on a 50 g/m^2 paper in an amount of 5.5 g/m^2. The characteristics of the two papers were compared to obtain the results given in the table below, which gives the color density. The smaller the color density, the better. It can be seen from these results that the strength of the capsule wall, impermeability and humidity resistance are markedly improved by employing the hardening agent of this process.

Comparative Data on Characteristics of Capsule Wall

	Example 2	Comparative Example
Strength of capsule wall		
Pressure resistance	0.13	0.15
Friction resistance	0.09	0.12
Humidity resistance	0.33	0.40
Permeability of wall	0.15	0.28

Glyoxal or Glutaraldehyde in Combination with Formaldehyde

K. Saeki and H. Matsukawa; U.S. Patent 3,956,172; May 11, 1976; assigned to Fuji Photo Film Co., Ltd., Japan provide a process whereby microcapsules which do not yellow are produced without an increase in viscosity with the passage of time and without the aggregation of capsules, even when a dialdehyde is used as a hardening agent. This is attained by using a dialdehyde and formaldehyde in combination as a hardening agent. It is surprising that, in spite of the fact that both a dialdehyde having no more than 5 carbon atoms such as glyoxal, glutaraldehyde, etc., and formaldehyde are known as hardening agents for use in a complex coacervation process wherein at least one of the colloids is gelatin, the objects of the process can successfully be attained by using both in combination.

In order to emulsify and disperse a hydrophobic liquid which is to be the nuclear material in water, an anionic, cationic or nonionic surface active agent is preferably used to prevent phase reversal (i.e., formation of an oil-in-water emulsion). Turkey red oil or sodium alkylbenzene sulfonates can be utilized. An oil-in-water emulsion can be obtained by emulsifying a hydrophobic oily liquid which is converted to the nuclear material in at least one hydrophilic colloid aqueous solution, the colloid becoming a wall material. The resulting emulsion is then subjected to water dilution and adjustment of pH to deposit the coacervate around the emulsified individual oil droplets.

The coacervate deposited on the surface of the oil droplets is cooled from outside the vessel to gel the wall film. Then, in order to harden the wall film, a dialdehyde, e.g., glutaraldehyde, is added to the system followed by adjusting the pH of the system to the alkali side, or the pH of the system is adjusted to the alkali side followed by adding a dialdehyde, e.g., glutaraldehyde, thereto.

Adding formaldehyde is not particularly limited and may be before, during or after the abovedescribed hardening procedure. The same effects of the combined use of the formaldehyde with a dialdehyde are obtained in any case.

In order to provide the capsule wall film with heat resistance, the system is left for a long period of time, such as a day, at a low temperature, e.g., room temperature, or, if short time processing is required, heated to 40° to 60°C.

The amount of formaldehyde to be added together with a dialdehyde used as a hardening agent is necessary to improve the stability with the passage of time after the hardening pretreatment step, and varies depending upon the amount of dialdehyde used.

When the dialdehyde is glyoxal, the minimum necessary amount of formaldehyde is preferably at least 0.05 part based on 100 parts of gelatin. When less than 5 parts, based on 100 parts of gelatin, of glutaraldehyde is used as the dialdehyde, it is preferred that at least 0.7 part of formaldehyde be added. When 5 parts or more, based on 100 parts of gelatin, of glutaraldehyde are used, it is preferred that the amount of formaldehyde added be at least 0.05 part.

Example 1: 6 parts of acid-processed gelatin having an isoelectric point of 7.8 and 6 parts of gum arabic was dissolved in 40°C water, and 0.5 part of Turkey red oil was added as an emulsifier. Then, 30 parts of diisopropylbiphenyl containing dissolved therein 2% of crystal violet lactone (CVL) was added to the colloidal solution under vigorous stirring for emulsification to form an oil-in-water emulsion. The stirring was discontinued when the size of oil droplets became 6 to 10 microns. All of the above operations were conducted at 40°C. 250 parts of warm water at 45°C was added thereto.

Thereafter, 50% acetic acid was added dropwise, while continuing the stirring, to adjust the pH to 4.5. After maintaining the system at 45°C for 15 minutes under stirring, the system was cooled from outside the vessel from 45°C to 15°C for gelling and to solidify the colloidal wall deposited around the oil droplets, the stirring being continued and when the liquid temperature reached 15°C, 1.0 part of a 40% aqueous glyoxal solution and 0.2 part of a 37% aqueous formaldehyde solution were added thereto at the same time. Stirring and cooling were continued, and when the liquid temperature reached 10°C, the addition of a 10% aqueous sodium hydroxide solution was started and the pH of the liquid was adjusted to 10. After allowing the system to stand for 30 minutes at 10°C the temperature of the liquid was raised to 50°C over 20 minutes to obtain highly heat-resistant, nonyellowed microcapsules containing diisopropylbiphenyl having CVL dissolved therein. The viscosity of the resulting capsule solution was 65 cp at pH 10 at 10°C and 15 cp after raising the temperature to 50°C.

Where formaldehyde was not added, the viscosity was 77 cp at pH 10 and 10°C, but the viscosity became 351 cp after raising the temperature to 50°C. Furthermore, the capsule solution yellowed and the microcapsules aggregated in the form of a giant flock.

Example 2: 6 parts of acid-processed gelatin having an isoelectric point of 7.8 and 6 parts of gum arabic were dissolved in 35 parts of warm water at 40°C. To this solution was added 0.3 part of sodium alkylbenzene sulfonate as an emulsifier. Then, 35 parts of xylylphenylethane containing dissolved therein 2% of

CVL was emulsified therein to prepare an oil-in-water emulsion. The size of the oil droplets produced was 8 to 12 microns. This emulsion was then poured into 200 parts of a 45°C aqueous solution containing 0.08% of sodium sulfate, and a 50% aqueous acetic acid solution was dropwise added thereto while stirring to adjust the pH to 4.3. Subsequently, 0.68 part of a 25% aqueous glutaraldehyde solution and 0.22 part of a 37% aqueous formaldehyde solution were simultaneously added thereto, followed by cooling from outside the vessel from 45°C to a liquid temperature of 8°C. Thereafter, 25 parts of a 7% aqueous CMC solution was added thereto and a 10% aqueous sodium hydroxide solution was added dropwise thereto to adjust the pH to 9.5. The viscosity at this time was 68 cp. The liquid temperature was then raised from 8°C to 50°C. At this time, the viscosity was 13 cp, the capsule solution was not tinged a skinlike color, and no abnormality was observed as to the form of microcapsules.

When the 0.22 part of the 37% aqueous formaldehyde solution was not used the viscosity of the liquid was 117 cp at pH 9.5 and 8°C and, after raising the temperature to 50°C, the viscosity sharply rose to 542 cp, the capsule solution was tinged a skinlike color, and there were produced microcapsules aggregating in the form of a giant flock.

OTHER MODIFIERS

Binding Heterocyclic Amine to Film-Former to Increase Capsule Strength

H. Matsukawa and K. Saeki; U.S. Patent 4,062,799; December 13, 1977; assigned to Fuji Photo Film Co., Ltd., Japan have developed a method for forming microcapsule films having low porosity which comprises chemically or ionically binding a water soluble or water dispersable heterocyclic amine to a microcapsule film-forming material, or depositing the heterocyclic amine solely or a water insoluble material formed by reaction with the heterocyclic amine onto the microcapsule films.

The term heterocyclic amine also includes derivatives. Suitable heterocyclic amines are symmetric or asymmetric spiroacetal heterocyclic diamines. Examples of the preferred spiroacetal heterocyclic diamines are represented by the following formula:

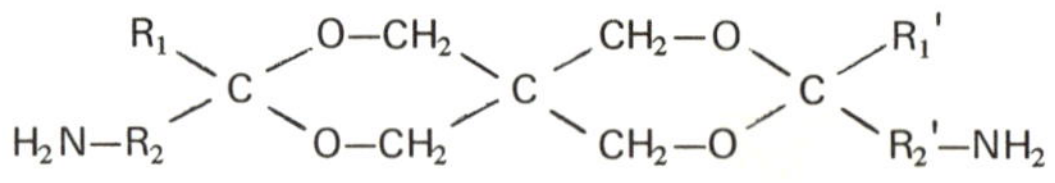

$$\begin{array}{ccccccc} R_1 & & O{-}CH_2 & & CH_2{-}O & & R_1' \\ & \diagdown C \diagup & & \diagdown C \diagup & & \diagdown C \diagup & \\ H_2N{-}R_2 & & O{-}CH_2 & & CH_2{-}O & & R_2'{-}NH_2 \end{array}$$

wherein R_1 and R_1' each represents a hydrogen atom or a lower alkyl group (e.g., a methyl group, an ethyl group and a propyl group), and R_2 and R_2' each represents a linear or branched chain alkylene group having 1 to 7 carbon atoms. Examples of suitable alkylene groups are methylene, ethylene, propylene, isopropylene, butylene, pentylene, hexylene and heptylene groups. Preferred alkylene groups are straight chain groups.

Preferred examples of derivatives of the above compound include the condensation products produced by reacting the amino groups of a diamine represented by the above formula with a compound containing at least one oxirane group;

the addition products produced by reacting the above amine with acrylonitrile; the reaction products produced by reacting the above amine with urea, thiourea or guanidine; and the reaction products produced by reacting the above amine with an alkylene oxide such as ethylene oxide, propylene oxide, octylene oxide, etc.

The method of forming microcapsule films can be applied to any microencapsulation process.

The heterocyclic amines are added to the system during a step for producing capsules or after formation of capsule films. However, it is preferred to add the heterocyclic amines as follows.

Interfacial Polymerization Process: It is preferred to add the heterocyclic amines during or after a dispersion step in the process comprising emulsification → dispersion → hardening → conclusion of encapsulation.

Coacervation Process: It is preferred to add amine during or after the cooling step which comprises cooling at a temperature below the gelling point of an ionizable hydrophilic colloid, particularly gelatin, in the process comprising emulsification → coacervation → cooling → prehardening treatment → hardening → conclusion of encapsulation, and particularly at the prehardening treatment step. The prehardening treatment step means the step prior to that step in which the hardening agent is added and an alkali is copresent in the same system.

In Situ Polymerization Process: It is preferred to add the heterocyclic amine during or after a dispersion step in the process comprising emulsification → dispersion → hardening → conclusion of encapsulation.

It is preferred that the amount of the amines be within a range of $\frac{1}{1,000}$ to $\frac{1}{2}$ more preferably $\frac{1}{100}$ to $\frac{1}{5}$, weight ratio based on the core (nucleus) material. It is especially effective to modify the capsule films formed from gelatin.

Heterocyclic Amine Synthesis: 6.8 g (0.05 mol) of pentaerythritol, 1 g of p-toluene sulfonic acid and 100 ml of toluene were mixed with 18.5 g (0.1 mol) of 5-cyanopentanal dimethylacetal. The mixture was refluxed by heating for 4 hours. The reaction mixture was filtered and the filtrate was condensed under vacuum to produce 17.9 g of 3,9-bis(4'-cyanobutyl)-2,4,8,10-tetraoxaspiro[5.5] undecane as a viscous liquid.

This viscous liquid was dissolved in 60 ml of ethanol and charged into an autoclave together with 100 ml of ethanol saturated with ammonia and 5 g of an activated alkali-treated Raney cobalt catalyst. Hydrogen was added at an initial hydrogen pressure of 107 kg/cm^2 at a reaction temperature of 120°C for 2 hours. After separating the catalyst by filtration, the filtrate was condensed and the condensate was distilled under vacuum to produce 8.2 g of 3,9-bis(5'-aminopentyl)-2,4,8,10-tetraoxaspiro[5.5]undecane as a distillate having a boiling point range of 217°-221°C /0.2 mm Hg.

33.1 parts by weight of the resulting 3,9-bis(5'-aminopentyl)-2,4,8,10-tetraoxaspiro[5.5]undecane were melted by heating. Then 13.0 parts by weight of butyl glycidyl ether were added dropwise with stirring while keeping the temperature at 60°C. After addition, the mixture was stirred for an additional 2 hours. The resulting reaction condensate was a colorless transparant viscous liquid.

Example: 6 parts of acid-treated gelatin (from pigskin) with an isoelectric point of 8.2 and 6 parts of gum arabic were dissolved in 30 parts of water at 40°C. As an emulsifier, 0.2 part of sodium nonylbenzene sulfonate was added.

30 parts of diisopropylnaphthalene containing 2.5% (by weight) of CVL and 2.0% (by weight) of benzoyl leucomethylene blue as a color forming oil were added to the colloid solution with vigorous stirring to produce an oil-in-water emulsion. Stirring was stopped when the oil drop size became 6 to 10 μ.

To this emulsion, 200 parts of warm water at 40°C were added. 20% hydrochloric acid was added dropwise while stirring to adjust the pH to 4.4. The mixture was cooled externally with stirring to gel the colloid films deposited on the oil drops. When the liquid temperature became 10°C, 2.0 parts of a 37% formaldehyde solution were added while stirring. Then 20 parts of a 7% solution of sodium carboxymethylcellulose (etherification degree, 0.75) were added.

A solution prepared by diluting 2.0 parts of the compound of the above Synthesis with 5 parts of water was added dropwise. A 10% solution of sodium hydroxide was added dropwise to adjust the pH to 10. The mixture was kept at 40°C for 1 hour by external warming to obtain color-former oil-containing capsules.

The capsules obtained by this example were useful for producing a pressure-sensitive copying paper. For example, 10 parts of a 10% solution of PVA-210 (a polyvinyl alcohol, average degree of polymerization 1,000, degree of saponification 87%, Kuray), and 3 parts of cornstarch were added to 100 parts of the resulting capsule slurry. The mixture was applied in a dry amount of 5.5 g/m^2 to a sheet of paper having a weight of 50 g/m^2 and dried to produce a coated paper. On the other hand, a mixture prepared by adding 7 parts of a 10% solution of PVA-210 and 3 parts of cornstarch to 100 parts of capsules which were produced without using the compound of the above Synthesis was applied in a dry amount of 5.5 g/m^2 to a sheet of paper a weight of 50 g/m^2 and dried to produce a copying paper comparison. When the characteristics of these coating papers were compared, the results showed that the strength permeability of the capsule films and the moisture resistance were remarkably improved.

Addition of Phenolic Compound Prior to Hardening Pretreatment to Reduce Aggregation

The work of *H. Matsukawa and K. Saeki; U.S. Patent 3,965,033; June 22, 1976; assigned to Fuji Photo Film Co., Ltd., Japan* relates to a process for microencapsulating an oily liquid by coacervation utilizing gelatin as at least one of the hydrophilic colloids, whereby oil-containing microcapsules, whose walls are less porous and thicker, can be obtained without aggregation. The process is conducted by the coacervation caused by the dilution with water and the addition of salt or pH adjustment, using the following procedure:

(1) dispersing a hydrophobic fine powder or emulsifying a hydrophobic liquid into an aqueous solution of at least one kind of high molecular weight electrolytic colloid which is used for forming the capsule wall (dispersing or emulsifying step);

(2) subjecting the dispersion or the emulsion obtained in step (1) to water dilution, and then salt addition and/or pH adjustment thereof. In this case, an aqueous solution of a high molecular weight colloid may be added thereto, if desired (coacervation step);

(3) cooling the formed coacervate to gell it (cooling step);

(4) adding a phenolic compound thereto at a temperature of above 5°C, preferably above 8°C, during the steps of (2) and (3);

(5) adding a hardening agent to the system;

(6) adding a shock-preventing agent at a temperature lower than the gelling point of gelatin; wherein by shock is meant such a phenomenon that the viscosity of the system elevates rapidly, i.e., at a pH not less than ~6, generally 6 to 13, when conducting the prehardening of the coacervation capsule liquid containing the gelatin, and by shock-preventing agent is meant a solution for preventing the shock;

(7) adjusting the pH of the system to the alkali side, (steps (5), (6) and (7)—prehardening treatment); and

(8) optionally elevating the temperature of the system to more effectively harden the coacervate (hardening step).

In the above method, the order of steps (5), (6) and (7) can freely be modified with respect to each other, and step (5) may also be conducted prior to step (4).

In the above procedure, even though the phenolic compound may be added to the system without using a prehardening treatment, some results are obtained, but, when the compound is added to the system at the step (4) and the shock-preventing agent is added at the prehardening treatment, more excellent results can be obtained. Both the phenolic compound and the shock-preventing agent can be simultaneously added at a temperature lower than the gelling point of gelatin and higher than 5°C, preferably higher than 8°C.

Examples of the hydrophilic colloids include gelatin, casein, alginate, gum arabic, carrageenan, maleic acid-styrene copolymer, maleic acid-methyl vinyl ether copolymer, maleic acid-ethylene copolymer and the like. In the process, gelatin must be used as one of the hydrophilic colloids.

Shock-preventing agents are disclosed in U.S. Patent Reissue 28,779.

The phenolic compound used in the process may be a phenol monomer or a phenol resin. The typical phenol monomer is an aromatic compound of which the hydrogen atom attached to the ring, is substituted with at least one hydroxyl group. The examples include substituted phenols, polyhydric phenols, phenol carboxylic acids, nitrophenols, and biphenols. They may usually be used as a solution after dissolving in water or in an alcohol.

As examples of the substituted phenols, there are phenol compounds having, as the substituent, an alkyl, an allyl, a halogen, a halogen-substituted alkyl, a cycloalkyl, a phenyl, a halogen-substituted phenyl, an alkyl-substituted phenyl, biphenyl, benzyl and α-alkylbenzyl groups.

Examples of the phenolic resin used in the process include phenol-aldehyde condensates which, in general, are called resol types or novolak types.

A water-soluble type of the phenolic resin is more suitable for the process, but a so-called alcohol-soluble novolak type can also be used after dissolving it in a water-compatible solvent.

Example: In 25 parts of water (35°C), 6 parts of acid-treated gelatin having an isoelectric point of 8.2, and 6 parts of gum arabic were dissolved. Then, 30 parts of chlorinated diphenyl in which 2.0% CVL and 2.0% of benzoyl leucomethylene blue were dissolved was added into the colloid solution and emulsified with vigorous stirring to form an oil-in-water type emulsion. When the drop size became 6 to 10 μ, the stirring was stopped, and then 170 parts of warm water at 35°C were added thereto.

Thereafter, 10 parts of a 5% aqueous resorcinol solution was added thereto while stirring, and the pH was adjusted to 4.4 with 50% acetic acid. Then the contents were externally cooled, with stirring, to gel the colloid wall, and when the temperature was 15°C, with stirring, 2.5 parts of 37% formaldehyde were added thereto. Further, 15 parts of a 10% aqueous solution of carboxymethylcellulose (degree of etherification: 0.73, average degree of polymerization: 220) was added thereto when the temperature of the system was 10°C (the viscosity of the capsule solution at 10°C was 35 cp), and the pH was then adjusted to 10.0 with 10% caustic soda.

The dropping time of the caustic soda was 5 minutes, and the viscosity at pH 8 was 48 cp. Subsequently, the system was heated to 50°C to harden the wall. The so-obtained capsules were mostly single nucleus capsules, and the dried capsules showed little release of the nucleus included therein in a deterioration test of heating to 100°C for 10 hours. The capsules obtained in this Example could be effectively utilized in pressure-sensitive copying paper. After the given capsule solution was coated onto a base paper of 40 g/m^2 and dried, it was contacted with a commercially available clay-coated paper for a pressure-sensitive copying paper and written on to obtain a distinct blue color image on the clay-coated paper.

Comparative Example 1: The same procedure as in the above Example was repeated except that neither resorcinol nor carboxymethylcellulose as the shock-preventing agent was used.

The capsule dispersion aggregated during the addition of alkali. The viscosity at pH 8.0 was over 3,000 cp.

Comparative Example 2: The same procedure as in the above Example was repeated except that resorcinol was not used. The viscosity at 10°C was 98 cp and that at pH 8.0 during the dropping of alkali was 205 cp.

Pearlescent Capsules

In accordance with the process of *N. Marinelli; U.S. Patent 4,115,315; September 19, 1978; assigned to NCR Corporation* pearlescent or nacreous particles are incorporated in the capsule walls during the formation thereof. The pearlescent particles are initially dispersed in the liquid internal phase material and then flushed out into the aqueous coacervation phase upon addition of the internal phase to the encapsulation media. The pearlescent particles remain embedded in the wall material during encapsulation, capsule hardening and capsule post-treatment steps, and thus become integral ingredients of the walls of the capsules. The finished capsules display pearlescent properties and resemble tiny pearls.

The use of white mineral oil as the internal phase for encapsulation is particularly preferred since the resultant pearlescent capsules of mineral oil can be added to various cosmetic products such as shampoos and hair conditioners. The addition of approximately 0.2 to 0.4% by weight of such capsules based upon the weight of the shampoo provides a formulation capable and useful for dispersing the mineral oil into the hair upon use by rupture of the mineral oil-containing capsules. The pearlescence in the capsules is visible throughout the shampoo and provides a product having a superior and aesthetic appearance.

The procedure for providing pearlescent capsules involves dispersing 0.5 to 6% by weight (preferably 1 to 2%), based upon the total amount of internal phase material, of pearlescent particles in the oil which is to become the internal phase in the capsules. The pearlescent particles employed are generally flat inorganic mica carrier materials coated with a titanium dioxide pigment. The particles, in the form of platelets, generally have a length of 5 to 35 microns along their longest dimension. The amount of titanium dioxide coated onto the mica is generally in the range of 15 to 50% of the total weight of the particles.

Capsules made according to the process are substantially spherical and have seamless walls. The usual size of capsules made is from 500 to 3,000 microns in average diameter with a preferred average diameter range of 800 to 2,500 microns. The most usual and preferred range for the amount of internal phase material within the capsules is 85 to 95% by weight of the capsule.

Example: An internal phase composition containing approximately 2% of pearlescent particles was prepared utilizing 588 g of white mineral oil (Blandol) and 12 g of mica particles coated with titanium dioxide (Flamenco Satina 100). The mica particles were first wet with a small quantity of the mineral oil and then the particles were added to the remaining mineral oil with stirring. Vigorous stirring was continued for 1 hour at ambient temperature.

Into a 4 liter beaker fitted with double 4 inch turbine blades were added 1,760 g of water, 40 g of gum arabic and 40 g of gelatin. The resulting mixture was heated to 50°C under agitation by adjusting the turbine to low speed to provide an aqueous manufacturing vehicle.

600 g of the mineral oil mica particle dispersion were added to the gelatin-gum arabic manufacturing vehicle and milled therein to give oil drops having an average size of 1,400 to 2,500 microns, care being taken to adjust the stirrer height and speed to eliminate layering of the oil drops on top of the batch. The pearl-

escent particles were found to flush out into the aqueous coacervation phase upon the addition of the oil internal phase to the encapsulation medium. The pH of the batch was adjusted to 4.3, and the batch cooled slowly to 27°C, whereby the coacervate enwrapped and encapsulated the oil droplets. The pearlescent particles formed a part of the capsule wall material. The batch was then chilled to 10°C in an ice bath. 10 ml of a 50% aqueous solution of glutaraldehyde was then added to the batch, and the mix was agitated overnight in order to harden the capsule walls.

A posttreatment with urea-formaldehyde was then conducted by washing the hardened capsules 2 times with deionized water to remove extraneous material such as free coacervate, each time replacing the supernatant with water, adding a solution of 24 g of urea in 50 ml of water thereto, adjusting the pH to 1.5 with a 10% volume aqueous solution of H_2SO_4 and adding 40 ml of an aqueous 37% formaldehyde solution to the batch. The batch was then stirred for an additional 5 hours. After washing the resulting capsules 2 times with water, the batch was passed through a No. 8-mesh sieve (2,380 μ) and a No. 16-mesh sieve (1,190 μ) to give a fraction containing wet capsules of 1,190 and 2,380 microns ready for shipment or storage.

The resulting capsules have a pearlescent glow resembling tiny pearls and may be incorporated into a shampoo formulation. As the shampoo is used the capsules rupture to release the mineral oil encapsulated therein.

Microscopic examination of the capsules and examination of the oil following rupture of the capsules clearly show that the pearlescent particles are disposed within the capsule walls and not in the internal phase material.

MICROENCAPSULATION USING SYNTHETIC FILM-FORMERS

IN SITU CONDENSATION IN PRESENCE OF SYSTEM MODIFIER

Urea-Formaldehyde Condensation Reaction

The process of *P.L. Foris, R.W. Brown and P.S. Phillips, Jr.; U.S. Patent 4,001,140; January 4, 1977; assigned to NCR Corporation* relates to the manufacture of minute capsules, en masse, in a liquid manufacturing vehicle. The process involves liquid-liquid phase separation of a relatively concentrated solution of polymeric material to be used in formation of walls for the minute capsules.

There is provided an encapsulating process wherein the capsule wall material includes a urea-formaldehyde polymeric material wherein the urea/formaldehyde wall material is generated by an in situ condensation reaction. The condensation reaction is conducted in the presence of a negatively-charged, carboxyl-substituted, linear aliphatic hydrocarbon polyelectrolyte material dissolved in the capsule-manufacturing vehicle.

The process provides for manufacture of capsule walls from the polymerization of urea and formaldehyde with the benefits of well-formed urea-formaldehyde polymer but without the disadvantages of required dilution and nugget formation, which plagued prior processes.

A system component material specially utilized in the process, which material is believed to be required for realizing any advantage of the process is negatively-charged polymeric polyelectrolyte material having a linear aliphatic hydrocarbon backbone with an average of about two carboxyl groups for every four backbone carbon atoms and having the backbone otherwise unsubstituted or having an average of about one methoxy group for every four backbone carbon atoms. Use of the proper kind and amount of this system modifier is necessary to permit the manufacture of microcapsules having urea/formaldehyde wall material in a high capsule concentration, a low vehicle viscosity, and at a beneficially high pH condition.

The system modifier takes some active part in the urea/formaldehyde polymerization reaction as evidenced by reduced viscosity of the system at increased polymer concentration and increased efficiency of the polymerizing component materials with increased optimum pH of polymerization. Nevertheless, the finished capsule walls retain only a minor residual amount of the system modifier. To be effective, the system modifier must be included in the encapsulating system before commencement of reaction between the urea and the formaldehyde.

Preferred poly(ethylene-maleic anhydride) should have a molecular weight of 1,000; poly(methyl vinyl ether-maleic anhydride) above about 250,000; and poly(acrylic acid) above about 20,000. As a general rule the encapsulating system should contain at least 0.75% system modifier.

The process specifically and preferredly includes the steps of establishing an aqueous, single-phase solution of the system modifier and urea into which is dispersed the intended capsule core material (substantially insoluble in the solution and substantially chemically unreactive with any of the solutes). The dispersing forces are maintained, formaldehyde is added to the system and, on reaction between the urea and the formaldehyde, a urea/formaldehyde polymeric material separates from the solution as a liquid solution phase, in its own right, relatively highly concentrated in urea/formaldehyde.

The separated liquid phase containing urea/formaldehyde wets and enwraps particles of the dispersed capsule core material to yield liquid-walled embryonic capsules. Agitation is continued to permit generation and continued reaction of urea/formaldehyde material to yield solid and substantially water-insoluble capsule walls. It is important to note that: (a) after make-up of the system and commencement of the capsule-wall-forming condensation reaction, there is no dilution step in the process; (b) the presence of the system modifier permits generation of a high concentration of urea/formaldehyde polymer at a relatively low viscosity; (c) the resulting high concentration-low viscosity system permits liquid phase separation and subsequent polymerization to a solid to produce capsules, en masse, in a by volume concentration in the manufacturing vehicle not before possible.

The polymerization reaction, even as altered by the system modifier is a condensation conducted in an acid medium. The condensation can be accomplished in an aqueous system having a pH of about 0 to 7, the time and temperature requirements being variable to optimize the reaction. As an effect of the system modifier and its relation to the condensation, the preferred pH for operation is from 2.5 to 5.0 and the most preferred pH is 3.5. As to amounts of urea and formaldehyde which should be used, it has been found that the molar ratio of formaldehyde to urea must be at least 1.6, preferably from 1.6 to about 3.

Individual capsules are substantially spherical and can be manufactured having diameters of less than 1 to about 100 microns, the preferred size range being from about 1 to 50 microns in diameter. Capsule aggregates can be made in sizes from a few microns in diameter to several hundred microns in diameter depending upon the size and state of the included core material.

Example 1: Preparation – (a) Negatively-charged poly(ethylene-maleic anhydride) is used to modify a urea/formaldehyde encapsulating system to yield capsules in the size range of 5 to 15 microns. The capsule contents is an oily solution of colorable dye materials for use in carbonless copying paper, as will be described below in relation to testing the capsule product of this example. The capsule contents is termed internal phase. A suitable poly(ethylene-maleic anhydride) includes approximately equimolar ethylene and maleic anhydride and has a molecular weight of about 75,000 to 90,000 such as, for example, the product EMA-31, (Monsanto Chemical Company).

Into a blending vessel having about a one liter capacity and equipped for agitation and heating are placed: 100 g of a 10% aqueous solution of hydrolyzed poly(ethylene-maleic anhydride) as the system modifier; 10 g of urea; 1 g of resorcinol; and 200 g of water, as the manufacturing vehicle. The pH is adjusted to 3.5 using 20% aqueous sodium hydroxide and 200 ml of internal phase is emulsified into the manufacturing vehicle to yield mobile internal phase droplets of an average size of less than about 10 microns in a single-phase solution of the manufacturing vehicle.

25 g of formalin (37% aqueous formaldehyde solution) is added to the system. The agitation is maintained, the system is heated to about 55°C, and under continued agitation, the temperature is maintained for about 2 hours and then permitted to decrease to ambient (about 25°C).

This example utilizes a molar ratio of formaldehyde/urea of about 1.9 and contains about 6% of urea and formaldehyde and 3% of system modifier in the manufacturing vehicle (excluding consideration of the internal phase). The capsules of oily dye solution are uniformly in a size range of about 1 to 15 microns and represent more than 40% by volume of the encapsulating system. The oily dye solution comprises 3,3-bis(4-dimethylaminophenyl) 6-dimethylaminophthalide (commonly known as crystal violet lactone) and 3,3-bis(1-ethyl-2-methylindol-3-yl)phthalide (sometimes known as Indolyl Red) in a mixture of solvents including a benzylated ethyl benzene and a relatively high boiling hydrocarbon oil, such as one having a distillation range of 400° to 500°F.

(b) This is identical with (a) with the exception that poly(acrylic acid) is substituted for the poly(ethylene-maleic anhydride). Poly(acrylic acid) is among the eligible system modifiers in providing the beneficial effect on the urea/formaldehyde condensation. Control of the capsule size range has been found to be more difficult using poly(acrylic acid), but the capsule quality is comparable with that of (a). The capsules range in size from about 1 to 100 microns. A suitable poly(acrylic acid) may have an average molecular weight of more than about 150,000 and less than about 300,000 such as, for example, the product Acrysol A-3 (Rohm and Haas).

Example 2: Evaluation – Because the size of capsules made in the above example is so small and because the intended capsule use is in carbonless copying papers, the capsules are tested by methods which relate to effectiveness in a copying paper use. As a general description, the capsules are coated onto a sheet termed a CB Sheet (sheet with coated back) and are tested in conjunction with a standardized sheet termed a CF Sheet (sheet with coated front). The coating of the CB Sheet includes about 75% capsules, 18% wheat starch and 7% of gum binder such as, for example, hydroxyethyl ether of corn starch or other water-soluble starch derivatives; and is made up by combining 100 parts of aqueous capsule slurry having 40% capsules, 125 parts of water, 10 parts of wheat starch and 40 parts of a 10% aqueous solution of the gum binder, all adjusted to about pH 9. The coating is cast using a wire-wound rod designed to lay a 20 lb per ream (3,300 ft^2) wet film coating.

The coating of an exemplary CF Sheet includes a metal-modified phenolic resin reactive with the dyes, kaolin clay and other additaments and binder material. A CF Sheet is described in U.S. Patent 3,732,120.

When a CB Sheet and a CF Sheet are placed in coated face-to-coated face relation and pressure is applied, capsules of the CB Sheet rupture and capsule-contained material is transferred to and reacted with the acid component of the CF Sheet to yield a color. A test associated with such capsule rupture and color formation is Typewriter Intensity (TI) and TI values indicate ratios of reflectances, the reflectances of marks produced on the CF Sheet by a typewriter striking two sheets together versus the paper's background reflectance. A high value indicates little color development and a low value indicates good color development.

$$\text{TI} = \frac{\text{Printed Character Reflectance}}{\text{Background Reflectance}} \times 100$$

Reflectances of a more-or-less solid block of print made with an upper-case X character and of the background paper are measured on an opacimeter within 20 minutes after the print is made, first, using freshly prepared CB Sheets and, then, using CB Sheets aged in an oven at 100°C. A small difference between the TI values indicates good capsule quality. After the oven aging, a TI value of 100 indicates complete loss of solvent from the capsules and a TI value less than 70 evidences acceptable capsules for these tests. When an initial TI value is less than 70, a TI value difference between initial and aged samples of less than 5 is acceptable for these tests; but, of course, a difference of less than 3 is much preferred.

TI Values

	Initial	Aged (time)
(a)	58	60 (one day)
(b)	47	47 (one day)

Example 3: Three series of different system modifiers are used in accordance with the procedure generally described in Example 1. When the capsules contain the oily internal phase of dye solution described above, and, when the capsule quality is tested as above, the test results are as shown on the following page.

The amounts and kinds of encapsulating system materials used in these examples are any of those previously disclosed. The pH of the encapsulating system can be pH 0 to 7 and the formaldehyde to urea mol ratio can be from 1.6 to 3. As the pH of the system is increased, it is helpful to increase the temperature of the encapsulating system also. Eligible temperatures of operation range from about 25° to 75°C or higher, about 50° to 55°C being preferred.

By adjusting the degree of agitation, droplets of liquid intended capsule core material can be produced of any size from a few to several hundred microns. Moreover, the amount of intended capsule core material can be altered to alter the amount of completed capsule which is internal phase as opposed to capsule wall material. Capsules can generally be made from less than 50 to 95% internal phase, or more.

System Modifier	Initial	Aged 100°C (one day)
Poly(ethylene-maleic anhydride), MW		
75,000-90,000	58	60
15,000-20,000	55	57
5,000-7,000	55	57
1,500-2,000*	54	61
Poly(methyl vinyl ether-maleic anhydride), MW		
1,125,000	55	56
750,000	61	62
250,000	64	94
Poly(acrylic acid), MW		
< 300,000	43	45
<150,000	47	47
< 50,000**	50	59

*To demonstate flexibility in the amount of system modifier used, only one-half as much is used as is used in the similar materials of higher MW.

**To demonstate flexibility in the amount of system modifier used, twice as much is used as is used in the similar materials of higher MW.

Polycondensation of Low MW Polymers of Dimethylolurea

In the processes of *P.L. Foris, R.W. Brown and P.S. Phillips, Jr.; U.S. Patents 4,087,376; May 2, 1978; and 4,089,802; May 16, 1978; both assigned to NCR Corporation* the capsule wall material comprises a polymer formed from a urea-formaldehyde, dimethylolurea or methylated dimethylolurea starting material wherein the wall material is generated by an in situ condensation reaction. The condensation reaction is conducted in the presence of a negatively-charged, carboxyl-substituted, linear aliphatic hydrocarbon polyelectrolyte material dissolved in the capsule manufacturing vehicle.

Examples of eligible carboxyl group system modifiers include hydrolyzed maleic anhydride copolymers, which are preferred, such as poly(ethylene-maleic anhydride) (EMA), poly(methyl vinyl ether-maleic anhydride) (PVMMA), poly(propylene-maleic anhydride) (PMA), poly(isobutylene-maleic anhydride) (iBMA), poly-(butadiene-maleic anhydride) (BMA), poly(vinyl acetate-maleic anhydride) (PVAMA), and polyacrylates, such as poly(acrylic acid). Preferred poly(ethylene-maleic anhydride) should have a molecular weight above about 1,000; poly-(methyl vinyl ether-maleic anhydride) above about 250,000; and poly(acrylic acid) above about 20,000.

The steps of the process have been described with reference to U.S. Patent 4,001,140 above. The pH of the encapsulating system can be pH 0 to 7 and the preferred temperature range is 50° to 55°C.

Example 1: 20 g of dimethylolurea (DMU) is dissolved in 200 cc of water by adding 200 cc of boiling water to the DMU in a beaker equipped with a magnetic stirrer. The solution is cooled to about 45°C and then about 2.7 cc of 20%

sodium hydroxide, 100 g of a 10% aqueous solution of hydrolyzed poly(ethylene-maleic anhydride) and 1 g of resorcinol are added thereto. The final pH is about 3.5. A standard internal phase as described in Example 1 of U.S. Patent 4,001,140 above in the amount of 180 g is emulsified into the solution as the capsule core material. The system is then heated to a temperature of 55°C in a water bath. After stirring and heating are continued for about 2 hours, the temperature is permitted to decrease to ambient conditions (about 25°C). The resulting capsules of oily dye solution have a uniform size range of about 1 to 15 microns and represent more than 40% by volume of the encapsulating system.

Example 2: A solution is prepared by combining 50 g of a 10% solution of poly(methyl vinyl ether-maleic anhydride) (Gantrez 149), 0.5 g of resorcinol, approximately 1.4 cc of 20% NaOH and 10 g of dimethylolurea dissolved in 100 g of hot (95°C) water. The pH is adjusted to 3.5. 90 g (100 cc) of standard internal phase (Standard IP) is emulsified into the solution, and the emulsion is placed into a water bath maintained at a temperature of 55°C. After 4 hours a draw-down of this emulsion on a CF test strip gave a reflectance value of 63%.

The CF draw-down test is a method of determining capsule wall formation. The encapsulation emulsion containing all of the capsule-forming ingredients is coated onto a reactive CF Paper. A color is formed by the reaction of the dye with the CF coating. Wall formation is demonstrated by the mitigation of the color when the emulsion is coated at a later time and is measured by an opacimeter to give the reflectance of the coated area.

Example 3: A solution of 50 g of a 10% solution of poly(propylene-maleic anhydride), 100 g of water, 10 g of methylated dimethylolurea resin (Beetle 65, 100% solid), and 0.5 g of resorcinol is adjusted to a pH of 3.5 with 20% NaOH. 90 g (100 ml) of Standard IP is emulsified in the solution, and the emulsion is placed into a 55°C water bath. After 2 hours, a sample of this emulsion coated on a CF test strip gave a reflectance of 60%. A sample coated on nonreactive paper gave a reflectance of 61%.

Melamine-Formaldehyde Condensation Reaction

In still another process described by *P.L. Foris, R.W. Brown and P.S. Phillips, Jr.; U.S. Patent 4,100,103; July 11, 1978; assigned to NCR Corporation* the capsule wall material comprises a melamine-formaldehyde polymeric material wherein the melamine-formaldehyde wall material is generated by an in situ condensation reaction in the presence of a negatively-charged, carboxyl-substituted, linear aliphatic hydrocarbon polyelectrolyte material dissolved in the capsule manufacturing vehicle.

In another modification, methylol melamines such as trimethylol melamine, or methylated methylol melamines may be employed in an in situ polymerization reaction to yield the desired condensation polymer. It is of significance to note that the reaction of melamine with formaldehyde to form capsule walls is conducted in the absence of urea.

The eligible carboxyl group system modifiers have been described above in U.S. Patent 4,087,376.

The polymerization reaction, even as altered by the system modifier, is a polycondensation conducted in an acid medium. The condensation can be accomplished in an aqueous system having a pH of about 4.3 to 6, the time and temperature requirements being variable to optimize the reaction. As an effect of the system modifier and its relation to the polycondensation reaction, the preferred pH for operation is from 4.5 to 6.0, the preferred pH being about 5.3 for the melamine-formaldehyde and methylol melamine systems. When methylated methylol melamine is used, a pH range of from 4.3 to 5.6 is suitably employed, the preferred pH being about 4.8.

Where melamine and formaldehyde are used as the starting reactant materials, it has been found that a wide range of molar ratio of formaldehyde to melamine can be utilized. However, a molar ratio of about 2-3:1 is advantageously employed. Eligible temperatures of operation range from about 20° to 100°C under ambient conditions, about 50° to 60°C being preferred.

Example 1: Poly(ethylene-maleic anhydride) is used to modify a melamine-formaldehyde encapsulating system. A suitable poly(ethylene-maleic anhydride) includes approximately equimolar amounts of ethylene and maleic anhydride and has a molecular weight of about 75,000 to 90,000 such as, for example, EMA-31 (Monsanto Company).

The capsule contents, termed the internal phase (IP) in this application, comprises an oily solution of a colorless chromogenic dye precursor material, such as described in U.S. Patent 3,681,390. The capsules of oily dye solution are generally in a uniform size range of about 1 to 15 microns. The standard IP used in the examples described herein comprises 1.7% of 3,3-bis(4-dimethylaminophenyl)-6-dimethylaminophthalide (commonly known as crystal violet lactone), 0.55% of (2'-anilino-3'-methyl-6'-diethylaminofluoran) and 0.55% of 3,3-bis(1-ethyl-2-methylindol-3-yl)phthalide (sometimes known as Indolyl Red) in a mixture of solvents including a benzylated ethyl benzene and a relatively high-boiling hydrocarbon oil, such as one having a distillation range of 400° to 500°F.

A solution is made of a mixture of 100 g of a 10% solution of the EMA-31 and 200 g of water. The pH of this solution is raised to 4.5 with 20% sodium hydroxide. Then into this solution is emulsified 200 ml of the IP. The emulsion is placed, with stirring, into a water bath at 55°C. A solution prepared by heating a mixture of 26.5 g of 37% formaldehyde and 20 g of melamine is added thereto. After 2 hours, the heating control is turned off and the capsule batch continues to stir in the cooling water bath overnight. Because the size of the resulting capsules is so small and because the intended capsule use is in carbonless copying papers, the capsules are tested by methods which relate to effectiveness in a copying paper use as described above in U.S. Patent 4,001,140.

A related test concerning capsule quality is the degree of loss of ability of capsule-coated paper to produce transfer prints in a typewriter test after storage of the coated paper in an oven at a specified temperature for a specified time. It is useful to perform a routine typewriter imaging transfer test with a CB/CF couplet, placing the CB in a 95°C oven for 18 hours and then reimaging the couplet after storage. This test has consistently shown that poor capsules will lose most or all of their ability to make a transfer print during such oven storage and that good capsules will withstand this storage with little or no loss in ability to give a print.

One of the significant advantages of the process is that good capsule quality is consistently obtained over a wide range of formaldehyde to melamine ratio. These satisfactory results are reflected in the table below where the F:M (formaldehyde to melamine) ratio, initial typewriter intensity, ITI (before oven storage) and typewriter intensity (TI) after oven storage are given for capsules made in accordance with the procedure described in this example:

F:M Ratio	ITI	TI After Overnight Storage at 95°C
2.06	63	66
4.14	54	59

Example 2: A solution of 50 g of a 10% solution of poly(methyl vinyl ether-maleic anhydride) (Gantrez AN-119, molecular weight approximately 250,000) and 100 g of water is adjusted to a pH of 4.5 with 20% NaOH. A 60% solution of methylol melamine in the amount of 35 g (Resimene 814) is added to the solution, and 150 cc of IP is emulsified therein. The emulsion is placed in a 55°C water bath with agitation. Successful capsules are obtained after 90 minutes as evidenced by an opacimeter reading of 71 obtained on a draw-down on a CF sheet.

Example 3: A solution of 50 g of a 10% solution of poly(propylene-maleic anhydride), as the modifier material, and 100 g of water is adjusted to a pH of 4.0 with 20% NaOH. Emulsified into this solution is 100 cc of standard IP as described in Example 1. Then, 25 g of 80% methylated methylol melamine resin (Resimene 714) is added thereto. The emulsion is placed in a 55°C water bath with agitation. Successful capsules are obtained after 25 minutes.

Example 4: A solution of 38 g of a 13% solution of poly(butadiene-maleic anhydride) in water (Maldene 285) and 77 g of water is adjusted to a pH of 4.0 with NaOH. To this solution is added 25 g of 80% methylated methylol melamine resin (Resimene 714) and 100 cc of standard IP is emulsified therein. The emulsion is placed in a 55°C bath. Successful capsules are obtained as evidenced by an opacimeter reading of 74 obtained by a draw-down on a CF sheet after processing for 40 minutes.

POLYMERIZATION REACTIONS

Polymerization of Reactants in Continuous Phase

M. Kiritani and Y. Ogata; U.S. Patent 3,981,821; Sept. 21, 1976; assigned to Fuji Photo Film Co., Ltd., Japan describe a process for preparing microcapsules having a very high ability to retain a material occluded therein, and a high stability to external forces such as pressure or friction.

This is achieved by a process for encapsulation which comprises emulsifying a hydrophobic liquid to be encapsulated as a disperse phase in a hydrophilic liquid immiscible therewith as a continuous phase, polymerizing at least one capsule wall-forming substance present in the hydrophilic liquid continuous phase, and depositing the resulting polymer around the droplets of the hydrophobic liquid thereby to envelope the hydrophobic liquid droplets from the outside. In the process a substance which has reactivity with at least one of the wall-forming substances in the continuous phase and consequently promotes the deposition of the polymer resulting in the continuous phase is caused to be present in the droplets of the hydrophobic liquid prior to the step of emulsifying the hydrophobic liquid.

It is not essential for the substance contained in the hydrophobic liquid droplets to react with the reactant in the continuous phase to form capsule walls. A part of the reactant in the continuous phase is trapped inside the droplets of the hydrophobic liquid, and the polymer formed in the continuous phase is deposited preferentially around the hydrophobic liquid droplets. Accordingly, the amount of the deposition promoting agent to be added to the hydrophobic liquid in the process is much less than that used in the interfacial polymerization method. In addition, since it is not essential for this agent itself to form capsule walls, this agent is not limited to substances having at least two functional groups as is required in the interfacial polymerization method.

In the process, when one wall-forming substance is used in the continuous phase, it is self-polymerized to form polymer walls, and when two or more wall-forming substances are used, they are copolymerized at least with each other to form polymer walls. The amount of the deposition promoting agent is about 0.05 to 10 parts (preferably 0.2 to 5 parts) per 30 parts by weight of the oily liquid. The weight ratio between the amount of the deposition promoting agent and the amount of the capsule wall-forming substance is 0.16 to 0.4.

The deposition promoting agent to be added to the hydrophobic liquid so as to trap the reactant in the continuous phase onto the surface of the hydrophobic liquid droplets can be any compound which is soluble in the hydrophobic liquid and reacts with at least one reactant in the continuous phase to form a bond.

Typical examples of the reactants which can be used in the continuous phase are a combination of an amino-containing compound and an epoxy compound, a combination of an amino compound and an aldehyde compound, a combination of a urea resin and an aldehyde compound, a combination of a urea resin and an amino compound, a combination of a melamine resin and an amino compound and a combination of a melamine compound and an aldehyde compound, and also compounds which self-polymerize, such as a urea resin or a melamine resin.

Typical examples of deposition promoting agents which can be used in the hydrophobic liquid to be occluded are compounds containing isocyanate groups, compounds containing amino groups, compounds containing acid chloride groups, compounds containing epoxy groups, compounds containing chloroformate groups, and compounds containing aldehyde groups, which are all soluble in the hydrophobic liquid.

Typical combinations of the deposition promoter and the reactant to be polymerized in the continuous phase which can be used are shown in the following table. The deposition promoting agent can be the same compound as or a different compound from the reactant. Any combination can be chosen, as desired.

The reactants used in the continuous phase can be added to the continuous phase prior to the emulsification of the hydrophobic liquid in the continuous phase, or after the emulsification. The deposition promoter used in the hydrophobic liquid should be dissolved in the hydrophobic liquid prior to emulsification.

Deposition Promoter in the Hydrophobic Liquid	Reactants to Be Polymerized in the Continuous Phase
Isocyanate compound	Amino compound and epoxy compound
Amino compound	Amino compound and aldehyde compound
Acid chloride compound	Urea resin and aldehyde compound
Epoxy compound	Urea resin and amino compound
Chloroformate compound	Melamine resin and aldehyde compound
Aldehyde compound	Melamine resin, urea resin

A suitable amount of the reactants in the hydrophilic liquid can range from about 0.1 to 20, preferably 0.2 to 10 parts by weight per 30 parts by weight of the hydrophilic liquid. To prepare the microcapsules, an oily liquid including a deposition promoter is added into the continuous phase optionally containing a reactant and emulsified. Alternatively, after emulsification a reactant can be added to the continuous phase. The temperature at which microencapsulation is performed is not limited in particular. Generally, a preferred range is from about room temperature (e.g., 20° to 30°C) to about 95°C.

The hydrophobic liquid to be encapsulated is an organic solvent which is immiscible with water. Specific examples include synthetic oils such as alkylnaphthalenes, alkylated diphenyls, alkylated diphenylalkanes, hexahydroterphenyl, triaryldimethanes, chlorinated paraffins, diethyl phthalate, dibutyl phthalate, dioctyl phthalate, dibutyl maleate, toluene, dichlorobenzene or benzyl alcohol, and natural oils such as cottonseed oil, soybean oil, corn oil, castor oil, fish oil or lard. Furthermore, it is possible to use the deposition promoter itself as the hydrophobic liquid and encapsulate the deposition promoter as the hydrophobic liquid.

In order to emulsify and disperse the hydrophobic liquid in an aqueous liquid, a protective colloid or a surface active agent can be used. Examples of protective colloids are natural or synthetic water-soluble polymeric substances such as gelatin, gum arabic, casein, carboxymethylcellulose, starch or polyvinyl alcohol. A suitable amount of the protective colloid can range from about 0.5 to 30% by weight, preferably 2 to 20% by weight.

Examples of surface active agents are anionic surfactants such as alkylbenzenesulfonic acid salts, alkyl naphthalenesulfonic acid salts, polyoxyethylene sulfuric acid salts or Turkey red oil; nonionic surfactants such as polyoxyethylene alkyl ethers, polyoxyethylenes, or sorbitan fatty acid esters; cationic surfactants such as alkylamine salts, quaternary ammonium salts or polyoxyethylene alkyl amines; and amphoteric surfactants such as alkylbetaines. A suitable amount of the surface active agent can range from about 0.02 to 1% by weight, preferably 0.05 to 0.5% by weight in the continuous phase.

The microcapsules produced by the process have a very high ability to retain the contents of the capsules and a very high mechanical strength. Accordingly, these advantages are especially significant when the microcapsules obtained by the process are utilized in pressure-sensitive copying paper.

Example: 1 g of crystal violet lactone (a color former for pressure-sensitive copying paper and used as an indicator for determining the ability of the capsules to retain the contents) was dissolved in 30 g of isopropyl naphthalene (a hydrophobic liquid to be occluded). In the resulting solution was dissolved 0.5 g of tolylene diisocyanate trimer as a deposition promoter. The hydrophobic liquid obtained was added with vigorous stirring to 50 g of water at 15°C containing 2 g of carboxymethylcellulose and 2 g of polyvinyl alcohol dissolved therein to thereby form droplets of the hydrophobic liquid each having a diameter of about 5 to 10 microns and then 100 g of water was added.

To the resulting system were added as reactants to be added to the continuous phase, 3 g of Epomate N-001 (an adduct of 1 mol of 3,9-bis-aminopropyl-2,4-8,10-tetraoxaspiro[5.5] undecane and 1 mol of acrylonitrile, a polyamine, active hydrogen equivalent 110, amine value 340) and 3 g of an aqueous solution of formaldehyde (47% by weight) gradually. At this time, the Epomate N-001 polymerized with the formaldehyde in the aqueous phase to form a water-insoluble polymer. The polymer deposited around the hydrophobic liquid droplets preferentially due to the action of the deposit-promoting agent present in the hydrophobic liquid, and formed the capsule walls.

The above steps were all conducted at 15°C. After stirring this system continuously for 4 hours at this temperature, the system was heated to 40°C to complete the reaction, and the encapsulation was completed. Microcapsules containing the solution of crystal violet lactone in isopropyl naphthalene, enveloped with a capsule wall of a polymer formed between the polyamine and formaldehyde, were obtained. The microcapsules so obtained had a very superior ability to retain the contents, and were stable to pressure or friction. In order to compare these microcapsules with microcapsules produced using other methods, microcapsules were prepared by the following two methods, and compared with the microcapsules obtained by the process.

Encapsulation by Method A – Encapsulation was performed only by a polymerization of reactants in the continuous phase without using a deposition promoter in the hydrophobic liquid to be occluded. In other words, the example was repeated except that the deposition promoter was not used.

Encapsulation by Method B – Encapsulation was performed only by the interfacial polymerization of the reactant in the hydrophobic liquid to be occluded with the reactant in the continuous phase. That is to say, the example was repeated except that the formaldehyde was not added to the continuous phase. In this case, the tolylene diisocyanate polymer in the hydrophobic liquid droplets and the Epomate N-001 (polyamine) in the continuous phase were reactants for forming the capsule walls by interfacial polymerization. Actually, however, capsules were not formed in this case.

Each of these three capsule solutions (the capsule solution obtained by the process, the capsule solution obtained by method A, and the capsule solution obtained by method B) was coated on a sheet of paper using a coating bar, and dried at 100° to 150°C to form a sheet coated with capsules. Since these capsules contained crystal violet lactone as a color former for a pressure-sensitive copying paper, the resulting sheet could be used as an upper sheet of a pressure-sensitive paper. The upper sheet immediately after coating was superimposed on a lower sheet of a pressure-sensitive copying paper. The lower sheet had been obtained by adding 8 cc of a 20% by weight aqueous solution of sodium hydroxide as a dispersing agent and 100 g of acid clay to 300 g of water, stirring the mixture vigorously to form a dispersion, then adding 40 g of a styrene-butadiene latex as a binder to form a color developer solution, coating the color developer solution on a sheet of paper using a coating bar, and drying it. A pressure of 600 kg/cm^2 was applied to the superimposed assembly to rupture all the microcapsules whereupon blue marks were obtained on the lower sheet of the pressure-sensitive copying paper.

When the upper sheet coated with each of the capsule solutions was first heated at 80°C for 24 hours and then pressure was applied to an assembly of the upper and lower sheet, no reduction in color-forming ability was observed with the upper sheet coated with the capsule solution obtained by the encapsulation method of this process. However, since the upper sheets coated with the capsule solution obtained using methods A and B had already released their occluded liquid due to the action of heat, no color was formed at all. It can thus be seen that with methods A and B, capsules were essentially not formed, but only an emulsion of the hydrophobic liquid resulted. The microcapsules obtained by the encapsulation method of this process have an excellent ability to retain the occluded hydrophobic liquid as compared with methods A and B.

Furthermore, the upper sheet immediately after coating was superimposed on the lower sheet, and the capsules were ruptured with a relatively weak pressure of 40 kg/cm^2. Then, the density of color contamination on the lower sheet was measured for comparison. It was found that when the upper paper coated with the capsules obtained by the process was used, the density of color contamination was far lower than in the case of using the capsule solutions obtained with methods A and B. This showed that the microcapsules obtained by the process are very resistant to slight pressures. Accordingly, when utilized in a pressure-sensitive copying paper, the microcapsules in accordance with the process have the advantage of giving products of a high commercial value because color is not formed due to weak pressures encountered during handling.

According to methods A and B, capsule walls were not at all formed, and the emulsion of the hydrophobic liquid was exposed. Consequently, even by mere contact with the lower sheet, color was formed on the lower sheet. As described above, the microcapsules obtained by the method were far superior to those obtained with methods A and B in respect to the ability to retain the occluded liquid and mechanical strength.

Emulsion Polymerization Using Copolymer of Sulfo Ester and n-Butyl Acrylate

The work of *D.S. Morehouse, Jr., and F.H. Bolton; U.S. Patents 4,075,134; Feb. 21, 1978; and 4,049,604; September 20, 1977; both assigned to The Dow Chemical Company* relates to the preparation of microspheres having liquid centers and seamless rigid walls of an organic polymer.

The method comprises the steps of: (1) dispersing an oil phase comprising at least one emulsion polymerizable monomer in an aqueous phase containing from about 0.5 to 4 wt % based on total monomer of a stabilizing emulsifier and from about 0.2 to 2 wt % based on total monomer of a polymer of a sulfo hydrocarbyl ester of an α,β-ethylenically unsaturated carboxylic acid, the polymer containing at least about 1 milliequivalent of sulfo groups (SO_3^-) per gram of polymer, the total monomer of the oil phase being capable of polymerization to form a water-insoluble polymer; and (2) subjecting the dispersion to emulsion polymerization conditions such that the total monomer polymerizes to form particles of water-insoluble polymer. Polymeric particles of these aqueous dispersions generally have average diameters ranging from about 0.5 to 20 microns, with some particles having diameters up to about 45 microns. The essence of this process resides in the use of a polymer of a sulfohydrocarbyl ester of an α,β-ethylenically unsaturated carboxylic acid as a coalescing aid in an emulsion polymerization process.

These microspheres can be utilized as expandable spheres in the fabrication of porous foams. Thermoplastic microspheres encapsulating liquids are also useful in the production of insecticides, pharmaceuticals, inks, fire retardants and the like. Additionally it is possible to remove the liquid by evaporation or a similar means, thus leaving a hollow microsphere which serves as an excellent lightweight filler for paints or paper coatings. Microspheres having polymeric liquid centers are useful in the production of multipurpose plastic materials.

Any emulsion polymerizable ethylenically unsaturated monomer which is inert to the copolymer of the sulfohydrocarbyl ester is suitably employed, provided that the total emulsion polymerizable monomer will polymerize to form a water-insoluble polymer.

Of the suitable monomers, particularly advantageous monomers include styrene and methyl methacrylate. Of the monomers often beneficially employed in small quantities, it is found that the use of divinylbenzene as a crosslinking agent in the monomeric mixture substantially increases the percent of liquid which can be encapsulated. However, the use of divinyl benzene and other crosslinking agents is preferably limited to concentrations up to about 3.0% by weight based on the monomer weight in order to avoid formation of significant amounts of coagulum during polymerization.

Liquids which are encapsulated by the process are substantially inert, i.e., non-reactive with the monomer or with the polymer formed. Liquids suitable for this purpose are nonpolymerizable and do not inhibit the emulsion polymerization of the monomeric components. Such liquids are generally soluble in the monomeric phase and insoluble in the resulting polymer.

Examples of suitable liquids include the inert hydrocarbons and halo-hydrocarbons, e.g., hexane, neopentane, carbon tetrachloride; the aromatic hydrocarbons and halogen-substituted aromatic hydrocarbons, e.g., benzene, toluene, chlorobenzene; the chlorofluorocarbons; and the tetraalkyl silanes. Also included are liquid polymers such as a low molecular weight polybutadiene.

Coalescing aids utilized are polymers of sulfohydrocarbyl esters of α,β-ethylenically unsaturated carboxylic acids. Such sulfohydrocarbyl ester polymers are at least inherently water-dispersible, and are preferably water-soluble. By "inherently water-dispersible" is meant capability of forming a colloidal dispersion in water in the absence of chemical dispersing aids such as surfactants, emulsifiers, etc. Sulfohydrocarbyl ester polymers usually contain from about 1 to 5.5, preferably from about 1 to about 2.6 milliequivalents of sulfo groups (SO_3^-), whether in form of the acid and/or salt, per gram of the sulfohydrocarbyl ester polymer. Normally, sulfohydrocarbyl ester polymers containing at least 10 mol % of the polymerized sulfohydrocarbyl ester, preferably at least about 15 mol %, are sufficient to provide the preferred proportion of sulfo (SO_3^-) groups. So long as the sulfohydrocarbyl ester polymer is at least inherently water-dispersible, molecular weight of the polymer is not particularly critical. Accordingly, polymers having average molecular weights from about 5,000 up to about 3 million are suitable, with polymers having average molecular weights in the range from about 10,000 to 200,000 being preferred. Of the sulfohydrocarbyl esters, those of the α-methylene carboxylic acids are preferred, especially 2-sulfoethyl methacrylate.

Preferred coalescing aids are the copolymers of the preferred ethylenically unsaturated monomers and the sulfoalkyl esters of α-methylene carboxylic acids, for example, copolymers of n-butyl acrylate and 2-sulfoethyl methacrylate, copolymers of styrene and 2-sulfoethyl methacrylate and copolymers of acrylonitrile and 2-sulfoethyl methacrylate and other copolymers wherein alkyl of the sulfoalkyl ester has from 2 to 12 carbon atoms. Especially preferred coalescing aids are the copolymers of the alkyl acrylates having alkyl moieties from 1 to 12 carbon atoms and the sulfoalkyl esters of α-methylene carboxylic acids, and in particular, a copolymer of 70 wt % of n-butyl acrylate and 30 wt % of 2-sulfoethyl methacrylate. Other preferred and suitable copolymers and methods for the preparation thereof are described in U.S. Patent 3,033,833.

Stabilizing emulsifiers suitable are the water-soluble anionic and nonionic surfactants, with anionic or mixtures of anionic and nonionic being preferred.

The choice of emulsifiers varies with the emulsion system, particle size desired, and so forth. In systems where a particle size ranging from about 4 to 5 microns is desired, sodium dodecylbenzenesulfonate is preferred.

In some instances it is preferable to include a small amount, i.e., up to about 1 wt % based on total monomer, of an electrolyte in the polymerization recipe in order to keep the formation of coagulum at a minimum and to increase the degree of liquid encapsulation.

The emulsion polymerization of one or more suitable monomers is carried out in the presence of from about 0.5 to 4 wt % (preferably 1 to 3%) of a suitable stabilizing emulsifier and from about 0.2 to 2 wt % (preferably 0.25 to 1%) of a suitable polymer of a sulfohydrocarbyl ester, both percentages being based on total emulsion polymerizable monomer (hereinafter referred to as total monomer).

If the method is carried out in the presence of an electrolyte in addition to an emulsifier and a polymer of a sulfohydrocarbyl ester, it is desirable that the electrolyte be present in concentrations from about 0.2 to 1 wt % based on total monomer, preferably from 0.25 to 0.5 wt %.

In preparing microspheres having liquid centers by the method, it is necessary to use concentrations of the liquid to be encapsulated less than about 50 volume percent based on the oil phase of liquid and monomer, with the best results being attained at concentrations from about 15 to 20 volume percent. In addition, the ratio of the volume of the oil phase to the volume of the aqueous phase also has a decided effect on the amount of liquid which is encapsulated in the microspheres. Total oil phase concentrations from about 33 volume percent to about 55 volume percent based on the total oil and aqueous phases are operable, with concentrations from about 44 to 55 volume percent being preferred.

The method is carried out by first dispersing an oil phase containing at least one emulsion polymerizable monomer in an aqueous phase containing a stabilizing emulsifier and a suitable coalescing aid. The dispersion is preferably achieved by subjecting the two phases to high-shear mixing conditions, for example, a homogenizing device, a Waring blendor and the like. In the preparation of microspheres, encapsulation of the liquid is not accomplished unless a dispersion of the phases is achieved.

The resulting dispersion of the oil and aqueous phases is charged to a suitable reaction vessel and subjected to conditions of emulsion polymerization, for example, initiation by a free-radical-type catalyst such as potassium persulfate at a temperature from about 60° to 100°C and agitation of the dispersion during the polymerization period. The emulsion polymerization is usually carried out in the presence of from about 0.01 to about 3 wt % based on the total monomer weight of the free-radical-producing catalyst. Suitable catalysts are the peroxygen compounds, especially the inorganic persulfate compounds such as sodium persulfate; the peroxides such as hydrogen peroxide; the organic hydroperoxides, such as cumene hydroperoxide; the organic peroxides such as benzoyl peroxide; and the other free-radical-producing materials such as 2,2'-azobisisobutyronitrile.

Example 1: 1.25 g of 2-hydroxyethyl acrylate and 98.75 g of methyl methacrylate were mixed in 25 g of neohexane. This oil mixture was mixed with an aqueous solution of 125 g of deionized water, 0.5 g of sodium sulfate, 0.5 g of potassium persulfate, 1.0 g of sodium dodecylbenzenesulfonate and 1.0 g of a copolymer of 30% (~22 mol %) of 2-sulfoethyl methacrylate and 70% (~78 mol %) of butyl acrylate. The mixture was passed through a hand homogenizer to obtain intimate mixing of the oil and aqueous media. The intimate mixture was poured into a citrate bottle and then was agitated by tumbling the bottle end-over-end at about 4.5 rpm for a period of 16 hours in a water bath at a temperature of 70°C. At the end of the sixteen hour period, 94% of the charge was recovered in addition to a small amount of coagulum.

Under an optical microscope the reaction product was shown to consist of microspheres having a uniform size of about 1 micron with only a few particles as large as 5 microns. In order to show the presence of a liquid inclusion, a film containing the microspheres was cast upon a flat surface and allowed to dry at room temperature overnight. By heating this film in a vacuum oven at 150°C and measuring the loss of weight, it was found that the dry film contained 12% neohexane. Inclusion of liquid in the microspheres was further confirmed by observation of the Brownian motion of a bubble on the surface of the encapsulated liquid.

Example 2: The following ingredients were placed into a 12-ounce citrate bottle.

	Amount, g
Styrene	50.0
Deionized water	150.0
Sodium sulfate	0.5
Potassium persulfate	0.5
Sodium dodecylbenzenesulfonate	3.0
Copolymer of 30% of 2-sulfoethyl methacrylate and 70% of n-butyl acrylate	0.5

The bottle and contents were cooled in ice and 50 g of liquid butadiene was added to the contents. The bottle was capped and tumbled in a 70°C water bath for 24 hours after which the bottle was opened and the contents filtered. The contents consisted of 20 g of coagulum and 235 g of an aqueous dispersion having 38.7% polymer solids. The particles of the dispersion were examined under an optical microscope and most were found to have diameters ranging from 6 to about 18 microns, with some particles having diameters as small as 1 to 2 microns. The aqueous dispersion was readily concentrated to high solids by evaporation.

Micelle Polymerization for Microcapsules in the Nanometer Range

A method of polymerization limited to the micellar region has been developed by *P. Speiser and G. Birrenbach; U.S. Patent 4,021,364; May 3, 1977* on the basis of the existing doctrine and knowledge of emulsion polymerization. This method leads to the microcapsules which consist of a polymeric material, preferably of a hydrophilic gel from polymerized acrylamides, acrylic acid and/or their derivatives and which have a diameter in the nanometer range of 20 to 200 nanometers, preferably 80 nanometers and are colloidally soluble in water, and contains active substances in a capsulated and/or adsorbed form. The polymer preferably has a porous structure.

These micellar capsules can be produced by genuinely or at least colloidally dissolving water-soluble, polymerizable molecules and the material to be encapsulated, for example, the biologically or pharmacodynamically active substance together in water. This aqueous solution is distributed while stirring, in a hydrophobic liquid, which constitutes a phase, in which the synthetic monomers and the active substances are difficultly soluble or insoluble, with the aid of boundary surface active auxiliaries (tensides).

Minute micelles containing the polymerizable monomers, active components and possibly other auxiliary agents, are solubilized in a relatively large volume of the hydrophobic phase and form extremely small reaction regions for ensuing polymerization of the monomers. This is induced by the methods already known (cf., for example, German Patent 1,081,288 or U.S. Patents 2,880,152 and 2,880,153). In this process, polymerization is restricted principally to the micellar regions, for the hydrophobic main phase contains no polymerizable material and even a diffusion of monomers in and through this phase is largely prevented.

To encapsulate water-insoluble materials the system can be modified in such a way that a lipophilic phase with the dissolved material and oil-soluble monomers are solubilized in a hydrophilic medium, usually water. In this case the diffusion of monomers through the hydrophilic phase is largely prevented.

In contrast to emulsion polymerization, in which in most cases water-insoluble monomers polymerize in water and in which the radical-containing, polymerizing emulsion droplets may swell to many times their original size, due to the diffusion of monomers from the stock of the emulsion droplets present into the growing polymer-monomer particles (latex particles), micelle polymerization, according to the process is limited strictly to the monomers contained in the micelles. For this reason the particles remain extremely small.

After completion of the polymerization, the solid residue is diluted with a suitable solvent, generally with an aqueous alcohol, e.g., methanol, by removal and concentration of the external phase, e.g., by distillation, ultrafiltration and centrifuging, and the polymer particles formed can usually be precipitated and extracted by the filtration or centrifuging of the soluble accompanying substances and the emulsifier. Relatively short-chained n-alkanes, preferably n-hexane and n-heptane are most suitable as liquid for the hydrophobic phase.

It has also been found that the combination of a suitable nonionogenic emulsifier with an ionogenic emulsifier leads to a substantially better solubilization of the aqueous phase. As nonionogenic emulsifiers, good results have been obtained with fatty alcohol polyglycol ethers, e.g., polyethylene lauryl ether with an average of 4 ethylene oxide units in the chain, and as an ionogenic emulsifier, alkaline salts of higher sulfosuccinic acid bisalkyl esters, e.g., sulfosuccinic acid bis-2-ethylhexyl ester sodium salt.

For the capsulation of lipophilic active materials good service has been given by a solubilized mixture in water of Tween 80, e.g., polyoxyethylene sorbitol monooleate, in, for example, ethyl oleate, paraffin, castor oil or other fatty acid esters with acrylic acid derivatives as monomers, preferably acrylic acid or acrylic acid methyl ester or, where appropriate, some vinyl derivatives.

Not every active material, protein, drug, pesticide, fertilizer, dye, is equally suitable for incorporation in the micellar reticular structures obtained according to the process. A particular molecular size and the ability to form at least colloidal, aqueous or oily solutions are essential conditions, for incorporation in the micelles occurs during the production only when the active substances are located in the micelles. Substances with a molecular weight up to about 150,000 and which are at least colloid water-soluble or oil-soluble are suitable.

In the case of radioactively tagged human gamma globulin in micelle capsules, kept in vitro for a period of 50 days at 37°C in an agitated phosphate buffer solution, only 20% of the gamma globulins were liberated unaltered from the time measurement was commenced, which shows that the largest part of the active substance had been well encapsulated. On the other hand, results with gamma globulin in an immunization test with guinea pigs in vivo show that high and relatively persistent titers are obtained very soon.

Example 1: Toxoid – 12.0 g sulfosuccinic acid bis-2-ethylhexyl ester as sodium salt (Aerosol OT), and 6.0 g polyoxyethylene(4)-lauryl ether with an average of 4 ethylene oxide units in the chain (tenside LA-55-4, Hefti AG) are dissolved in 20.0 g n-hexane; the solution is filtered until sterile. While stirring, from this point onwards under sterile conditions, 10.0 g aqueous toxoid solution (diphtheria or tetanus toxoid with 100 Lf/ml) is added, care being taken to add the toxoid slowly in order that the solution remains clear. After a further 20.0 g n-hexane have been added, the monomers are stirred in, viz, 0.250 g N,N'-methylene bisacrylamide and 2.000 g acrylamide. Once the crystalline components have been completely dissolved, the total weight is brought up to 110.0 g with n-hexane.

The solution is covered with a layer of nitrogen, sealed tight, and exposed continuously to the radiation of a cobalt 60 source at about 20° to 30°C. A dose of 0.3 Mrad is sufficient to ensure polymerization. The end of polymerization, i.e., the disappearance of the monomers can be checked with an acidimetric color titration method to determine α,β-unsaturated compounds by means of a reaction with morpholine (F.E. Critchfield, G.L. Funk, J.B. Johnson; *Analyt. Chem.* 28, 78–79, 1956).

After polymerization is complete the n-hexane hydrophobic phase is removed by gentle distillation at room temperature under a vacuum created by a water jet pump. From the remaining concentrated aqueous solution of product and tenside, the tensides are removed by ultrafiltration with distilled water (diaphragm—Amicon PK 30) under an excess pressure of nitrogen (approximately 2 to 4 atm). A colloidal aqueous solution of the product of microcapsules having a diameter in the range of 20 to 200 nanometers is obtained and can be lyophilized (freeze-dried). The mean diameter of the microcapsules is less than about 50 nanometers.

Example 2: Gamma Globulin – 45.0 g Aerosol OT and 25.0 g LA-55-4 are dissolved in 215.0 g n-hexane. 2.5 g ethanol, 2.5 g methanol, 40.0 g of distilled water, 1.000 g N,N'-methylene bisacrylamide and 8.000 g acrylamide are then added in that order and dissolved until the solution is clear. The solubilized mixture is filtered until sterile, and the weight made up to 340.0 g with n-hexane. While stirring, and under sterile conditions from this point onwards, 10.0 g of a gamma globulin solution (aggregate-free in tris-HCl + NaCl 0.100 g; approximately 1.4% human IgG) are solubilized drop by drop.

The polymerization was carried out by gamma irradiation, as described in Example 1. The isolation of the micelle capsules having diameters in the range of 20 to 200 nanometers can take place, corresponding to Example 1.

Example 3: Enzyme – 12.0 g Aerosol OT and 6.0 g LA-55-4 are dissolved in 80.0 g n-hexane; 35.0 g distilled water is slowly solubilized, while the solution is being stirred, and the crystalline monomers 0.500 g N,N'-methylene bisacrylamide and 4.000 g acrylamide are dissolved therein. The solution is filtered until sterile and 0.300 g urease (freeze-dried product, water-soluble, Merck) is introduced to form a micellar solution.

The solution obtained is irradiated from the inside by an ultraviolet dipping lamp (quartz burner 70 W) for 45 minutes in the cylindrical reaction vessel, while stirring and at a temperature constancy of 35±5°C and with a nitrogen stream continuously bubbling through the solution until the monomers disappear.

After polymerization is complete the solution is mixed in excess with methanol containing not less than 80% alcohol. The product of microcapsules having a diameter in the range of 20 to 200 nanometers is precipitated and can be extracted by centrifuging or filtered under pressure and washed.

Example 4: Insecticide – 50 g water was added, while stirring, to a solution of 5.0 g toluene, 50 mg diethyl-p-nitrophenyl monothiophosphate and 10 g polyoxyethylene sorbitan monooleate (Tween 80). 1.5 g acrylic acid methyl ester was stirred into this solution.

In this solution, placed in a cylindrical, double-walled, thermostable reaction vessel of pyrex glass (internal diameter of 6 cm) 0.2 mg riboflavin 5'-sodium phosphate and 0.2 mg $K_2S_2O_8$ are dissolved, while stirring. While stirring constantly and at a constant temperature of 35°±5°C the solution is continuously perfused with a stream of nitrogen bubbles, and irradiated from outside, halfway up the column of liquid at a distance of 15 centimeters with a light bulb, type Osram (300 W), for seven hours until the monomers disappear.

The isolation of the micelle capsules having diameters in the range of 20 to 200 nanometers with the insecticide was accomplished according to Example 3.

PHASE SEPARATION

Partially Hydrolyzed Poly(Ethylene-Vinyl Acetate) Sheath

The method of producing microcapsules having a capsule core material surrounded by a protective wall described by *R.G. Bayless; U.S. Patent 4,107,071; Aug. 15, 1978; assigned to Capsulated Systems, Inc.* is practiced by forming an agitated system which includes (a) a liquid vehicle as a major component of the system and constituting a continuous first phase; (b) a plurality of discrete capsule core material entities dispersed in the liquid vehicle and constituting a discontinuous second phase; and (c) a film-forming, crosslinkable, polymeric base material, such as partially-hydrolyzed poly(ethylene-vinyl acetate) containing about 60 to 85 mol % ethylene, having a melt index of about 18 to 50, that ultimately provides the protective wall for the core material.

The polymeric base material is selected so as to wet the capsule core material, i.e., to microencapsulate an aqueous solution a hydrophilic polymeric base material is used. To microencapsulate, a sheath of the crosslinkable polymeric base material and liquid vehicle entrapped therein (i.e., an embryonic microcapsule wall) is formed about the capsule core material entities by inducing liquid-liquid phase separation within the aforesaid system. To this end, a phase separation-inducing material in an amount sufficient to separate the crosslinkable polymeric base material from the continuous first phase can be used, or phase separation can be induced by adjusting the system temperature so that the crosslinkable polymeric base material is rendered less soluble in the liquid vehicle and separates out as a distinct liquid phase.

Thereafter at least the major portion of the entrapped liquid vehicle is extracted from the sheath, reducing the thickness and increasing the density thereof, and the densified polymeric base material in the embryonic capsule wall is crosslinked to form a densified protective wall around the capsule core material. The produced microcapsules can then be recovered from the system, washed, and dried to produce a freely-flowing particulate mass.

The quantitative relationships of the wall-forming material and the phase separation-inducing material depend on the particular materials that are used and also on the thickness of the protective wall desired for the capsule core material. In general, the wall-forming material constitutes about 0.5 to about 5% (preferably about 1 to 2%) of the total system volume, the phase separation-inducing material constitutes about 1 to 15% (preferably about 8 to 12%) of the total system volume, and the discrete capsule core material entities constitute about 2 to 30% (preferably about 15 to 20%) of the total system volume.

Microcapsule size can extend from an average diameter of about 1 micron and less to about several thousand microns and more. The usual size for the produced microcapsules is about 1 to about 15,000 microns in average diameter, and is generally in the range of about 5 to 2,500 microns. Similarly, the microcapsules can be manufactured containing varying amounts of core material which can constitute up to about 99% or more of the total weight of each microcapsule. Preferably the core material constitutes about 50 to 97% of the total weight of each microcapsule.

The encapsulation method is particularly useful for the production of microcapsules containing aqueous solutions and dispersions, water-soluble compounds such as hydroxy-containing organic compounds, polyhydroxy-containing organic compounds, and the like. The method also lends itself very well to the production of pharmacological preparations having controlled or slow-release properties, e.g., microencapsulated potassium penicillin, microencapsulated aspirin, and the like.

Example 1: Manufacture of Microcapsules Having Densified Walls of Cross-Linked Hydrolyzed Poly(Ethylene-Vinyl Acetate) – Poly(ethylene-vinyl acetate) which is about 44 to 52% hydrolyzed and having a melt index of about 35 to 37 is dissolved in hot trichloroethylene (about 500 ml; about 80°C) to produce a solution containing about 2 wt % hydrolyzed poly(ethylene-vinyl acetate)(HEVA). The obtained solution is then cooled to room temperature with stirring. An aqueous citric acid solution (about 80 ml; about 20 wt % citric acid) is then added to the cooled trichloroethylene solution of HEVA and emulsified to about 100 to 500 micron droplets.

Cottonseed oil (about 90 ml) is then added to the produced emulsion, followed by toluene diisocyanate (about 5 ml) dissolved in trichloroethylene (about 30 ml) and more cottonseed oil (about 500 ml). The thus produced admixture is then stirred for about 24 hours at ambient temperature, and subsequently discrete microcapsules having a size of about 100 to 500 microns are recovered from the admixture, washed with trichloroethylene and dried. The microcapsules contain aqueous citric acid solution as the core material, surrounded by a relatively nonporous, densified protective wall.

Example 2: Manufacture of Microcapsules Utilizing Silicone Oil as Phase Separation-Inducing and Wall Densifying Agent – Microcapsules containing an aqueous citric acid solution as the core material are prepared in a manner similar to Example 1 except that polydimethylsiloxane L-45, (Union Carbide Corporation) is used in lieu of cottonseed oil to induce the phase separation and to densify the capsule walls. The prepared microcapsules are of good quality and have a relatively nonporous protective wall around the core material.

Example 3: Preparation of Microcapsules Using a Densifying Agent That Is Different than the Phase Separation Inducing Agent – Poly(ethylene-vinyl acetate) which is about 44 to 52% hydrolyzed and has a melt index of about 35 to 37 is dissolved in hot toluene (about 500 ml; about 80°C) to produce a solution containing about 2 wt % HEVA. The obtained solution is then cooled to about 50°C with stirring and an aqueous citric acid solution (about 80 ml; about 20 wt % citric acid) is added thereto and emulsified to aqueous droplets of about 50 to about 200 microns in size. Thereafter cottonseed oil is added to the produced emulsion and the resulting admixture is cooled in an ice bath to about 20°C as a HEVA sheath forms about the aqueous droplets.

Polydimethyl siloxane (L-45, about 200 ml) is slowly added to the cooled admixture to permit a slow shrinkage of the HEVA sheath. After the addition of polydimethylsiloxane is completed, a toluene diisocyanate adduct of trimethylol propane (Mondur CB-75, about 10 ml) dissolved in toluene (about 30 ml) is added with agitation to crosslink the HEVA sheath that has been densified by the addition of polydimethylsiloxane.

To effect crosslinking of the HEVA-sheath, the produced admixture is stirred for about 18 hours, and thereafter about 50 to 200 micron microcapsules, having a densified wall are recovered from the admixture, washed in toluene, and then dried. The dried capsules are of high quality and exhibit no tendency toward exudation of the core material.

Example 4: Preparation of Microcapsules Utilizing Malonyl Chloride as Cross-Linking Agent – Microcapsules are prepared in a manner similar to Example 3 except that malonyl chloride dissolved in toluene (about 4 wt % solution; about 50 ml) is utilized in lieu of the toluene diisocyanate adduct of trimethylol propane. To effect crosslinking, the produced admixture is stirred for about 10 minutes, and thereafter high quality microcapsules are recovered, washed, and dried.

Critical Combination of Polymer, Solvent, Vehicle and Nonsolvent

M. Morishita, Y. Inaba, M. Fukushima, S. Kobari, A. Nagata and J. Abe; U.S. Patent 3,943,063; March 9, 1976; assigned to Toyo Jozo Company, Ltd., Japan found that microcapsules can be made easily by effecting a phase separation between the three elements of a polymer, a solvent and a nonsolvent in the fourth element of a vehicle. That is, microcapsules can be made by dispersing or dissolving a core substance into a polymer dissolved in a solvent, emulsifying this dispersion or solution in fine droplets in a vehicle which is poorly miscible with the solvent and then adding a nonsolvent which is miscible with the solvent, poorly miscible with the vehicle and does not dissolve the polymer, to the emulsion system, whereby the solvent is removed by being absorbed by the nonsolvent emulsion droplets to precipitate the polymer around the cores.

By a suitable combination of a polymer solvent, a nonsolvent and a vehicle, a core substance, whether it may be in a state of liquid or solid, may be formed into microcapsules. In addition, it is also found that a polymer, whether it may either be hydrophilic or hydrophobic, natural or synthetic, may be used as a film-forming polymer. The core can be hydrophilic or hydrophobic, unstable to heat or pH, soluble or insoluble in a polymer solvent, and in any state, including liquids, solutions, pastes and solids.

In order to conduct encapsulation operation easily and also to obtain microcapsules with tough films, it is desirable to use a core substance in an amount from 0.2 to 20 times the amount of a film-forming polymer.

It is critical that a combination of the four elements, i.e., polymer, solvents, vehicle and nonsolvent, should be restricted by the following requirements: (a) polymer solvents should be poorly miscible with vehicles; (b) nonsolvents should not dissolve polymers; (c) polymer solvents should be miscible with nonsolvents; (d) nonsolvents should be poorly miscible with vehicles; and (e) vehicles should not dissolve polymers.

For example, when a solvent and a nonsolvent are hydrophilic and a vehicle is lipophilic, a solvent is preferably selected from water, acidic water, alkaline water, acetone, methanol, ethanol, isopropanol, dimethylformamide, formic acid, acetic acid and dimethylsulfoxide, while the nonsolvent is preferably selected from water, acidic water, alkaline water, acetone, methanol, ethanol, isopropanol, n-butanol, ethylene glycol, dimethylformamide, tetrahydrofuran and aqueous formalin solution. In this case, a vehicle is preferably a liquid paraffin or a silicone oil. The most preferable result is obtained when water or an aqueous solution is used as a nonsolvent.

On the other hand, when a solvent and a nonsolvent are lipophilic and a vehicle is hydrophilic, a solvent is preferably selected from ethylene chloride, chloroform, methyl acetate, ethyl acetate, benzene, toluene, xylene and carbon tetrachloride, while the nonsolvent is preferably selected from hexane, petroleum ether and toluene. In this case, a vehicle is preferably ethylene glycol, propylene glycol, formamide or an aqueous gelatin solution.

Example 1: 5 g of a cellulose acetate phthalate (product of Wako Junyaku Co.) are dissolved in 60 ml of dimethylsulfoxide to prepare a solution. Into this solution are dispersed 10 g of pancreatin powders of the Japanese Pharmacopoeia (product of Iwashiro Seiyaku Co.). This dispersion is emulsified under stirring with a propeller in 300 ml of the liquid paraffin of the Japanese Pharmacopoeia (19 cp, 25°C) in fine droplets (200 to 500 μ). Stirring is continued for several minutes until the state of emulsion is stabilized. Then, 100 ml of a mixed solvent of water-acetone (4:1) is added as a nonsolvent to the emulsion, whereby microcapsules are formed. The microcapsules are collected by filtration by using a filter cloth, washed thoroughly with n-hexane and dried.

The product obtained is an intestine soluble microcapsule, which on administration is disintegrated not in the stomach, but in the intestine. Hence, this method is suitable for encapsulation of core substances which are unstable in gastric juice.

Example 2: 2 g of a vinyl chloride-vinyl acetate copolymer (product of Denki Kagaku Kogyo KK) are dissolved in 20 ml of ethylene chloride to prepare a solution. Into this solution are dispersed uniformly 4 g of alkali phosphatase powders (1 to 5 μ, product of Seikagaku Kogyo Co.). This dispersion is added dropwise into 200 ml of ethylene glycol containing 0.5% of a surface active agent Lanex (product of Croda Nippon Co.), to prepare an emulsion containing 100 to 150 μ of emulsified droplets. Then, 100 ml of n-hexane are added slowly to the emulsion, whereby polymer films are precipitated around the cores to give microcapsules containing alkali phosphatase. After filtration, the microcapsules are washed with n-hexane and dried.

The films of the microcapsules obtained are semipermeable membranes, which hydrolyze p-nitrophenyl phosphate in an aqueous p-nitrophenyl phosphate solution of pH 9.0. This method of microcapsule preparation may therefore be utilized for production of insolubilized enzymes.

Example 3: 4 g of polyacrylonitrile (product of Asahi Kasei Kogyo KK) are dissolved in 20 ml of dimethylsulfoxide to prepare a solution, into which 1 g of urease powders is dispersed. This dispersion is emulsified under stirring in 200 ml of a liquid paraffin of the Japanese Pharmacopoeia containing a surface active agent, 0.25% of Span 85, to form emulsified droplets with sizes 150 to 200 μ.

Then, 50 ml of water is added to the emulsion as a nonsolvent, drop-by-drop in 30 minutes to obtain microcapsules containing urease. The polymer films of the microcapsules obtained are excellent semipermeable membranes, which hydrolyze urea at high efficiency to release NH_3 and CO_2.

OTHER WALL-FORMING MATERIALS

Polyacrolein-Bisulfite with Crosslinking Constituents

M. Kuhn and M. Harris; U.S. Patent 4,003,846; January 18, 1977; assigned to Ciba-Geigy Corporation describe a process in which the substance to be encapsulated is dispersed in a distribution medium in the presence of an aqueous solution of a polyacrolein or acrolein copolymer present as a hydrate or bisulfite adduct, which aqueous solution is capable of forming a compound insoluble in the distribution medium; and the hydrate or the bisulfite adduct is reacted in the resulting dispersion with a water-soluble, polyfunctional, monomeric or polymeric hydrophilic compound and, optionally, additionally with a curing agent or an aminoplast precondensate to form an insoluble capsule material.

Suitable monomeric or polymeric hydrophilic reagents are, in principle, polyfunctional compounds which can be reacted in aqueous solution with the carbonyl groups of the polyacrolein constituent, and which contain as reactive groups preferably amino, hydroxyl or mercapto groups, especially, however, primary and/or secondary amino groups.

Reactive amino, hydroxyl and mercapto group, as used here, denotes every amino, hydroxyl or mercaptan group in the hydrophilic compounds which can participate in the reaction with the polyacrolein constituent.

Preferably employed polyfunctional hydrophilic polymers are albuminous substances, particularly scleroproteins such as gelatin or gelatinous products.

The distribution medium used is preferably an aqueous medium, for example, water, in which the polyacrolein component and, optionally, further substances are dissolved. Suitable substances for fine dispersion in the process are solid, liquid or gaseous substances, and also solutions of substances, which are insoluble in water and which do not react with water and with the substances forming the wall of the capsule. Solids must become dispersed in the presence of the polyacrolein component and, optionally, they are to be pulverized by grinding to such a degree that a stable dispersion can be obtained.

As dispersible solids, it is possible to use the widest range of active substances, for example: pharmaceutical products including growth hormones and vitamins, cosmetics, pigments, dyestuffs, color-formers, optical brighteners, textile auxiliaries, textile protective agents or finishing agents, fillers, waxes, fertilizers, agents regulating plant growth, pest-control agents, such as insecticides, fungicides, antimicrobics, biocidal agents, such as e.g., agents exterminating ticks, also synthetic polymers usable as adhesives, perfumes and aromatics, photochemicals, water-insoluble metal oxides, e.g., magnetic iron oxide, water-insoluble salts, etc.

For the encapsulating of liquid substances, it has proved advantageous to use 33.5 to 335 parts by weight, preferably 67 to 200 parts by weight of 15% aqueous polyacrolein-bisulfite solution to 100 parts by weight of liquid. This corresponds to a solids content of polyacrolein of 5 to 50 parts by weight, preferably 10 to 30 parts by weight, per 100 parts by weight of liquid to be encapsulated.

By a 15% polyacrolein-bisulfite solution is meant a solution containing 15% by weight of polyacrolein, exclusive of the amount of SO_2 necessary for the preparation of the solution, which amount is to be just sufficient for the obtainment of clear solutions. In general, this amount varies between 1 and 16% by weight of SO_2 in the solution. Preferably, however, it is between 2 and 10% by weight.

The amount of polyfunctional hydrophilic compound is advantageously likewise 5 to 50 parts by weight, preferably 10 to 30 parts by weight, to 100 parts by weight of liquid to be encapsulated. In the case of solid substances to be encapsulated, the lower limits of the applied amounts of the two constituents, i.e., of the polyacrolein constituent and of the hydrophilic polyfunctional compound, is, as a rule, somewhat higher than for liquids. To 100 parts by weight of solid substance, there are used, e.g., about 35 to 335 parts by weight, preferably 80 to 200 parts by weight of the 15% polyacrolein-bisulfite solution, which corresponds to a solid content of polyacrolein of 6 to 50 parts by weight, preferably 12 to 30 parts by weight.

The amount of hydrophilic polyfunctional compound varies between 6 and 50 parts by weight, preferably between 8 and 30 parts by weight, per 100 parts by weight of solid substance. The proportion of substance to be encapsulated with respect to the total mass of the capsule can be 50 to 95% by weight, preferably 60 to 90% by weight.

To effect encapsulation, the substrate intended as the content of the capsule is emulsified in the polyacrolein-bisulfite solution or polyacrolein-hydrate solution; the whole is diluted with water, and an aqueous solution of the hydrophilic polyfunctional compound, acting as a crosslinking agent, is substantially added. Encapsulation is performed advantageously with pH values in the range of 2 to 10, preferably, however, with pH values between 5 and 8. With the system polyacrolein-bisulfite-gelatin, encapsulation is preferably performed in the pH range of 8 to 10, whereby in this case the polyacrolein-bisulfite solution is brought to the given pH value advantageously with triethylamine, and this solution is used preferably immediately for the preparation of the emulsion. The polyacrolein-bisulfite solutions usable according to this process are stable at pH values of below 10 and up to 80°C. The reaction temperature is generally between 5° and 80°C. Encapsulation should preferably be performed at 20° to 60°C.

The polyacrolein-bisulfite solutions prepared with sulfur dioxide are, when stored in sealed containers, storage-stable for a practically unlimited length of time, and have, depending on the content of SO_2, a pH value of between 1 and 4. Suitable for the adjustment of the pH values desired for encapsulation are, in particular, alkali metal hydroxides, alkali metal bicarbonates and alkali metal carbonates. In particular, however, there are used, inter alia, tertiary bases, e.g., tertiary amines, such as triethylamine, triethanolamine and pyridine.

The formation of the capsule material occurs directly after the adding together of the polyacrolein-bisulfite substrate emulsion and the hydrophilic polyfunctional crosslinking constituent, with the sequence in which the two constituents are combined having no effect. The formation of the capsule is the result of a precipitation reaction in which the polyacrolein-bisulfite or polyacrolein-hydrate is reacted with the crosslinking constituent to form a polymeric compound that is insoluble in the external phase as in the internal phase. Insofar as the hydrophilic polyfunctional compound is likewise polymeric, there is formed, with cocrosslinking, a composite polymer forming the wall of the capsule. The crosslinking reaction can be catalyzed by the addition of small amounts of aliphatic carboxylic acids having 1 to 6 carbon atoms, such as, e.g., formic acid, acetic acid, oxalic acid or citric acid. Also suitable are salts which produce an acid reaction when hydrolysis is performed.

The capsule material obtained as dispersion can optionally be postcured or reinforced by subsequent encapsulating. For the additional postcuring, halogenated aliphatic carbonyl compounds having preferably 1 to 6 carbon atoms can be optionally used as curing agents. Suitable carbonyl compounds are, for example, monoaldehydes such as formaldehyde, acetaldehyde, propionaldehyde or acrolein, as well as dialdehydes such as glyoxal, methylglyoxal, glutardialdehyde and mucochloric acid.

The capsule material present in aqueous dispersion can, if desired, be after-reinforced. Suitable for this purpose are the aminoplast precondensates, particularly urea-formaldehyde condensates or melamine-formaldehyde condensates.

The capsules are as a rule colorless and have a long storage life. Even temperatures of about 100°C have no harmful effect on the quality of the capsules, provided that the substances encapsulated are not sensitive to heat. The microcapsules produced by the process have as a rule a particle diameter of 1 to 500 μ, preferably 1 to 20 μ. They are suitable, in particular, for the manufacture of heat-sensitive and pressure-sensitive copying papers and recording materials.

Preparation of Polyacrolein-Bisulfite Solutions: 328.4 g of polyacrolein (91.1% of polyacrolein, 8.9% of water) having a mean molecular weight of 24,500 and a reduced viscosity η_{spec}/c = 0.203 dl/g determined according to R.C. Schulz, H. Cherdron, and W. Kern, *Makrom. Chem.* 24 (1957) 141, obtained by redox-polymerization of acrolein with potassium persulfate ($K_2S_2O_8$) and silver nitrate ($AgNO_3$), is suspended in 1,671.6 g of distilled water, and dissolved in the course of 3 hours, with stirring, by the introduction of 110 g of sulfur dioxide gas. After filtration through a glass filter under reduced pressure, there is obtained a slightly yellow-colored polyacrolein-bisulfite solution containing 16.35% of polyacrolein and 5.6% of sulfur dioxide.

Example 1: 50 g of the polyacrolein-bisulfite solution obtained by the preparation above is brought to pH value of 6.5 with 5% aqueous sodium hydroxide solution. There is then stirred in to form an emulsion, by means of a high-speed stirrer, 50 g of an insecticidal mixture consisting of 25 g of a compound of the following formula and 25 g of paraffin.

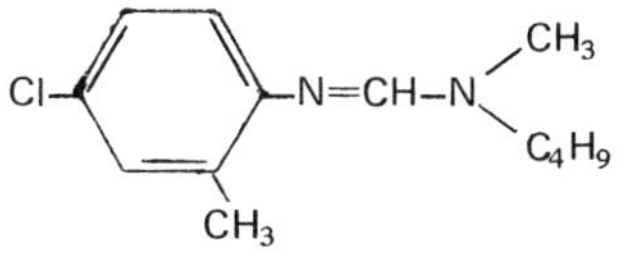

CH_3
Cl– (benzene ring) –N=CH–N
C_4H_9
CH_3

With continuous stirring, the emulsion is diluted with 500 ml of distilled water and an addition is made of 500 g of a 1.2% gelatin solution. The resulting dispersion is transferred to another vessel; it is further stirred and 8 ml of a 37% aqueous formaldehyde solution is added. The pH value is adjusted to 6.0 by the addition of glacial acetic acid. The reaction mixture is thereupon heated to 60°C, and cured for 24 hours at this temperature. After the addition of 0.25 g of sodium lauryl sulfate, the capsule mixture is isolated by spray-drying at an inlet temperature of 120°C and an outlet temperature of 50°C. There is obtained a colorless powder which can be readily dispersed in water. The capsule material dispersed in water does not settle out.

95% of the capsule material has a particle size of 1 to 10 μ; the main proportion is within the range of size of between 1 and 5 μ. The capsule material consists to the extent of 95% of particles having a density of $<$1.0 g/cc and to the extent of 80% of particles having a density of $>$0.96 g/cc.

Example 2: 114.5 g of the same polyacrolein-bisulfite solution used in Example 1 is brought to a pH value of 6.5 with 5% sodium hydroxide solution. There is then stirred in to form an emulsion, with a high-speed stirrer, 100 g of a 4% color-former solution, obtained by the dissolving of 18 g of crystal violet lactone and 12 g of benzoyl-leucomethylene blue in 360 g of chlorinated diphenyl and 360 g of paraffin oil. The emulsion is diluted with 1,000 ml of water, and the pH value thereof is adjusted, while stirring is maintained, with 1,000 g of a 1.5% edible gelatin solution.

The capsule mixture obtained is then heated to 40°C; it is held for one hour at this temperature, and an addition is thereupon made of 8 ml of a 24 to 26% glutardialdehyde solution and 6 ml of 37% formaldehyde solution. After a curing time of 24 hours, the capsule material is isolated by spray-drying. There is obtained 119 g of a colorless, finely pulverulent capsule material, which is usable for pressure-sensitive copying paper and which exhibits an excellent duplicating effect. An aging test at 105°C produces after 24 hours a capsule material displaying an unchanged copying effect.

Example 3: 50 g of the same polyacrolein-bisulfite used in Example 1 is adjusted with 5% sodium hydroxide solution to have a pH value of 6.4. There is then stirred in to form an emulsion, by means of a high-speed stirrer, 50 g of an insecticide mixture of the composition given in Example 1; and the emulsion is subsequently diluted with 500 ml of water. An addition is made thereto of 100 g of a 9% solution of a condensation product from 42 g of dicyanodiamide, 121.6 g of a 30% formaldehyde solution and 25.8 g of diethylenetriamine in 937 g of water; and the pH value is adjusted to 6.0 with acetic acid.

Capsule formation occurs as a result of precipitation of a polymeric compound. The reaction mixture is held at 60°C for 18 hours; the capsule material is filtered off, washed with 1,000 ml of water and dried in air. There is obtained 63 g of microencapsulated insecticide. The capsule material is microporous; the contents of the capsule have a retarded release.

Example 4: 113.3 g of the same polyacrolein-bisulfite solution used in Example 1 is adjusted with 10% sodium hydroxide solution to have a pH value of 6.5. There is then stirred in to form an emulsion, by means of a high-speed stirrer, 100 g of a mixture consisting of 130.2 g of an insecticide of the formula given in Example 1 and 119.8 g of paraffin; and the emulsion is subsequently diluted with 1,000 ml of water. There is then added, with further stirring, a solution, adjusted to have a pH value of 6.5, consisting of 5 g of a polyethyleneimine having a viscosity of 20°C of 10,000 to 20,000 cp in 1,000 ml of water, whereupon capsules are formed as a result of precipitation of a composite polymer.

An addition is subsequently made of a precondensate from 30 g of melamine and 62 g of a 37% formaldehyde solution, and the whole is further condensed at 60°C. The reaction mixture is held at 60°C for 20 hours, and then cooled to room temperature. The capsule material is afterwards filtered off, washed with 1,000 ml of water and finally dried at 40°C. There is obtained 158 g of a lemon colored, readily agglomerated capsule material.

Example 5: 114.5 g of the same polyacrolein-bisulfite solution used in Example 1 is brought with 10% sodium hydroxide solution to a pH value of 6.5. There is then stirred in to form an emulsion, by means of a high-speed stirrer, 100 g of a mixture consisting of 312.5 g of an insecticide of the formula given in Example 1 and 187.5 g of paraffin; and the emulsion is subsequently diluted with 1,000 ml of water.

An addition is then made with further stirring of a solution of 51.5 g of melamine-formaldehyde precondensate in 1,000 ml of water at 60°C, and the pH value of the reaction mixture is adjusted to 6.5 with glacial acetic acid. After 20 hours of curing at 60°C, the resulting capsule material is filtered off, washed with 1,000 ml of water and dried at 40°C in a light stream of air. There is obtained 152.6 g of a capsule material having a good chemical stability.

Film-Forming Polycarbodiimide with Terminal Isocyanate Groups

The process of *G. Baatz, M. Dahm and W. Schäfer; U.S. Patent 4,119,565; October 10, 1978; assigned to Bayer AG, Germany* relates to the production of microcapsules, wherein a film-forming polycarbodiimide having functional terminal isocyanate groups is dissolved in the core material or in an inert solvent or solvent mixture, and a core material which is miscible with it, is added. The resulting organic phase, subsequently termed inner phase, is introduced into a liquid phase immiscible with the organic phase such as water, subsequently termed outer phase, which contains a dissolved catalyst for isocyanate reactions, and the microcapsules formed are isolated.

In order to carry out this reactive process, i.e., an encapsulation, by polyreaction at the organic phase interface in a dispersion, the polycarbodiimide is dissolved in the core material or in an inert solvent or solvent mixture and subsequently mixed with the core material.

In a shear gradient, which is preferably generated by intensive mixing with small mixers or mixing machines, the resulting organic phase is introduced into a liquid phase immiscible with it, for example, water which contains a component which is catalytically active towards isocyanate groups. The catalyst may also be added after dispersion. The encapsulation may be carried out continuously and discontinuously. The turbulence level during mixing determines the diameter of the microcapsules obtained. This may be approximately 5 to 5,000 μ according to the mixing conditions. The weight ratio of core material to shell material in the finished microcapsules is normally in the range of from 50:50 to 90:10.

Polycarbodiimides which are used preferably have free isocyanate terminal groups, and thus the idealized structure:

$$OCN-(R-N=C=N)_x-R-NCO$$

in which R represents alkylene, cycloalkylene and arylene groups and x is a whole number of from 2 to 40, wherein partially functional carbodiimide- and/or isocyanate groups formed as a result of dimerization may be present as uretidione- or uretone-imine groups, etc. R is preferably a C_{2-6} alkylene, C_{5-7} cycloalkylene, or a C_{6-12} arylene radical.

The production of polycarbodiimides is known and is described, for example, in the *Encyclopedia of Polymer Science and Technology,* Vol 7, pages 751 and 754. The polycarbodiimides are obtained in the simplest case by adding phospholine oxides to the isocyanates and by crushing the foam-like material obtained.

Example 1: (a) Production of the Polymer (H-PCD) – 134 g of hexamethylene-1,6-diisocyanate are mixed with 2 g of 1-methylphospholine-1-oxide and heated to 50°C for 15 hours. An exceptionally viscous product is produced with slow evolution of carbon dioxide, this product being soluble in the following solvents: methylene chloride, chloroform, chlorobenzene, toluene, solvent naphtha, Chlophene A 30, tri-n-butyl phosphate, trichloroethyl phosphate, ethylene chloride, 1,3-dichloropropane, cyclohexane, diphenyl ether, methyl ethyl ketone, acetone, ethyl acetate, pyrrolidone, N-methylpyrrolidone, dimethylformamide, benzene, dioxane and tetrahydrofuran. The polycarbodiimide should be kept at temperatures of below 5°C.

(b) Encapsulation – 1.1 g of crystal violet lactone and 0.5 g of N-benzoyl leucomethylene blue are dissolved in 25 g of solvent naphtha (aromatic mixture of xylene, cumene, toluene and other naphthene oils of the BV Aral) while stirring and heating to about 70°C. After cooling the solution, 5 g of the polycarbodiimide described in (a) were added and dissolved.

The homogeneous mixture was subsequently dispersed in 300 ml of water, in which 1.5 g of polyvinyl alcohol (Moviol 70/98) is dissolved as an emulsifying agent. A Kotthoff mixing siren is used for dispersing (6,500 rpm, 1 liter beaker about 10 seconds). A solution of 0.5 g of N-dimethylaminoethyl-N'-methylpiperazine in 70 g of water was subsequently added under similar dispersion conditions. The dispersion apparatus (after about 50 to 60 seconds) is then replaced by a simple laboratory stirrer of the Lenart-Rapid-type (500 rpm). The contents were rapidly heated to 80°C and kept at this temperature for 2 hours, with continuous stirring. The diameter of the capsules obtained is in the size range from 5 to 20 μ.

Example 2: 25 g of the herbicide methyl parathion [O,O-dimethyl-O-(4-nitrophenyl)monothiophosphate] are mixed as an 80% solution in solvent naphtha with 5 g of the polycarbodiimide described in Example 1a. The resulting homogenous organic phase was subsequently dispersed in water by using a Kotthoff mixing siren (8,900 rpm, about 60 seconds). In the water are dissolved 2 g of polyvinyl alcohol (Moviol 50/98) as an emulsifying agent. During the emulsifying period, 0.5 g sodium hydroxide (dissolved in 69.5 g water) are added to the aqueous phase.

The Kotthoff mixing siren is then replaced by a simple laboratory stirrer of the Lenart Rapid-type (500 rpm) and the mixture is kept for 2 hours at 60°C with continuous stirring. The resulting slurry was neutralized by adding acetic acid. The diameter of the capsules obtained is in the size range of from 1 to 12 μ.

Polycarboxylate Polymer Containing Carboxylic Amide Groups

The process of *P.J. Allart and H.B. May; U.S. Patent 4,124,526; November 7, 1978; assigned to Monsanto Company* comprises forming a dispersion of droplets of an oil in an aqueous alkaline liquid medium containing in solution a water-soluble salt of a polycarboxylate polymer having the structure of an ethylene-maleic acid copolymer wherein a proportion of the carboxylic acid groups are replaced by carboxylic amide groups, (hereinafter referred to as the encapsulating polymer), and acidifying the aqueous liquid medium to a pH in the range of 5 to 8 while maintaining the droplets in dispersion, whereby the encapsulating polymer is precipitated to form walls around the droplets.

Preferred amide groups in the polycarboxylate polymer are secondary amide groups, especially secondary amide groups having the formula –CONHR, where R represents an aliphatic or cycloaliphatic group, for example an alkyl or alkenyl group of up to 6 carbon atoms, for instance ethyl, n-propyl, isopropyl, n-butyl, t-butyl, n-amyl, isoamyl or allyl, or a cycloalkyl group of 5 or 6 ring carbon atoms and a total of up to 10 carbon atoms, for example, cyclopentyl, cyclohexyl or methylcyclohexyl. R may also be a group derived from a polyamine of the formula:

$$H_2N(CHRCH_2NH)_nCHRCH_2NH_2$$

where R is hydrogen or methyl and n is an integer from 1 to 4, or from a diamine of the following formula where m is an integer from 2 to 8:

$$H_2N(CH_2)_mNH_2$$

In the aqueous alkaline medium in which the oil droplets are dispersed, a sufficiently high proportion of the carboxylic acid groups of the encapsulating polymer exist as carboxylate anions to render the polymer water-soluble, while during acidification of the aqueous medium, carboxylate anions are converted to carboxylic acid groups. It is believed that acidification of the aqueous medium to a pH in the range of 5 to 8 does not result in a complete conversion, but that carboxylate ions may still exist in the wall polymer, especially adjacent to the oil droplet. The aqueous medium is preferably acidified to a pH in the range of 5 to 6, preferably using an acid having a dissociation constant not greater than 2×10^{-3} in an aqueous solution at 25°C. The acid is usually added as an aqueous solution.

Encapsulating polymers can be prepared by the partial amidation of an ethylene-maleic acid copolymer, by the partial hydrolysis of an ethylene-maleamide copolymer or by the copolymerization of the required proportions of ethylene, maleic acid and maleic amide monomers.

The process can be carried out by dissolving an encapsulating polymer in an aqueous alkaline medium wherein the alkalinity is preferably provided by the presence of an alkali metal hydroxide, for example, sodium hydroxide, or alternatively, and in some instances more conveniently, a solution of a water-soluble salt of an encapsulating polymer can be formed in situ from a precursor or precursors.

In a preferred process for the preparation of an encapsulating polymer, an ethylene-maleic anhydride copolymer is added to a solution of an amine in dilute sodium hydroxide solution, which results in the formation of a solution of the sodium salt of the maleic acid half-amide.

The alkali metal hydroxide and aliphatic amine may be used in a molar ratio of hydroxide to amine of from 3:5 to 5:3, giving an encapsulating polymer containing relatively more alkali metal carboxylate groups than carboxylic amide groups or vice versa.

If desired, the encapsulating polymer forming the capsule walls can be hardened by treatment with a crosslinking agent. When the process is applied to the production of transfer copy systems, the oil that is encapsulated is a solution of a dye precursor or chromogen.

Example: 7.5 g of an ethylene-maleic anhydride copolymer having a molecular weight of 20,000 to 30,000 were added with stirring to a solution of 4.3 g of n-butylamine and 2.4 g of sodium hydroxide in 100 g of water at room temperature.

The copolymer dissolved to form a clear solution which was then stirred with a high speed agitator while 100 g of a 3% by weight solution of crystal violet lactone in an oil consisting of 2 parts by weight of partially hydrogenated terphenyls and 1 part by weight of kerosene was added slowly. Emulsification of the oil solution occurred readily. The high speed agitator was replaced by a slowly rotating paddle stirrer, and a 10% by weight aqueous acetic acid solution was added slowly until the pH had fallen to about 5. 5 g of a 60% by weight solution of methylolated melamine were then added and, with continued stirring, the emulsion was heated to and held at 65°C for 2 hours. Microscopic examination of the sample of the emulsion at this time showed the oil droplets coated with a distinct wall of polymer material.

A coating of the emulsion was applied by brushing to one side of a sheet of paper, and dried to give a colorless layer. The paper was superimposed, coated side downwards, on a clay-coated receiver sheet. Pen and type markings made on the top sheet were reproduced quickly and clearly on the receiver sheet.

OTHER ENCAPSULATION TECHNIQUES

CELLULOSE DERIVATIVES

Cyclohexane-Free Ethylcellulose Microcapsules

A commonly used microencapsulation system involves the release of ethylcellulose from cyclohexane to form a liquid envelope on a solid core. It then is converted into a hard-walled microcapsule. However, when ethylcellulose is precipitated by cooling or coacervation, it comes out solvated with cyclohexane. In such case, the final washed and filtered cakes of microcapsules are difficult to dry. Tray drying leads to dry cakes of microcapsules. Breaking the cakes into lumps, followed by drying, leads to dry lumps of microcapsules.

L.D. Morse, M.J. Boroshok and R.W. Grabner; U.S. Patent 4,107,072; August 15, 1978; assigned to Merck & Co., Inc. were able to improve the drying methodology of microcapsules by displacing from ethylcellulose capsules, phased out of cyclohexane, the solvated cyclohexane with pentane, hexane, heptane or octane or mixtures thereof such as petroleum ether (i.e., C_{5-8} alkanes). The microcapsules thus obtained do not aggregate or clump up and even very small microcapsules are maintained as discrete dry particles.

The displacement of the cyclohexane by pentane, hexane, heptane or octane can be done in one of several ways. The cyclohexane slurry can be decanted and the residual mass can be reslurried at least once with the pentane, hexane, heptane and/or octane, followed by decanting and then finally filtering. Alternatively, the cyclohexane suspension can be filtered into cake and this can be reslurried at least once in the C_{5-8} alkane and refiltered.

Example: (a) The following are dispersed in 5 liters cyclohexane: 280 g ethylcellulose (47.5% ethoxy content by weight; viscosity 45 cp) and 520 g niacinamide. The mixture is heated with stirring to 78°C. At that temperature the ethylcellulose has dissolved in the cyclohexane. Stirring is continued while the system is allowed to cool. As the temperature drops solvated ethylcellulose develops as a separated phase due to the poor solvent characteristics of cyclohexane at lower temperatures (cf U.S. Patent 3,531,418). The solvated ethylcellulose, distributed in the cyclohexane as droplets, tends to wet the niacinamide particles and to envelop them. As the droplets coalesce, they lose solvent and develop into solid encapsulating walls. The mixture is then cooled to 10°C and filtered, washed twice with 1.5 liters hexane and dried in a fluid bed to achieve discrete capsules as a free flowing powder.

(b) The procedure of (a) is used substituting pentane for hexane. The results are the same as in (a).

(c) The procedure for (a) is used substituting heptane for hexane. The results are the same as in (a).

Insoluble Complex of Acetate Sulfates of Polyglycosides and Polycations

In a process developed by *T. Sakai, T. Kagaya, K. Yokota and K. Hata; U.S. Patent 3,994,827; November 30, 1976; assigned to Jujo Paper Co., Ltd., Japan* microcapsules are formed by providing a coating of capsulating agents comprising acetate sulfate of polyglycosides on the core substances. Aqueous solutions of the salt of cellulose acetate sulfate, starch acetate sulfate or dextran acetate sulfate are used as the acetate sulfate of polyglycosides and the oily substances such as alkyl biphenyl, liquid paraffin, fat and higher alcohol, and pulverulent substances such as active carbon and yeast are used as the core substances.

According to the method, the core substances are added to aqueous solutions of the polyglycosides to be emulsified and dispersed therein, and then aqueous solutions of polycations are added to form an insoluble complex comprising the polyglycosides and polycations, and as a result, the core substances are coated by insoluble complex. Thereafter the insoluble complex is stiffened by stiffening reagents or dispersed in aqueous solutions of polyvinyl alcohol, thus producing stable microcapsules.

The polyglycosides are first acetylated to contain 10 to 40% of acetyl group as acetic acid and then further reacted to contain at least 4%, preferably 7 to 15% of sulfuryl group as sulfuric acid. The resultant products may be further converted into salts such as sodium, calcium and ammonium.

Preferred polycations include cationic surfactants, such as hexadecyldimethylammonium chloride, hexadecyltrimethylammonium chloride, hexadecyldimethylbenzylammonium chloride, dodecylpyridinium chloride, polyoxyethylenelaurylamine and the like. Other polycations include polycationic materials having weak surface activity, such as polyethyleneimine, weak cationic derivatives of polyacrylamine, cationic derivatives of polyvinylpyridine, chitosan and the like.

Further, since acetylated and sulfated polyglycosides bring forth a superior surface activity effect, they are readily dissolved together with many polyanionic materials including carboxymethylcellulose, polyacrylic acid and polystyrene sulfonic acid to form a mixed aqueous solution superior in the surface activity effect.

Example 1: 7 g of sodium salts of cellulose acetate sulfate [acetyl and sulfuryl (38% CH_3COOH, 9% H_2SO_4)] was dissolved in 100 ml of 20% aqueous solution of methanol to prepare a solution to be used as the encapsulating agent.

Then, 1 ml of 0.5% aqueous solution of nonionic surfactant Tween-80 was added to the solution and admixed therein. The resultant admixture was gently agitated while adding thereto 30 ml of alkyl biphenyl, causing the formation of an oil in water type emulsion. Thereafter, 25 ml of 5% aqueous solution of polyethyleneimine was slowly added to the emulsion while continuing the agitation, to cause the complex of cellulose acetate sulfate and polyethyleneimine to be formed. A microcapsule dispersion was obtained by adding 300 ml of 0.5% aqueous solution of polyvinyl alcohol to the solution containing the complex and then diluting the resultant solution.

Example 2: 7 g of sodium salts of cellulose acetate sulfate (containing 38% of CH_3COOH and 9% of H_2SO_4) was dissolved in 150 g of 20% methanolic aqueous solution. To the solution, 15 g of pulverized active carbon (100 to 200 mesh) was added to the core substance and admixed therewith, and then the admixture was continuously agitated to obtain a uniform dispersion of the core substance.

While continuing the agitation and heating the dispersion to 60°C, 20 g of 5% aqueous solution of polyethyleneimine having its pH adjusted to 8.0 was slowly added thereto, and the resultant mixture was further agitated. Thereafter, 15 g of 5% aqueous solution of polyethyleneimine having its pH adjusted to 6.0 was slowly added thereto and the agitation was continued until an insoluble complex of cellulose acetate sulfate and polyethyleneimine was formed. After lowering the temperature of the solution system, 300 ml of 0.5% aqueous solution of polyvinyl alcohol was added to the solution to dilute the latter, consequently obtaining a stable dispersion of microcapsules.

Example 3: 6 g of sodium salts of starch acetate sulfate (containing 36% of CH_3COOH and 11% of H_2SO_4) was dissolved in 100 g of water. To the resultant solution, 10 g of dry yeast was added as the core substance and the resultant mixture solution was agitated continuously until a uniform dispersion of the yeast was obtained. After permitting the dispersion to stand for a time, 150 ml of 3% aqueous solution of hexadecyldimethylammonium chloride, which is a cationic surfactant, was added thereto slowly and the resultant dispersion was continuously agitated until an insoluble complex was obtained. Thereafter, 3% aqueous solution of acetic acid was added to adjust the system pH to 4.0 and the system was heated to 40° C and then left as it stands. After lowering the temperature to room temperature, 2 g of glyoxal was added to further stiffen the insoluble complex. A dispersion of the microcapsules was obtained by adding thereto 5 ml of 2% aqueous solution of polyvinyl alcohol.

Example 4: 7 g of sodium salts of cellulose acetate sulfate (containing 38% of CH_3COOH and 9% of H_2SO_4) was dissolved in 150 ml of 20% methanolic aqueous solution and 5% aqueous solution of sodium hydroxide was added thereto to raise the pH above 10. To the solution, 25 g of 5% aqueous solution of polyethyleneimine and 12.5 g of 10% aqueous solution of cationic derivative of polyacrylamide (PAA-N-aminomethyl derivative, tertiary amine) were added and mixed therewith.

To the mixture solution, 40 g of liquid paraffin was added under a hard and continuous agitation to cause emulsion of oil in water type to be formed. After adding thereto 200 ml of diluent water, the pH of the system was lowered to 4 or 5 by using 5% aqueous solution of acetic acid, consequently causing a complex of cellulose acetate sulfate, polyethyleneimine and the cationic derivative of polyacrylamide to be formed.

MISCELLANEOUS PROCESSES

Centrifugal Encapsulating Apparatus

The process of *C.C. Dannelly; U.S. Patent 4,123,206; October 31, 1978; assigned to Eastman Kodak Company* relates to an apparatus and method for forming capsules using centrifugal force developed by a rotating nozzle to extrude material encapsulation.

The process is described with reference to Figure 3.1a through 3.1g. Referring to Figure 3.1a, nozzle **10** is fixed to shaft **12** which is mounted for rotation about a generally vertical axis. Vessel **14** is provided for placement under nozzle **10** to maintain a body of liquid **16** in contact with a portion of the nozzle. The nozzle may be fabricated from any suitable material such as metal, ceramic, plastic, wood, or the like which is capable of withstanding centrifugal forces of rotation. The nozzle is generally circular in cross section along a plane perpendicular to shaft **12** as shown in Figure 3.1b. Shaft **12** may be fixed to the nozzle by any convenient means such as, for example, threading, press fit, key, etc.

The nozzle is provided with a generally conical, or truncated conical outside circumferential surface **20** inclined upwardly as the radius increases. The circumferential surface extends from the bottom or closed end of the nozzle, to a circumferential ring **22** on the sidewall of the nozzle. The inclination of circumferential surface **20** is such that when the nozzle is rotated about a generally vertical axis with the lower portion submerged in a body of liquid **16**, centrifugal force and surface tension of the liquid combine to impel a sheet or spray **24** upwardly along the surface thereof. The nozzle is partially submerged in the liquid. That is, the liquid level, while the nozzle is at rest, would extend at least one-quarter of the axial distance from the bottom of the nozzle to the orifices, and no higher than the outer ports of the orifices.

The inclined circumferential surface **20** is generally smooth and may assume a variety of shapes, one of which is shown in Figure 3.1c. For example, this surface need not extend to the axis of rotation and terminate at a point **26**. The inclined section may be somewhat concave or convex. The nozzle should be designed with regard to intended speed of rotation, diameter, viscosity and surface tension of liquid **16**, such that upon rotation of the nozzle, sheet of liquid **24** will be impelled along the inclined surface **20** to separate leading tips of extruded material from the outer ports of the orifices.

The nozzle is provided with at least one, and preferably a plurality of spaced orifices **34** extending generally radially through the wall and usually on a circumferential line. Orifices **34** provide for the capsule material **13** to be extruded by centrifugal force when the nozzle is rotated. Inside ports are therefore positioned at, or near, the portion of greatest inside diameter. The inside wall **18** of the nozzle is preferably tapered inwardly toward the open end to reduce the likelihood of material to be encapsulated from escaping as the container **10** is rotated.

Figure 3.1: Centrifugal Encapsulating Apparatus

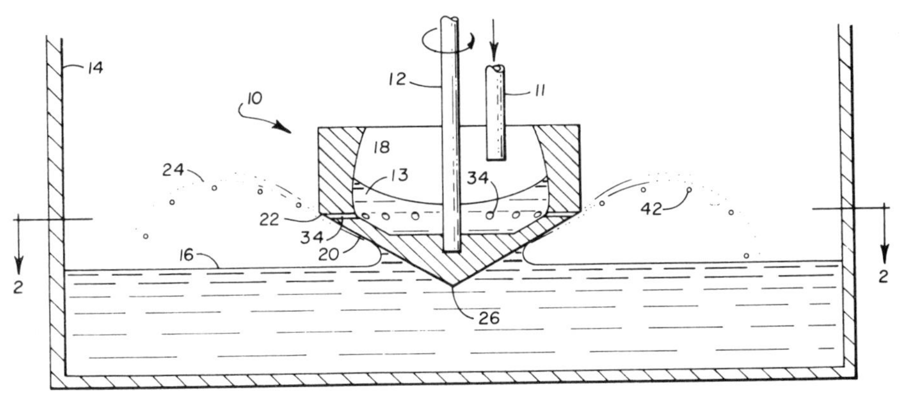

a.

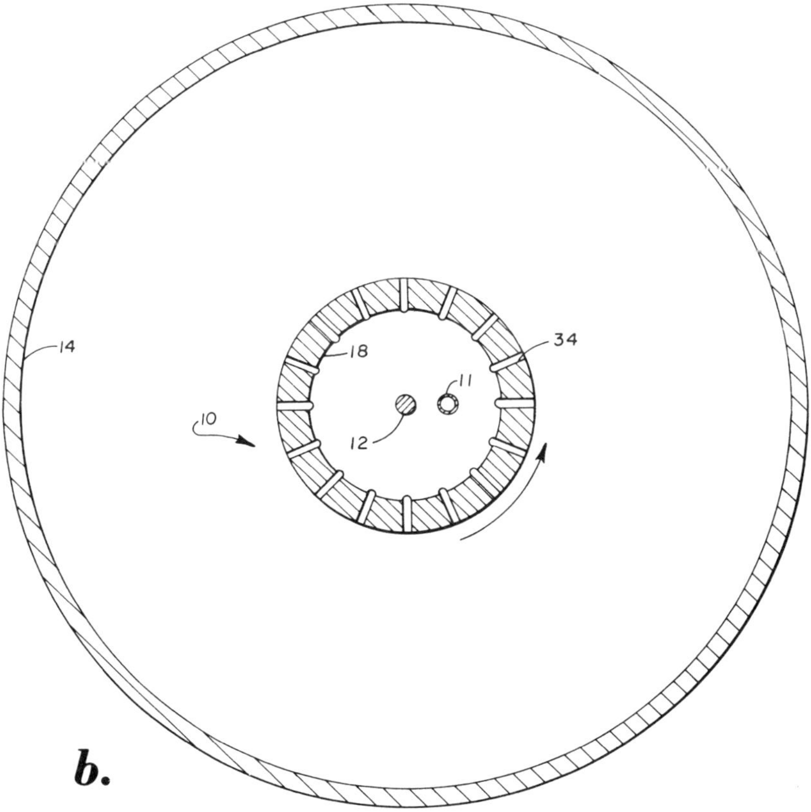

b.

(continued)

Figure 3.1: (continued)

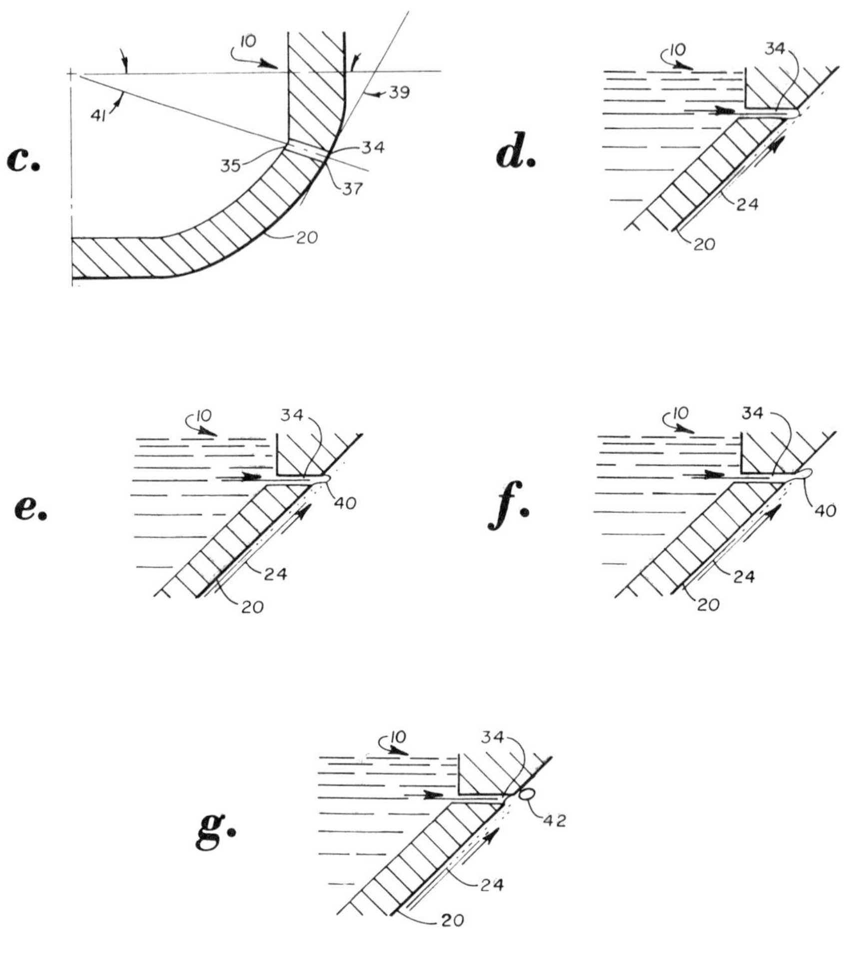

(a) Plan view of apparatus
(b) Cross sectional elevational view along **2-2** of Figure 3.1a
(c) Possible shape for circumferential surface
(d)-(g) Formation of capsules

Source: U.S. Patent 4,123,206

Material to be encapsulated may be conveyed to nozzle **10** continuously or batchwise through line **11**. The orifices must at least have a substantial radial component, and preferably extend generally in a radial direction from the axis as shown in Figure 3.1c. The interior port **35** of the orifices must be positioned to communicate with the material **13** when nozzle **10** is rotated at operating speed. The orifices may be positioned to have an axial component, i.e., inclined downwardly in the radial direction in its operating position. Such inclination (angle **41**) should not be greater than about 70° from horizontal. Preferably, angle **41** is near zero, but angles up to about 30° have no substantial adverse effect on performance. The outer port **37** of the orifices must be positioned such that the sheet of liquid moving across the surface **20** intercepts the capsule during formation and separates it from the outer port **37**. Thus, the plane in which the outer port generally lies should make an angle (angle **39**) of between about 70° and 90° with the horizontal when the nozzle is in operating position.

Figures 3.1d through 3.1g illustrate the formation of capsules. Centrifugal force exerted on liquid material **13** causes such material to be extruded through the orifices **34** as nozzle **10** is rotated. Simultaneously, centrifugal force and surface tension of liquid **16** cause a sheet **24** of such liquid to be impelled along the inclined surface **20** as indicated by the arrow. In Figure 3.1e the leading tip **40** of material **13** is being deformed by the sheet of liquid.

In Figure 3.1f force of the sheet of liquid is about to separate the leading tip **40**. In Figure 3.1g the leading tip has been separated and is being carried away as a separate capsule **42**. The next leading tip of the extrudate is approaching a point where the sequence will be repeated. Completed capsules may be allowed to fall by gravity back into the vessel **14** containing liquid **16** for recovery.

The material **13** to be encapsulated must be capable of flowing through the orifices **34** and forming droplets (leading tips **40**) held intact by surface tension until separated by sheet **24**. Liquid **16** must be capable of being impelled along inclined surface **20** past the orifices **34** to separate successive leading tips **40** of extrudate. Also, contact of the material **13** with air and/or liquid **16** must harden the surface of the formed capsules. Such hardening may be accomplished by either physical or chemical means.

Some of the variables within the control of the operator which may affect the characteristics of the finished capsules as well as a summary of certain of the inherent operational characteristics of the apparatus follow. The speed of rotation of the nozzle affects the size and rate of capsule formation. Rim speeds within the range of about 2,000 to about 50,000 in/min are normal.

The capsule size is affected by the size of the encapsulating orifices. Smaller orifices result in smaller sized capsules, while larger orifices result in larger sized capsules. Generally, orifices will be about 0.05 to 0.5 inch. The capacity of this apparatus can easily be increased by increasing the number of encapsulating orifices.

Higher viscosities tend to reduce both the size and the rate of production, while lower viscosities tend to increase both the size and the rate of production. Normally, the viscosity of material **13** will be about 50 to 30,000 cp. Normally, the surface tension of material **13** will be about 26 to 100 dynes/cm.

Example: Apparatus similar to that illustrated in Figure 3.1a and Figure 3.1b is used. The nozzle, made of a ceramic material, has an outside diameter of 3.0 inches, an inside diameter at the ring of orifices of 2.75 inches, an angle of orifice to horizontal of 0° (angle **41** in Figure 3.1c). The plane in which outer port **37** lies makes an angle of 80° with horizontal (angle **39** in Figure 3.1c). The nozzle contains 36 orifices of 1/16 inch diameter equally spaced circumferentially around the nozzle. The nozzle is submerged 0.5 inch in a body of butyl acetate such that the liquid level at rest is about half-way between the extreme bottom of the nozzle and the ring of orifices. The butyl acetate has a viscosity of 0.7 cp, 24.7 dynes/cm surface tension, and a temperature of 25°C. The nozzle is rotated at a rim speed of 9,000 inches per minute, and a 4% solids solution of agar in water heated to 60°C is charged into the nozzle.

The agar solution has a viscosity of 2,450 cp, a surface tension of 73.4 dynes/cm, and a temperature of 60°C. The butyl acetate is impelled along the inclined surface as a sheet and intercepts the tips of material being extruded to separate them. Capsules are formed by their contact with the butyl acetate and/or the surrounding atmosphere. In this case, a self-supporting film of the agar gels upon contact with matter of a cooler temperature. Capsules of 0.12 inch diameter are formed at a rate of >10,000/min.

Outer Paraffin Layer Destroyed and Intermediate Layer Hardened

Y. Hagiwara, T. Suzuki and A. Imai; U.S. Patent 3,962,383; June 8, 1976 describe a method and apparatus for manufacturing seamless material-filled capsules. A capsule filler material, a sol solution and a water-insoluble solution in the form of a continuous jet are fed from a triple orifice of the same core into a stream of hardening solution.

The spherical drops consisting of the abovementioned three layers are completed due to their interfacial surface tensions. Then the water-insoluble solution of the outermost layer is caused to strike several interrupting plates to have the water-insoluble layer destroyed and separated from the sol solution as a second layer to react the sol solution with the hardening solution at this instant for forming a water-insoluble film. The diameter of the wall thickness of the spherical drop can be changed easily by modifying the flow speed of the hardening solution and the diameter of the orifice.

The process is described with reference to Figure 3.2. Purified vegetable oil was used as a capsule filler material. The sol solution was made up of 1.6% sodium alginate, 3.0% polyvinyl alcohol, 1.0% gelatin, 4.4% glycerin and 90% purified water. The water-insoluble solution used was liquid paraffin, and the hardening solution was an aqueous solution of 10% calcium chloride.

First of all, refined vegetable oil as a capsule filler material contained in the tank **1** was jetted through the innermost pipe **3** by means of the pump **2** for feeding a predetermined amount of the purified vegetable oil, and the sol solution described above was jetted through the intermediate pipe **6** around the innermost pipe. Liquid paraffin as a water-insoluble solution was jetted through the outermost pipe **9** around the intermediate pipe whereby a multilayered continuous jet of the same core was caused to jet from the triple-orifice **N** of the same core and was discharged into the capsule-drop forming cylinder **12b** of the tower **12** for capsule-drop forming and hardening purpose.

An aqueous solution of 10% calcium chloride is adapted to flow upwards through tower **12** at definite speeds with the result that due to interfacial tension between the multilayered jet and the aqueous solution of 10% calcium chloride, the vegetable oil jetted from the innermost pipe **3** becomes a component of the content of the multilayered jet. This component is enclosed in the sol solution jetted from the intermediate pipe **6** and then the sol solution enclosing the vegetable oil as the active component is enclosed in the liquid paraffin jetted from the outermost pipe **9**, thereby forming a constricted portion **X** at the top of the jet assembly. Thereafter, this constricted portion **X** becomes a separated drop **Y** which is adapted to float up in the capsule-forming cylinder **12b**. The separated drop **Y** is destined to continue its spherical formation before it reaches the upper chamber **12c**.

Tower **12** is of such length, that it is possible to obtain a spherical drop of the three layers of the same core (see Figure 3.2b). The spherical drop **A** of the three layers continues ascending while floating in the hardening solution of 10% calcium chloride flowing up at definite speeds in the upper chamber **12c** and is caused to rise up and pass among six interrupting plates **13** formed with many piercing holes **13a** respectively. The spherical drop hits the six interrupting plates **13** which are secured to the internal wall surface in the upper part of upper chamber **12c**.

Figure 3.2: Encapsulation Apparatus Containing Triple Orifice

a.

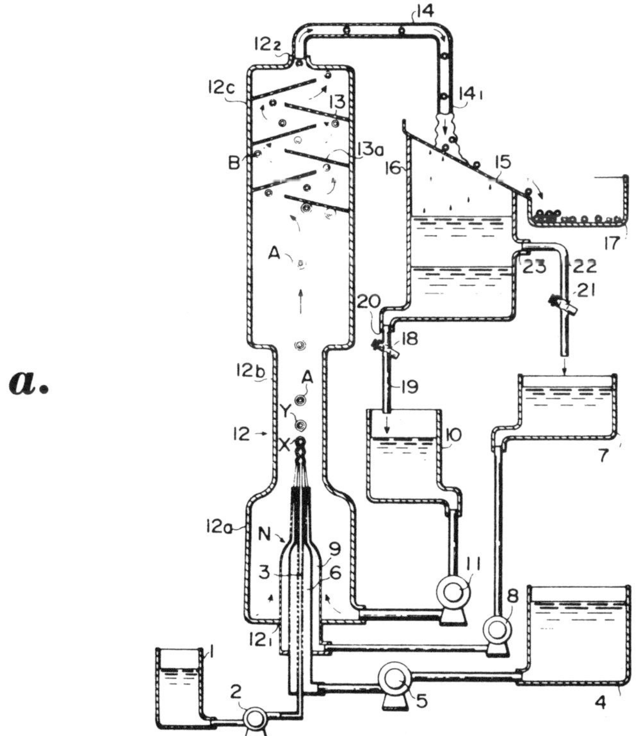

(continued)

Figure 3.2: (continued)

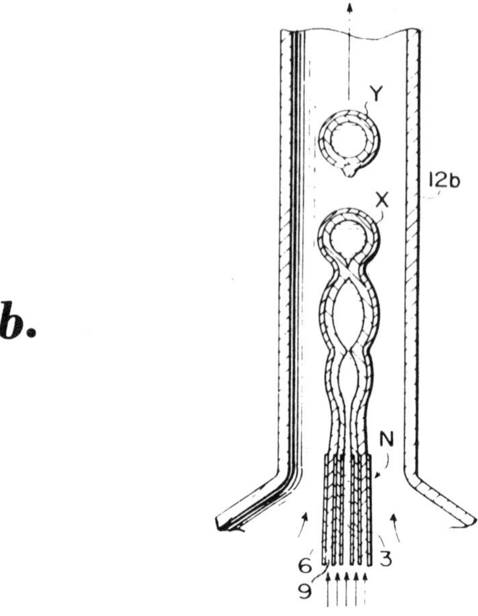

(a) Apparatus
(b) Enlarged view of triple orifice

Source: U.S. Patent 3,962,383

At the instant that the spherical drop **A** of the three layers, hits the interrupting plates **13**, its outermost layer, i.e., the layer of liquid paraffin is destroyed and separated. That is to say, the spherical drop **A** occurs in such condition as one shell is taken off so that the second layer (intermediate layer) consisting of sodium alginate, polyvinyl alcohol, gelatin, and glycerin as the sol solution is allowed to come in direct contact with the aqueous solution of calcium chloride as the hardening solution, whereby both these solutions begin to react at this point of time to form a water-insoluble film of calcium alginate.

Thus, by this method, a perfect, seamless and material-filled capsule **B** can be obtained, the capsule **B** containing the vegetable oil as its content, and its outer layer being enclosed in the film of calcium alginate, as mentioned above.

At this stage, it is very important to control the flow speed of the hardening solution, i.e., the aqueous solution of 10% calcium chloride which is kept flowing from below to upward in the tower **12** for capsule-drop forming and hardening purposes. In effect, it is possible to adjust at will the diameter of the continuous jet of the three layers by changing the abovementioned flow speed of the hardening solution. This accounts for the fact that it is possible to manufacture spherical material-filled capsules, having approximate diameters ranging from 1 to 7 mm by the use of one orifice. At the same time, the thickness of the film of the capsule can be made uniform when manufacturing it.

The solution delivered from the feed pipe **14** of the tower **12** is adapted to drop downwardly through the multihole catch plate **15** disposed on the upper part of the recovering tank **16** so that it can remain as recovered in the recovery tank **16.**

Then, due to a difference in specific gravity, the water-insoluble solution remains in the upper part of the recovering tank **16** and the hardening solution remains in the lower part thereof, that is to say, both solutions are allowed to remain in two different layers. Thus, the hardening solution can flow through water-discharge outlet **20** at the bottom of tank **16** into tank **10** for storage, and the water-insoluble solution can flow through water-discharge outlet **23** on the side wall of tank **16** into tank **1** for storage, thereby enabling all the solutions to be recovered without waste.

PHARMACEUTICALS AND HEALTH-RELATED PRODUCTS

CONTROLLED RELEASE SYSTEMS

Sustained Release Propranolol Hydrochloride

Propranolol hydrochloride is an important medicament which is widely used throughout the world. It is a β-adrenergic blocking agent which is mainly used for the treatment of angina pectoris, cardiac arrhythmias and hypertension. The chemical name for propranolol is dl-1-isopropylamino-3-(1-naphthoxy)-2-propanol.

According to *J. McAinsh and R.C. Rowe; U.S. Patent 4,138,475; February 6, 1979; assigned to Imperial Chemical Industries Limited, England* there is provided a sustained release pharmaceutical composition consisting of a hard gelatin capsule containing film coated spheroids, the spheroids comprising, prior to coating, 40 to 65 wt % of propranolol or a pharmaceutically-acceptable acid-addition salt thereof in admixture with non-water-swellable microcrystalline cellulose, and the spheroids having a film coat comprising ethylcellulose optionally together with hydroxypropyl methylcellulose.

The term "spheroid" is known in the pharmaceutical art, and means a spherical granule having a diameter of approximately 0.5 to 2 mm. A suitable microcrystalline cellulose is the material sold as Avicel-PH-101. The uncoated spheroids may contain 50 to 60 wt % of propranolol hydrochloride and 50 to 40 wt % of microcrystalline cellulose, respectively.

A preferred form of ethylcellulose is that having a viscosity of 50 cp at 20°C (content of ethoxy groups 48 to 49 wt %). A suitable form of hydroxypropyl methylcellulose is that having a viscosity 3 to 6 cp at 20°C (U.S. National Formulary XIII). The film coat preferably comprises 90 wt % of ethylcellulose and 10 wt % of hydroxypropyl methylcellulose. In addition, the film coat may optionally contain up to 20 wt % of a plasticizer, e.g., a vegetable oil, or glycerol, or a glyceryl ester of a fatty acid. The film coat preferably comprises 9 to 10 wt % of the coated spheroids.

Example: Propranolol hydrochloride (60 kg) and microcrystalline cellulose (Avicel-PH 101, 40 kg) were blended together in a 450 liter planetary mixer. Water (50 kg) was added, and the mixer was run for 10 minutes until a homogeneous, plastic mass was obtained. The mass was extruded under pressure through a perforated cylinder to give cylindrical extrudates of nominally 1 mm diameter.

The damp extrudates (in batches of 15 to 20 kg) were placed in a spheronizer in which the rotating disc (diameter, 68 cm) rotated at 300 to 400 rpm. The rotation was continued for 10 minutes, and the resulting spheroids were then dried at 60°C in a fluidized bed drier. The dried spheroids were passed over a 1.4 mm screen, and those which passed through were subjected to a 0.7 mm screen. The over- and undersized spheroids were discarded.

Acceptable spheroids (100 kg) were placed in a perforated coating drum fitted with a 0.5 mm screen and rotating at 17 rpm. A film formulation consisting of ethylcellulose (9 kg) and hydroxypropyl methylcellulose (1 kg) dissolved in a mixture of dichloromethane (100 liters) and methanol (100 liters) was sprayed onto the rotating spheroids at 750 milliliters per minute using a standard airless spray system. The resulting film coated spheroids were passed over a 1.4 mm screen to remove any aggregates, and then filled into hard gelatin capsules using a conventional encapsulation machine, such that each capsule contained 160 mg of propranolol hydrochloride. There was thus obtained a sustained release composition containing propranolol hydrochloride.

Controlled Release Liquid Medicament Entrapped in Phospholipid Spherules

According to *A. Suzuki, H. Miura, S. Matsuda and T. Ohsawa; U.S. Patent 4,016,100; April 5, 1977; assigned to Tanabe Seiyaku Co., Ltd., Japan* a controlled release pharmaceutical composition can be prepared by dispersing a phospholipid uniformly in water to produce an aqueous phospholipid dispersion, adding a medicament to, or dissolving it in, the aqueous phospholipid dispersion, freezing the thus-obtained medicament dispersion, thereby entrapping the medicament in the lipid spherules, and then thawing the frozen dispersion to give an aqueous suspension of the medicament entrapped in the lipid spherules.

Suitable phospholipids which can be used include egg yolk phospholipids, soybean phospholipids, phosphatidyl choline, phosphatidyl ethanolamine, sphingomyelin, phosphatidyl serine, dipalmitoyl lecithin and mixtures thereof. The preferred amount of the phospholipid used is 0.001 to 0.2 g, especially 0.005 to 0.08 g/ml of water.

In order to produce lipid spherules or particles having a diameter of less than 5.0 μ, it is preferred to carry out the process under a pressure of more than 200 kg/cm^2, especially 350 to 550 kg/cm^2. The freezing step is preferably carried out at a temperature below -5°C (i.e., -5° to -40°C), especially -10° to -30°C.

Thawing or liquefaction is carried out by allowing the frozen phospholipid dispersion to stand at a temperature of 5° to 40°C, especially about 15° to 25°C. The aqueous suspension thus obtained comprises finely divided spherules of the phospholipid, the medicament entrapped in the lipid spherules thereof, and water. The lipid spherules in the aqueous suspension have a substantially uniform diameter of less than 5.0 μ, preferably 0.1 to 2.0 μ. If required, the medicament containing phospholipid may be further separated from the aqueous suspension. The separation of the entrapped medicament from the aqueous suspension is carried out in a conventional manner such as by centrifugation thereof.

As is illustratively shown in the following examples, the larger the amount of the entrapped medicament, the slower the rate of release of the medicament. Moreover, the rate of release of the medicament from the aqueous suspension (i.e., the aqueous suspension of the medicament entrapped in the lipid spherules) can be easily controlled by changing the amount of the medicament added to the aqueous phospholipid dispersion (i.e., the dispersion which is obtained by dispersing the phospholipid in water).

When the aqueous suspension of the process is administered to gastrointestinal tracts, muscles, blood vessels or other tissues, the medicament is released therefrom into the tissues constantly for a period as short as 30 minutes, or as long as 40 hours or longer according to a preselected release pattern. In view of the foregoing, the aqueous suspension can be used per se as a controlled or sustained release liquid pharmaceutical composition which is suitable for injection or oral administration.

Example 1: Sufficient water is added to 60 g of egg-yolk phospholipids to bring the total volume to 1.5 liters. The mixture is stirred with a homomixer. Then, the mixture is homogenized with an emulsifier under a pressure of 400 kg/cm^2 for 30 minutes, whereby an aqueous phospholipid dispersion is obtained. 10 g of tretoquinol hydrochloride are dissolved in enough water to bring the total volume to one liter. 950 ml of the aqueous phospholipid dispersion is mixed with 950 ml of the tretoquinol solution.

The aqueous dispersion thus obtained is allowed to stand at -20°C for 20 hours in a freezer. Then, the frozen dispersion is thawed by allowing it to stand at room temperature. An aqueous suspension of tretoquinol hydrochloride entrapped in phospholipid spherules is thereby obtained. The size of the spherules of egg-yolk phospholipids in the suspension is within the range of 0.1 to 2.0 μ in diameter.

Example 2: Sufficient water is added to 100 g of egg-yolk phospholipids to bring the total volume to one liter. The mixture is stirred with a homomixer. Then, the mixture is homogenized with an emulsifier under a pressure of 300 kg/cm^2 for 30 minutes, whereby an aqueous phospholipid dispersion is obtained. 20 g of diphenhydramine hydrochloride and 18 g of sodium chloride are dissolved in enough water to bring the total volume to one liter. 850 ml of the aqueous phospholipid dispersion is mixed with 850 ml of the diphenhydramine solution.

The aqueous dispersion thus obtained is filtered through a membrane filter (pore size 0.45 μ in diameter). The filtrate is sterilized at 120°C for 20 minutes and then allowed to stand at -20°C for 20 hours in a freezer. The frozen dispersion thus obtained is thawed by allowing it to stand at room temperature. An aqueous suspension of diphenhydramine hydrochloride entrapped in phospholipid spherules is thereby obtained. The size of the spherules of the egg-yolk phospholipids in the suspension is within the range of 0.1 to 2.0 μ in diameter.

Multilayered Tablet Containing Medial Layer of Controlled Release Microcapsules

Y.F.M.J. Estevenel, M.H. Thely and W.A. Coulon; U.S. Patent 4,113,816; September 12, 1978; assigned to Choay SA, France describe the production of tablets containing, in their mass, controlled release microcapsules, characterized in that they are constituted by the association of a plurality of superposed layers, of which the medial layer is essentially constituted by microcapsules containing an active substance, while the exterior layers, which may possibly also contain identical or different active substances and which have a composition usual for the making of tablets, constitute means of protecting the microcapsules of the medial layer, particularly against the shock of compression.

The tablets have a hardness of the order of 10 to 20 kg on their surface and of the order of 8 to 16 kg on their periphery. The ratio between the sum of the thicknesses of the external layers and the thickness of the medial layer containing the microcapsules is between 0.8 and 4 and preferably between 1 and 2.4. Tests have shown that for a medial layer thickness of between 0.6 and 3 mm, and preferably between 1 and 2 mm, the thickness of each of the external layers must be between 0.8 and 2 mm and preferably between 1 and 1.2 mm. The tablets obtained are advantageously flat and bevelled having a diameter of the order of 11 mm, a final weight of between 0.360 and 0.660 g, and a final total thickness of between 3.3 and 5.65 mm.

Example: (1) A composition adapted to form the external layers of the final tablet is prepared by mixing the following constituents in the proportions stated: hesperidin methyl-chalcone, 0.065 g; aspirin, 0.100 g; 4-chloro-1-dehydromethyl-testosterone, 0.00165 g; and excipients: lubricants, such as, e.g., a mixture of mono-, di- and tripalmitostearic esters of glycerol, 0.00175 g; cornstarch, 0.050 g; and filler excipient, such as, e.g., microcrystalline α-cellulose, qsp, 0.260 g.

This mixture is put into the form of granules of a grain size identical to that of the microcapsules, in such a manner that the dispersion in the tablet making machine of this composition is identical to that of the microcapsules. In practice, the granules obtained have a grain size less than 1,000 μ.

(2) A composition adapted to form the medial layer of the final tablet is prepared by mixing the following constituents in the proportions stated: microcapsules enclosing papaverine chlorhydrate, 0.097 g and filler excipient favoring free flow, qsp, 0.140 g.

(3) 0.130 g of the composition described in (1) is placed into the matrix of a tablet machine, and is subjected to a pressing, by levelling, e.g., with the aid of the suitable means such as the punch of the machine, without, however, supplying a compressive force to the latter. On the external layer thus produced, the composition described in (2) is superposed and this is also subjected to a pressing, by levelling, e.g., with the aid of suitable means such as the punch of the machine, in such a manner that the punch only exerts the compressive force exercised by its own weight.

On the microcapsule layer is then superposed 0.130 g of the composition described in (1). The multilayer composition thus obtained, comprising a medial layer of microcapsules protected by two external layers, is submitted to a suitable compressive force in a tablet machine in such a manner as to obtain tablets having a hardness sufficient to be pharmaceutically satisfactory while nevertheless, permitting a disintegration conforming to the standards laid down in the French Pharmacopoeia and preserving the programmed controlled release of the active constituents.

The tablet obtained by using the method which has just been described is a flat tablet, chamfered, having a diameter of 11 mm, a final thickness of 3.8 mm and a final weight of 0.400 g. This disintegrates in a period of 35 minutes. The thickness of each of the external layers is 1.07 mm while the thickness of the microcapsule layer is 1.65 mm. The hardness of this tablet measured on Stokes apparatus is 10 kg on its surface and 5 kg on its periphery.

The processing of the tablets as described causes the immediate liberation of the therapeutic agents contained in their external layers and the controlled release, over a prolonged period of time, up to 8 hours, of the papaverine contained in the microcapsules of the medial layer.

Medicant Release at Constant Rate in GI Tract

G. Benedikt; U.S. Patent 4,083,949; April 11, 1978; assigned to Byk Gulden Lomberg Chemische Fabrik GmbH, Germany describes an oral medicament form which comprises active-substance-containing spheroidal particles provided with a dialysis membrane, whose film former comprises (a) a cellulose ether which is insoluble in the pH range of the gastrointestinal tract and which cannot be enzymatically degraded and (b) one or more organic compounds which are essentially only soluble in the alkaline part of the intestinal tract. The active-substance-containing spheroidal particles are preferably collected together to form a unit dosage.

The cellulose ethers used are rather low-molecular-weight polymers which do not swell to form a gel in an aqueous medium, which have an alkoxy group content of from 43 to 50 wt % and which have a viscosity of from about 7 to 100 cp. Methyl, ethyl and propylcelluloses are particularly preferred. The viscosity data refer to solutions of cellulose ethers containing 5 wt % of cellulose ether in toluene:ethanol mixtures (80:20 parts by weight) measured at 25°C.

In accordance with the process the cellulose ether solutions with a relatively low viscosity range, i.e., from about 7 to 20 cp, are particularly preferred. The organic compounds, substantially only soluble in the alkaline part of the intestinal tract, are characterized by a content of from 5 to 40 wt % of free carboxyl groups.

The film-forming component of the dialysis membrane comprises (according to the particular active substance used) from 15 to 70 wt % of cellulose ether and from 30 to 85 wt % of the alkali-soluble compound. The following table enumerates preferred alkali-soluble compounds together with their physical characteristics, their content of free carboxyl groups and their preferred proportion by weight in the dialysis membranes; see H.P. Fiedler, *Lexikon der Hilfsstoffe für Pharmazie, Kosmetik und angrenzende Gebiete*, Editio Cantor KG (1971).

Compound	Viscosity (cp)	Melting Point (°C)	Carboxyl groups (% by wt)	Percent by Weight of Dialysis Membrane
Cellulose acetatephthalate	70-80*	–	9-13	30-85
Hydroxypropylmethyl-cellulose phthalate	450±90**	–	6-8	30-85
Hydroxypropylmethyl-cellulose phthalate	150±30**	–	8-12	30-85
Shellac	–	115-120	8-10	30-85
Sandarac	–	135	–	30-85
Methacrylic acid-methacrylic acid ester copolymer	–	–	36-37	30-85
Methacrylic acid-methacrylic acid ester copolymer	–	–	22-23	30-85
Ethyl ester of poly(methyl-vinyl ether/maleic acid)***	–	–	34-40	20-85
Stearic acid***	–	71	16	15-40
Palmitic acid***	–	62	18	15-40
Myristic acid***	–	54	20	15-40

*10% in acetone, 20°C.

**15% in acetone:ethanol 1:1, 20°C.

***This alkali-soluble compound is preferably used in combination with one or more other alkali-soluble compounds listed in this table.

The incorporation of the compound (which is water soluble in the alkaline range and is water insoluble in the acidic range) into the dialysis membrane of the medicament form makes precise control of the release of active substance possible, since permeability of the dialysis membrane is adapted in each respective case to the solubility of the active substance in the individual ranges of the gastrointestinal tract. Very many medicaments are salts of weak bases. Such substances have excellent solubility in the acidic range; however, in the neutral or alkaline range the solubility of these materials decreases by several powers of 10, i.e., several orders of magnitude.

The concentration of active substance within the dialysis membrane for these medicaments is substantially greater in the acidic range of the stomach than in the alkaline range of the intestine. The concentration gradient of the drug constituent often changes to a great extent during passage of a medicament form through the stomach and intestine. However, since the permeability of the dialysis membrane adapts itself to the respective and changing pH range during passage through the stomach and intestine, variations in the concentration gradient are compensated for accordingly and essentially the same quantity of active substance is released per unit time during the whole passage through the stomach and intestine.

In the acidic range of the stomach the concentration gradient of a weakly basic medicinal substance is admittedly high in the dialysis membrane, but the permeability of the membrane is low. Although the concentration gradient in the membrane decreases in the alkaline intestinal tract owing to decreased solubility of the active substance, the alkaline-soluble component of the membrane dissolves and the permeability of the membrane is increased at the same time. Preferred forms of medicament of the process are characterized by an active substance which is a nitrogen-containing organic base or a salt of such a base, with a pK_B value of the base below 14.

Example: (A) Delayed Release of an Analgesic Medicament – 14 kg of sugar spherulets with a diameter of 0.6 mm are evenly moistened in a rotating dragée-forming vessel with approximately 500 g of a 10% ethanolic ethyl cellulose solution (ethoxyl content of 45 to 46%, 10 cp) and, following this, 500 g of finely powdered sodium salicylate are applied to the thus-moistened spherulets. This operation is repeated until 38 kg of sodium salicylate have been applied. For this purpose 30 kg of the abovedescribed 10% ethanolic ethylcellulose solution are used. The size of the active substance pellets so produced lies between 1.4 and 1.6 mm, and they comprise an amount of sodium salicylate equal to 84% of their weight.

These pellets are sprayed in a fluidized bed apparatus with a solution of 3.8 kg of shellac (with a carboxyl group content of 6 wt %) and 700 g of ethylcellulose (having a viscosity of 10 cp in 10% ethanolic solution and an ethoxy-group content of about 48 to 49.5 wt %) in a mixture made up of 38 liters of denatured ethanol and 38 liters of dichloromethane.

The active substance release figures, as determined according to the half-change method, are as follows: 1 hr, 25.6%; 2 hr, 40.8%; 3 hr, 55.3%; 4 hr, 65.1%; 5 hr, 83.2%; 6 hr, 95.4%; and 7 hr, 103.5%. The figures for the release of active substance in accordance with the half-change method as determined in the Sartorius solution model of H. Stricker do not depart therefrom by more than ±3%.

(B) Comparative Example – The pellets produced according to (A), first paragraph, are sprayed with a solution of 3.8 kg of methacrylic acid-methacrylic acid ester copolymer having a carboxyl group content of 36 to 37% (Eudragit L) and 700 g of methacrylic acid-methacrylic acid ester copolymer having a carboxyl group content of 22 to 23% (Eudragit S) in 38 liters of denatured ethanol and 38 liters of dichloromethane.

The active substance release figures, as determined according to the half-change method, are as follows: 1 hr, 0%; 2 hr, 2%; and 3 hr, 100%. These results show that, by the sole application of film formers which are soluble in intestinal juices, the release of active substance readily occurs at or approaching the neutralization point. This medicament form acts as a stomach-resistant form and is not apt to achieve constant blood level values.

Bioerodible Delivery System for Sustained Administration of Ophthalmic Drugs

A.S. Michaels; U.S. Patent 3,962,414; June 8, 1976; assigned to Alza Corporation describes a bioerodible device for the sustained administration of a therapeutically effective predetermined dosage of drug to a patient comprising one or more reservoirs each of which comprises a drug formulation confined within a polyvalent metal ion crosslinked anionic polyelectrolyte which bioerodes in the body in response to the biological environment therein by a process of polyvalent metal ion displacement.

One aspect of the process relates to a bioerodible ocular insert for the controlled continuous administration of a predetermined dosage of drug to the eye over a prolonged period of time, comprising a matrix polyelectrolyte having distributed throughout a plurality of reservoirs, each of the reservoirs comprising a drug formulation confined within a drug release rate controlling material, the reservoirs characterized by being either (1) a microcapsule of an initial size and configuration such as to be capable of being eliminated from the ocular cavity through the punctum with ear fluid, or (2) a microcapsule of biodegradable material; the matrix material being permeable to the passage of drug at a higher rate than through the drug release rate controlling material, the latter material metering a therapeutically effective amount of drug from the reservoir to the eye at a controlled rate over a prolonged period of time, the insert being of an initial shape which is adapted for insertion and retention in the eye and wherein the materials comprising the insert are eliminated from the ocular cavity by bioeroding or biodegrading in the environment of the eye or the reservoir material eliminated by passage through the punctum, the eliminations taking place concurrently with the dispensing or at a point in time after the dispensing of the therapeutically desired amount of drug.

Figure 4.1 illustrates an ocular insert **50** of this process particularly suited for administering a water-soluble drug. The drug delivery device **50** is comprised of a bioerodible matrix **22** of polyvalent cation crosslinked anionic polyelectrolyte material having dispersed therethrough a plurality of drug reservoirs **51**. The reservoirs **51** are microcapsules comprised of a water-soluble drug whether in solid form, liquid form or in admixture with a carrier, confined within a drug release rate controlling material.

Figure 4.1: Bioerodible Drug Delivery System for Sustained Administration of Ophthalmic Drugs

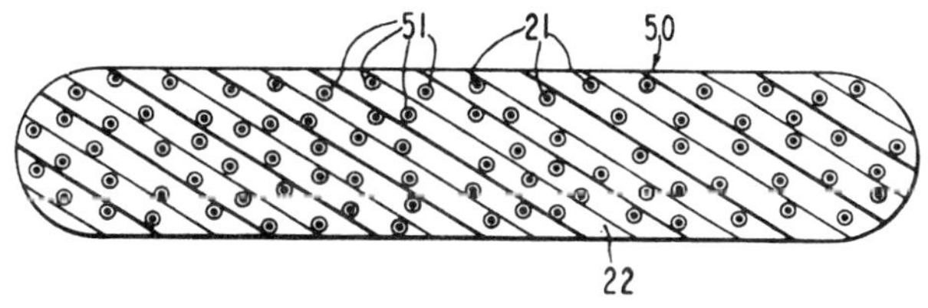

Source: U.S. Patent 3,962,414

Drug molecules released from the reservoirs **51** pass into the matrix **22** and then migrate through the matrix **22** for administration of drug to the eye. Release of drug from the reservoir is the rate controlling step for release of drug from the device. In construction, the device can be viewed as a single unit device comprising two structures acting in concert for effective drug administration to the eye. One structure pertains to the reservoirs **51** which are microcapsules comprising a microbody of drug release rate controlling material having drug **21** confined therein, and the other structure relates to the bioerodible matrix **22** housing the reservoirs and is formed of a material permeable to the passage of drug.

The reservoirs **51** can be formed as a hollow container having a drug therein formed from drug release rate controlling material. Additionally, the reservoirs **51** can be a solid particle having a drug distributed therethrough and formed of a drug release rate controlling material. Alternatively, the reservoir **51** can be a porous structure formed of a material possessing drug release rate controlling properties. It can be aggregate or particulate and geometrically shaped. By controlling the structure of the reservoirs of the drug delivery device, the process makes possible a drug time pattern of release, including a zero order drug release.

Thus, in the preferred modifications for obtaining a constant rate of release, the reservoir is formed as a capsule containing the drug therein and surrounded by a rate controlling membrane, or the reservoir is a solid matrix with a limited number of discrete particles of drug contained therein.

The materials suitable for fabricating the reservoir **51**, whether of hollow, solid, porous, semiporous or the like structures, are generally those materials capable of forming membranes with or without pores or voids, or coating through which the drug can pass at a controlled rate by the process of diffusion. Suitable materials for forming the reservoirs are naturally occurring or synthetic materials that are nontoxic and which preferably have a low solubility and/or low diffusivity to water. In general, these qualities will be possessed by rate release controlling materials that are hydrophobic in nature.

The rate controlling materials used for the reservoir **51** can be biodegradable, biodegradation in the environment of the eye taking place concurrently with the dispensing or at a point in time after the dispensing of the therapeutically desired amount of drug. Alternatively, when the reservoir **51** is of an initial size and configuration such as to be capable of being eliminated from the ocular cavity through the punctum with tear fluid it can be made of nonbiodegradable material. Microcapsules, preferably of approximately 100 micron size or less, will be of suitable dimension for proper punctum passage.

Exemplary nonbiodegradable materials suitable for fabricating the microcapsules when of an initial size such as to pass through the punctum are drug release rate controlling materials such as hydrophobic polymers, e.g., polyvinyl chloride, nylon, silicon rubber, cholesterol; substituted alkyl celluloses such as hydroxypropyl methylcellulose, methylcellulose, ethylcellulose, cellulose acetate, waxes, e.g., paraffin, ethylene wax, hydrogenated castor oil; $C_{10\text{-}20}$ fatty acids, e.g., stearic acid, palmitic acid; hydrophilic polymers, e.g., polymerized esters of methacrylic acid (Hydron), etc.

Biodegradable materials suitable for preparing the microcapsule reservoirs have the characteristics below. The actual material selected for fabricating the microcapsule reservoir is one that can slow down the rate of release of the water-soluble drug to the desired level. Preferred are the hydrophobic materials. Although hydrophilic type materials can sometimes be employed for fabricating the reservoir in cases where the water-soluble drug is not too highly permeable therein, in most cases thicker coatings of microcapsule material and larger microcapsule diameters will be required than for hydrophobic type microcapsule materials.

In this regard, among other factors which must be considered, in addition to the nature of the reservoir rate controlling material, and which affect the rate of release of drug from the microcapsule, are the microcapsule size, the density of the drug and the thickness of the reservoir wall. Qualitative guides in this regard are that the rate of release of drug will decrease with the corresponding increasing values for each of these parameters as will be appreciated by those skilled in the art.

Any of the standard encapsulation or impregnation techniques known can be used to prepare the microcapsules **51** to be incorporated into the matrix material **22**. Thus, the drug, admixture of drug, or drug solution can be added to the encapsulating material in liquid form and uniformly distributed therethrough by mixing; or solid encapsulating material can be impregnated with the drug by immersion in a bath of the drug to cause the drug to diffuse into the material. Subsequently, the solid material can be reduced to fine microcapsules by grinding, each of the microcapsules comprising the drug coated with and distributed throughout the encapsulated material. Alternatively, fine particles or solutions of the drug can be encapsulated with a coating. One suitable technique comprises suspending dry particles of the drug in an air stream and contacting that stream containing the encapsulating material that coats the drug with a membrane permeable to the drug.

Another standard method of microencapsulation suitable for the purpose is the coacervation technique. The coacervation technique of fabrication as conventionally employed consists essentially of the formation of three immiscible phases, a liquid manufacturing phase, a core material phase and a coating phase with deposition of the liquid polymer coating on the core material and rigidizing the coating, usually by thermal, crosslinking or desolvation techniques to form microcapsules.

Although the device in Figure 4.1 is particularly well suited to the administration of water-soluble drugs it is equally well adaptable to the administration of drugs which are non-water-soluble. Devices of the type shown can be designed by first selecting the drug to be used, its dosage, and the period of therapy. This establishes the required drug release rate and amount of drug to be incorporated in the device. Materials having the appropriate drug release rate characteristics and erosion rates can then be correlated with the effective surface release reas to fabricate a device which meters the desired rate of the drug to the eye over the established period of time. A particular added advantage of a device illustrated is the fact that the number of reservoirs employed can be varied in order to achieve the desired drug release rate from the device.

Any of the drugs used to treat the eye and surrounding tissues can be incorporated in the ocular insert. Also, it is practical to use the eye and surrounding tissues as a point of entry for systemic drugs or antigens that ultimately enter circulation in the blood stream, or enter the nasopharyngeal area by normal routes, and produce a pharmacologic response at a site remote from the point of application of the ocular insert. Thus, drugs or antigens which will pass through the eye or the tissue surrounding the eye to the blood stream or to the nasopharyngeal, esophageal or gastrointestinal areas, but which are not used in therapy of the eye itself, can be incorporated in the ocular insert.

Suitable drugs for use in therapy of the eye with the ocular insert consistent with their known dosages and uses are without limitation, e.g., antibiotics, antibacterials, antivirals, antiallergenics, anti-inflammatories, decongestants, miotics and anticholinesterases, mydriatics and sympathomimetics.

To provide compatibility with the eye and surrounding tissues, at least for the initial period after insertion, the surfaces of the ocular insert in contact with the eye can be coated with a thin layer, e.g., from 1 to 2 microns thick, of biodegradable hydrophilic material. Exemplary of the suitable materials for this purpose are gelatin, noncrosslinked polysaccharides, and biodegradable materials such as glycerinated gelatin, collagen, gum acacia, polyvinyl alcohol, polyvinyl pyrrolidone, alginic acid and alkali metal salts of alginic acid, starch phosphate, starch, e.g., agar or gum arabic.

Example: 500 g of chloramphenicol of a particle size of 50 microns is encapsulated with polylactic acid polymer of molecular weight 50,000, according to the following procedure. 250 g of the polylactic acid is dissolved into two liters of chloroform. The chloramphenicol particles are coated by polylactic acid using Wurster air suspension technique. The coat thickness is determined to be 30 microns thick. Separately, in a Waring blender, 10 g of sodium alginate is vigorously stirred with 300 ml of deionized water to yield a slightly viscous solution.

Stirring is stopped and 3 g of the chloramphenicol microcrystals are thoroughly dispersed in the sodium alginate solution. The final mixture is then cast on a clean glass plate leveled with a doctor blade to a thickness of 80 mils, and dried for 24 hours in a stream of circulating 35°C air. The resulting film is removed from the glass plate by stripping, and immersed in a 6 wt % zinc chloride solution (pH 5.0) for 12 hours. The film is then repeatedly washed until a washing gives a negative chloride test.

The film is then air dried at room temperature and punch-cut into elliptically shaped ovals 8 mm in major axis and 5 mm in minor axis. When these ovals are placed in the sacs of eyes, they release chloramphenicol for a prolonged period of time at a rate controlled by the polylactic acid microencapsulation polymer. The metal ion linked polyelectrolyte which functions as a matrix for the microcapsules, completely bioerodes in the environment of the eye at the termination of the therapeutic program.

Zein-Shellac Coating for Digitoxin

A. Pescetti; U.S. Patent 3,939,259; February 17, 1976 describes a therapeutic preparation consisting of particles containing a therapeutically active material which are coated with a disintegratable coating comprising zein and shellac. A first group of particles contains no coating or a coating subject to rapid disintegration upon ingestion to release an initial dose of therapeutic material and remaining groups of particles are coated with increasingly thicker coatings for delayed disintegration to release subsequent doses of therapeutic material. The coating composition may include disintegration modifiers so that thinner coatings of the zein-shellac coating material can be employed than would be required for zein-shellac alone to obtain the delayed disintegration of the coating.

Example: 40 kg of neutral particles (50 wt % starch, 50 wt % sugar pellets) having a 24 mesh particle size were placed in a 42-inch coating pan. The pan was rotated at between 28 and 30 rpm and 500 cc of a simple syrup solution containing 10 g of digitoxin were distributed over the particles. Following addition of the digitoxin solution, the particles were dried in warm air and assayed for digitoxin content per particle. The digitoxin containing particles were weighed and one-third of the particles, on a weight basis, were set aside and identified as group 1 particles. The remaining quantity of particles was re-placed in the 42-inch coating pan. A coating solution was prepared in accordance with the following formula:

Composition A

Zein, 10 wt % in alcohol, cc	2,000
Shellac (6 lb cut), cc	2,000
Ethylcellulose, 2 wt % in alcohol, cc	1,000
Beeswax, g	2
Castor oil, cc	10

The alcohol solvent utilized was 45 volume percent ethyl alcohol in water. The coating pan was set in rotation and a sufficient portion of the coating solution to cover the particles was distributed over the particles in the revolving coating pan. The particles were then dried in hot air until traces of the coating solution had disappeared and the particles were freely flowing in the pan. This procedure was repeated an additional seven times to build up the coating on the particles. The coated particles were weighed and one-half of the particles on a weight basis were separated and identified as group 2 particles. The remaining particles were returned to the 42-inch revolving coating pan and the coating procedure repeated as set forth above using the following coating compositions:

Composition B

Zein, 10 wt % in alcohol, cc	2,000
Shellac (6 lb cut), cc	2,000
Ethylcellulose, 2 wt % in alcohol, cc	1,000
Polyvinylpyrrolidone, 10 wt % in alcohol, cc	1,000
Beeswax, g	5
Dibutyl phthalate, cc	5

Ten applications of the coating solution were applied to the particles in the manner described above. These particles were identified as group 3 particles. A sufficient number of particles to provide a 0.1 mg dose of digitoxin were selected from each of the groups, 1, 2 and 3 of particles and placed in a number 0 gelatin capsule. The capsule contained a total dosage of 0.3 mg of digitoxin.

The capsule was subjected to a disintegration test in accordance with the U.S. Pharmacopoeia. In accordance with this test the capsule was first placed in simulated gastric juice and maintained therein for a period of one hour with constant shaking. The gastric juice was prepared by dissolving 7.0 ml of hydrochloric acid USP, 2.0 g of sodium chloride and 3.2 g pepsin USP in sufficient distilled water to make one liter (pH approximately 1.2). The simulated gastric juice was maintained at a temperature of 37°C. Following this period the remaining particles were removed from the simulated gastric juice and 100 cc of the gastric juice was extracted and assayed for digitoxin content in accordance with the method described in the U.S. Pharmacopoeia.

The remaining pellets were then placed in simulated intestinal juice and shaken for a period of three hours. The intestinal juice was prepared by adding 10.0 g of pancreatin USP to a mixture of 250 ml of 5 M potassium biphosphate, 190 ml of 5 M sodium hydroxide and 460 ml of distilled water. The pH was adjusted to 7.5 and sufficient distilled water was added to make one liter. At the end of the 3 hour test period 100 cc of the intestinal juice was extracted and assayed for digitoxin content. The test was continued for an additional 4 hours and a second 100 cc was extracted and assayed for digitoxin content.

In accordance with the test results, it was determined that the capsule had released 0.1 mg of digitoxin in the gastric juice at the end of one hour, 0.1 mg digitoxin at the end of four hours of testing and 0.1 mg of digitoxin was released after eight hours of testing.

Microparticulate Carrier Comprising Ionically Bonded Reaction Product of Piperazine and Acacia

The process of *T.J. Speaker and L.J. Lesko; U.S. Patent 3,959,457; May 25, 1976; assigned to Temple University* pertains to a microparticulate (microspheroid) material which may serve as a carrier for diffusible reactants such as pharmaceuticals and which therefore constitute a new form of sustained release medicaments.

The microparticulate material is comprised of the reaction product produced in a finely dispersed emulsion of a water-immiscible solution of (a) an organic polyfunctional Lewis base, in a (b) low boiling point, polar, organic solvent, and an aqueous solution of a (c) partially hydrophilic, partially lipophilic, polyfunctional Lewis acid. Suitable acidic materials (c) which have been found to be useful are: agar, acacia gum, arabic acid, carboxymethylcellulose, ghatti gum, guar gum, methylcellulose, oxidized cellulose, pectin, tragacanth or polyethylene glycol. Suitable polar solvents (b) found useful are: bromoform, chloroform, dichloromethane, dichloroethane, diethyl ether, methyl ethyl ketone or nitrobenzene. As basic materials (a), the following have been used: hexylamine, isopentylamine, N-methylpiperidine, piperidine, dimethylethylenediamine, hexanediamine, piperazine, ethylenediamine, hexamethylrosanilinium cation as chloride, rosanilinium cation as chloride, melamine or tetraethylpentamine.

Preferably, a solution of a polyamine, such as piperazine, triethylenediamine, or ethylenediamine, in chloroform, is added to an aqueous solution of a vegetable gum, such as acacia, with rapid stirring to produce a finely dispersed emulsion. The severity and time of stirring will determine the droplet size of emulsion particles and ultimately the particle size of the microparticulate product. A material for which the microparticulate product is to serve as a carrier is also included in the organic phase of the mixture.

Such a material must of course be substantially nonreactive with the other components in the reaction media and must also be substantially immiscible in the aqueous phase and soluble in the organic phase. For purposes of release of such material it must also be of such molecular size that it will be able to diffuse out of the individual microspheroids of the microparticulate material.

In each organic phase droplet of this finely dispersed emulsion the polyfunctional Lewis base is drawn to the surface of the droplet by the polar attraction of the surrounding aqueous phase. In the aqueous phase, the partially hydrophilic, partially lipophilic, polyfunctional Lewis acid is drawn, due to its partially lipophilic characteristic, toward the interface between the organic droplet and the surrounding aqueous phase where it reacts, presumably through dipole and/or ionic bonding, with the polyfunctional Lewis base concentrated on the outer surfaces of the organic phase droplets adjacent the interface, to produce a shell-like, insoluble particle generally corresponding in shape and size to the organic droplets. Each of these shell-like particles is thought to consist of an open network, or lattice, of molecules of a dipole and/or ionic salt.

Example: (A) Preparation – A solution of 10 g of finely divided acacia powder (USP) in 50 cc of distilled water and a second solution of 0.05 g of anhydrous piperazine and 50 cc of chloroform are prepared at room temperature. To the latter solution is added 100 mg of a selected drug, namely Quinacrine HCl. While stirring the acacia vigorously with a magnetic stirrer, the chloroform solution is added slowly and steadily so that the chloroform solution is emulsified in the aqueous solution. Stirring is continued for about 3 minutes to produce emulsion droplets about 5 microns in diameter. The organic phase, now consisting of emulsified microspheres, is then allowed to settle to the bottom of the container and the supernatant clear, aqueous layer is decanted. The organic phase is then washed with water to remove excess chloroform, piperazine and acacia. On exposure to the atmosphere, the microspheres lose their chloroform by evaporation leaving a microparticulate material comprised of microspheroids made up of wrinkled, continuous shell-like films, surrounding the drug, Quinacrine HCl.

(B) Evaluation – Such a microparticulate material has been injected directly into the blood stream of a frog and circulation of the microspheroids in the blood stream of the frog has been proven by microscopic observation of these microspheroids subsequently flowing in the capillary network of the web of the frog's foot. No adverse effect on the frog was observed. The sustained release of drug from the microparticulate material has been observed generally in dogs in vivo and has been studied in detail in vitro. The continued circulation of intravenously injected radionuclide-bearing microparticles has, in separate experiments, been demonstrated in rats.

OTHER PHARMACEUTICALS AND DRUGS

Aspirin Encapsulated in Ethylcellulose

M. Kitajima, A. Kondo and F. Arai; U.S. Patent 3,951,851; April 20, 1976; assigned to Fuji Photo Film Co., Ltd., Japan describe a process for the encapsulation of aspirin with a cellulose derivative. The steps of the process are as follows:

(1) As the capsule wall-forming substance, a cellulose derivative (an alkyl cellulose, preferably ethylcellulose) having an ethoxyl content of from 40.8 to 49.5%, is used. The term "cellulose derivative" means cellulose in which a hydrogen atom of at least one hydroxyl group of the cellulose molecule has a substituent.

(2) A solution of the cellulose derivative is prepared by dissolving it in an organic solvent which is a solvent for the cellulose derivative and is properly miscible with water (at least about 1 wt %); the maximum preferred degree of miscibility is about 35 g per 100 g of water. Then, aspirin particles are dispersed in the solution to form a dispersion. In this case, aspirin can be dissolved in the solution of the cellulose derivative, but it is preferred to choose an organic solvent that dissolves a low amount of aspirin. The cellulose derivative is completely dissolved by the organic solvent. The resulting solution contains the cellulose derivative in from about 1 to 10 wt % (i.e., concentration of the solution).

(3) As the encapsulation medium, water having dissolved therein about 1 wt % to the almost saturated amount (see table) of an organic solvent partially miscible with water (which may be same or different from the solvent(s) of step (2), water having dissolved therein at least about 0.01 wt % aspirin, or water containing the organic solvent and aspirin as described above is prepared. While the maximum amount of aspirin is not overly important, the maximum

amount of aspirin dissolved in 100 g of water at 20°C is about 0.6 g. It is thus seen the variation is relatively small.

(4) The aspirin-containing dispersion prepared in step (2) is added to the encapsulation medium maintained at any desired temperature not over 25°C (preferably not over 18°C) but above the freezing point thereof, and the mixture is stirred to divide the aspirin-containing dispersion into the particles of a size of about 0.1 to 2 mm. By evaporating off the organic solvent while stirring, the cellulose derivative is deposited around aspirin particles as walls, whereby a great number of capsules containing aspirin are prepared simultaneously. The process is completed in about 1 to 4 hours. The pressure used is preferably somewhat lower than atmospheric pressure, e.g., about 750 to 500 mm Hg.

It is desirable to use aspirin having a particle size of about 50 to 500 microns as listed in Japanese Pharmacopoeia. As the cellulose derivative, ethylcellulose having an ethylation degree of about 47 to 50% (N-100, Hercules Co., Ltd.), is convenient. Typical organic solvents partially miscible with water include alcohols, ethers, ketones, esters, etc., which are exemplified in the table below. From the viewpoint of the dissolving of the cellulose derivatives (especially ethylcellulose) and aspirin, ease of evaporation, cost, ease of recovery, etc., esters or mixtures of the solvents described above are preferred.

Solvent	Boiling Point (°C)	Amount Dissolved in 100 g of Water*
Alcohols		
Isobutanol	104	9(20)
sec-Butanol	99	22(20)
Amyl alcohol	130	2.6(20)
Ethers		
Ethyl ether	34	10(10)
Ketones		
Methyl ethyl ketone	80	26(22)
Esters		
Ethyl formate	54	10(18)
Methyl acetate	57	33(22)
Ethyl acetate	77	9(15)
Propyl acetate	101	1.9(20)
Isopropyl acetate	90	3.2(20)

*(Temperature in °C in parentheses).

The amount of cellulose derivative employed as the wall substance of the aspirin-containing capsules can be freely selected in the range of about ⅕ to 1/100 (by weight) of the aspirin to be dispersed in the organic solvent(s), but is preferably about 1/20 to 1/50 the weight of the aspirin. The solution in which aspirin is dispersed is preferably used in a concentration of about 1 to 10 wt % of the cellulose derivative. The amount of the encapsulation medium used can be about 3 to 19 (preferably 5 to 7) times the amount of aspirin dispersed in the organic solvent.

Example: Into a solution of 1.5 g of ethylcellulose N-100 in 35 ml of ethyl acetate were dispersed 28.5 g of aspirin particles of about 300 μ to about 50 μ in particle size. The dispersion thus obtained was added to 200 ml of aspirin-saturated water as an encapsulation medium while maintaining all components at 15°C, and the mixture was stirred to form small droplets of 300 to 500 μ (aspirin:cellulose ratio about 1:19). By continuing the stirring, ethyl acetate was evaporated off over about 1 hour at atmospheric pressure to provide 30 g of ethylcellulose-encapsulated aspirin. 95 wt % of the total aspirin particles were encapsulated in walls about 1 to about 2 μ thick, as commonly the process provides walls of about 1 to 3 μ thick containing about 10 to 30 times the capsule weight of aspirin.

1 g of the thus obtained aspirin-containing capsules was incorporated in one liter of artificial gastric juice at 37°C and the time required for dissolving one-half of the total weight of the encapsulated aspirin was measured. The time was found to be 60 minutes. On the other hand, the time required for dissolving the same total amount of aspirin which was not encapsulated was about 15 minutes.

Palatable Cholestyramine Coacervate Composition

The process of *G.P. Polli and C.E. Shoop; U.S. Patent 3,974,272; August 10, 1976; assigned to Merck & Co., Inc.* relates to the preparation of palatable coacervate compositions containing cholestyramine and a modified gum colloid of cellulosive material and charged anionic gum in an aqueous medium. The pharmaceutical compositions are useful in the treatment of hypocholesteremia and biliary cirrhosis.

Representative modified gums which can be employed include hydrophilic colloid of cellulosive materials such as methylcellulose, ethylcellulose, sodium carboxymethylcellulose, hydroxyethylcellulose and hydroxypropyl cellulose and charged anionic gums such as carrageenan, sodium alginate, potassium alginate and propylene glycol alginate. Of particular preference is sodium carboxymethyl cellulose or sodium alginate.

Optionally, either a water-insoluble or soluble dispersing agent may be employed. Representative water-insoluble dispersing agents are cornstarch, dibasic calcium phosphate and potato starch and representative water-soluble dispersing agents are Primojel, sucrose and dextrose. Of particular preference is Primojel or cornstarch.

To each part by weight of modified gum are added from about 4 to 10 parts by weight of cholestyramine and from about 4 to 10 oz of aqueous medium. Of particular preference is a combination of 1 part modified gum, from about 6 to 8 parts cholestyramine and from about 5 to 8 oz of aqueous medium. Optionally, a water-insoluble or soluble dispersing agent can be added to the composition at about 0.5 to 1.5 parts per part by weight of modified gum. Of particular preference is a combination of about 8 to 10 parts by weight cholestyramine, about 0.8 to 1.3 parts by weight of water-insoluble or soluble dispersing agent and from about 5 to 8 oz aqueous medium per part by weight of modified gum.

The dry reagents, cholestyramine, sodium carboxymethylcellulose, Primojel and lactose are mixed thoroughly into a powdered blend. An aliquot sample from the dry mixture is removed, mixed with flavor and then remixed with the original blend. The resulting powder blend mixture is then passed through a No. 80 mesh screen. The palatable cholestyramine-coacervate composition is obtained when mixed with 4 to 10 oz of aqueous medium. Of preference is a cholestyramine-coacervate composition containing 5.0 g of the palatable powder composition mixed with approximately 6 ounces of an aqueous medium prior to administration. Representative aqueous media which can be employed are water, milk and fruit juices such as orange, grapefruit, tomato, pineapple, apple, apricot and the like.

Encapsulation of Water-Insoluble Medicaments with Gastric- or Enteric-Soluble Wall Material

M. Morishita, Y. Inaba, M. Fukushima, Y. Hattori, S. Kobari and T. Matsuda; U.S. Patent 3,960,757; June 1, 1976; assigned to Toyo Jozo Co., Ltd., Japan provide a process for encapsulating various water-insoluble or slightly water-soluble medicaments. A suitable wall material for capsules is selected so as to make them gastric-soluble, enteric-soluble, gastric/enteric-soluble or slow release.

This process for preparing encapsulated medicaments comprises dissolving or dispersing a water-insoluble or slightly water-soluble medicament into a solution of a hydrophobic wall material in at least one organic solvent poorly miscible with water which has a boiling point of not more than 100°C (preferably 40° to 80°C), a vapor pressure higher than that of water and a dielectric constant of not more than about 10, dispersing the resulting solution or dispersion to the form of fine drops in a vehicle, and then vaporizing the organic solvent. It has also been found that when two or more of such organic solvents as mentioned above are used in admixture, more fine and excellent encapsulated medicaments can be obtained.

Typical examples of water-insoluble and slightly water-soluble medicaments are as follows: (A) Medicaments soluble in organic solvents–kitasamycin, acetylkitasamycin, spiramycin, acetylspiramycin, estradiol, erythromycin, erythromycin ethyl succinate, cortisone acetate, hydrocortisone acetate, prednisolone acetate, diazepam, triacetyl oleandomycin, chloramphenicol palmitate, phenacetin, progesterone, testosterone propionate, hexobarbital and methyl testosterone. (B) Medicaments insoluble in organic solvents–ampicillin trihydrate, chloramphenicol, chlorodiazepoxide, cyclobarbital, strychnine nitrate, dexamethazone, tetracycline, nalidixic acid, barbital, hydrocortisone, prednisolone, bromvalerylurea and folic acid.

Examples of poorly miscible organic solvents include ethyl ether, isopropyl ether, methylene chloride, ethylene chloride, chloroform, carbon tetrachloride, methyl acetate and ethyl acetate. Alternatively, a mixture of two or more organic solvents may be used. Preferably, the organic solvents used in admixture have a difference in boiling point of not less than 10°C. The wall material used to form wall films of microcapsules may be any material so far as it is hydrophobic and does not react with the medicaments.

Examples of the gastric-soluble wall material, which is a high molecular synthetic polymer, are cellulose acetate dibutylaminohydroxypropyl ether and polyvinyl acetal diethylamino acetate. An example of the gastric- and enteric-soluble wall material, which is a high molecular synthetic polymer is a 2-methyl-5-vinylpyridine methacrylate-methacrylic acid copolymer. An example of the enteric-soluble wall material, which is a high molecular synthetic polymer, is hydroxypropyl methylcellulose phthalate. Examples of the semipermeable wall material, which is a high molecular synthetic polymer, are ethylcellulose, cellulose acetate, cellulose propionate, cellulose butyrate, cellulose valerate, cellulose acetate propionate, polyvinyl acetate, polyvinyl formal, polyvinyl butyral, ladder polymer of sesquiphenyl siloxane, polymethyl methacrylate, polycarbonate, polystyrene, polyester, coumarone-indene polymer, polybutadiene, vinyl chloride-vinyl acetate copolymer, ethylene-vinyl acetate copolymer and vinyl chloride-propylene-vinyl acetate copolymer.

Further, examples of natural wall materials, which are soluble at the duodenum and which soften at elevated temperatures, preferably at 50°C or more, are waxes such as beef tallow, whale wax, beeswax, paraffin wax and castor wax, and higher fatty acids such as myristic, palmitic, stearic and behenic acids and esters thereof. The abovementioned hydrophobic wall materials may be used in the form of a mixture of two or more. In order to enhance the water repellency of the resulting microcapsules, it is particularly preferable to use the aforesaid high molecular synthetic polymer in admixture with the abovementioned wax or higher fatty acid.

The vehicle used is an aqueous solution of a hydrophilic colloid or surface active agent, in which an organic solvent solution of the hydrophobic wall material containing medicament can be dispersed to the form of fine drops, and in which the fine drops are stable. As the aqueous solution of hydrophilic colloid, there is used an aqueous solution containing 0.05 to 5% w/v, preferably 0.5 to 2% w/v, of gelatin, gelatin derivative, polyvinyl alcohol, polystyrene-sulfonic acid, hydroxymethylcellulose, hydroxyethylcellulose, hydroxypropyl cellulose, sodium carboxymethylcellulose or sodium polyacrylate.

As the aqueous solution of surface active agent, there is used an aqueous solution containing 0.01 to 2% w/v, preferably 0.1 to 1% w/v, of a water-soluble anionic or nonionic surface active agent having an HLB of not less than 10. Alternatively, a mixture of aqueous solutions of the hydrophilic colloid and surface active agent may also be used. In this case, it is preferable to use a 0.5 to 2% w/v aqueous solution of hydrophilic colloid in admixture with a 0.05 to 0.5% w/v aqueous solution of anionic surface active agent.

Example 1: A solution of 4 g of kitasamycin and 1 g of ethylcellulose in 20 ml of methylene chloride was dispersed with stirring at 300 rpm in 100 ml of a 1% w/v aqueous gelatin solution. Subsequently, the stirring was continued at 18°C for 60 minutes and then at 30°C for 60 minutes to obtain 3.8 g of kitasamycin-containing microcapsules of 140 to 300 microns in particle size. The thus-obtained microcapsules had been enhanced in slow release of kitasamycin by the ethylcellulose.

Example 2: A solution of 4 g of chloramphenicol and 1 g of beef tallow in 25 ml of ethyl acetate was dispersed with stirring at 400 rpm in 100 ml of a 1% w/v aqueous gelatin solution. Subsequently, the stirring was continued at room temperature for 2 hours to obtain 3.5 g of microcapsules of 240 to 530 microns in particle size. The thus-obtained microcapsules had been shielded from bitter taste of the chloramphenicol.

Example 3: 4 g of a fine powder (0.5 to 5 microns) of ampicillin trihydrate was dispersed in a solution of 1 g of hydroxypropyl methylcellulose phthalate (HP-50, Shintetsu Chemical Co.) in 20 ml of methylene chloride containing 0.5 ml of acetone. The resulting dispersion was dispersed with stirring at 280 rpm in 100 ml of a 1% w/v aqueous gelatin solution. Subsequently, the stirring was continued at room temperature for 2 hours to obtain 3.7 g of microcapsules of 700 to 1,200 microns in particle size. The thus-obtained microcapsules were not inactivated even when used in combination with dicloxacillin or ampicillin trihydrate.

Example 4: A solution of 4 g of kitasamycin and 1 g of polyvinyl acetal diethylamino acetate (AEA, Sankyo Co.) in 400 ml of a mixed organic solvent of chloroform-methylene chloride (1:1) was dispersed with stirring at 400 rpm in 100 ml of a 1% w/v aqueous gelatin solution. Subsequently, the stirring was continued at room temperature for 5 hours to obtain 3.5 g of microcapsules of 30 to 70 microns in particle size. The thus-obtained microcapsules were so stable as not to be inactivated in fodder.

Example 5: A solution of 4 g of chloramphenicol palmitate, 2 g of HP-50 and 2 g of beeswax in 30 ml of a mixed organic solvent of benzene-methylene chloride (1:2) was dispersed with stirring at 400 rpm in 100 ml of a 1% w/v aqueous gelatin solution. Subsequently, the stirring was continued at 45°C for 4.5 hours to obtain 5.4 g of microcapsules of 30 to 80 microns in particle size.

Example 6: A solution of 6 g of spiramycin, 2 g of AEA and 2 g of Lubri Wax 101 in 40 ml of a mixed organic solvent of chloroform-methylene chloride (1:2) was dispersed with stirring at 600 rpm in 200 ml of an aqueous solution containing 1 g of sodium laurylbenzene sulfonate and 2 g of gelatin. Subsequently, the stirring was continued at room temperature for 3.5 hours to obtain 8.0 g of microcapsules of 10 to 50 microns in particle size.

Pepstatin Floating Minicapsules

The process of *H. Umezawa; U.S. Patent 4,101,650; July 18, 1978; assigned to Zaidan Hojin Biseibutsu Kagaku Kenkyu Kai, Japan* relates to the formulation of pepstatin in a long-acting minicapsule and to its use for the treatment of gastric and duodenal ulcers. This minicapsule, in which carbon dioxide gas is produced by gastric acid floats, stays in the stomach and releases pepstatin continuously. It has been shown that when these minicapsules are given immediately after a meal, this capsule stays for 3 to 5 hours in the stomach and releases enough pepstatin to suppress the pepsin activity.

The composition in oral dosage form comprises minicapsules having a diameter in the range of 0.1 to 2 mm in which the center comprises a granule of sodium bicarbonate admixed if desired with at least one conventional solubilizing diluent, preferably lactose, and/or at least one water-soluble and solvent-soluble binder such as polyvinylpyrrolidone. The granule is coated with a conventional water-soluble, film-coating agent such as hydroxypropylmethylcellulose and the center is coated with pepstatin. The sodium bicarbonate is present in a weight in the range of 2 to 10, and preferably about 5, times the weight of the pepstatin. The minicapsule is further coated on the outside with a conventional water-soluble film-coating agent such as hydroxypropylmethylcellulose.

Example 1: Fine granules of 943.4 g of sodium bicarbonate, 37.7 g of lactose and 18.9 g of povidone (polyvinylpyrrolidone) were placed in a coating pan (the diameter was 60 cm) and spray-coated with 2% methanol solution of hydroxypropylmethylcellulose by the use of Airless-Spray. This coating procedure was repeated several times. The granules thus coated were screened by 100 to 150 mesh screen to remove the finer coagulated powders of the coating agents which passed through the screen.

Finely powdered pepstatin of 180 g was mixed with 10 liters of 2% solution of hydroxypolypropylmethylcellulose in methanol and this pepstatin suspension was sprayed on the granules described above. In this case, the spraying procedure was repeated until all of the pepstatin-hydroxypropylmethylcellulose mixture solution was used up. Thereafter, the minicapsules thus prepared were dried under reduced pressure at room temperature. When the minicapsules were added to artificial human gastric juice the time to release 50% of the pepstatin was 2.5 hours.

Example 2: Fine granules of 943.4 g of sodium bicarbonate, 37.7 g of lactose and 18.9 g of povidone were mixed and this mixture (1.0 kg) was mixed with fine granules of 200 g of pepstatin. This mixture was placed in a coating pan and coated with 2% methanol solution of hydroxypropylmethylcellulose by Airless-Spray. This coating procedure was repeated several times. The coated granules were screened by 100 to 150 mesh screen to remove the coagulated coating agents which passed through the screen. Thereafter, the pepstatin minicapsules were dried under reduced pressure. When these minicapsules were added to an artificial human gastric juice, the time taken to release 50% of the pepstatin was 3 hours.

Example 3: Administration of Pepstatin Floating Minicapsules – The minicapsules prepared above are now called pepstatin-floating minicapsules. The minicapsules prepared by the method described in Example 2 contained 10% pepstatin. When 1.0 g of this minicapsule was given to two volunteers immediately after a meal and 3 hours thereafter the gastric juice was taken, the gastric juices showed almost no pepsin activity.

The pepsin activity was tested by the method using hemoglobin as the substrate as described in the following paper: I. Aoyagi, S. Kunimoto, H. Morishima, T. Takeuchi and H. Umezawa, *Journal of Antibiotics*, 24, 687-694 (1971). When 1.0 g of the pepstatin-floating minicapsule was given to two volunteers immediately after a meal and the gastric juice was taken 5 hours thereafter, the pepsin activity was 30 to 60% of the control gastric juice taken without administration of pepstatin-floating minicapsules.

Process for Preparing β-Lactam Antibiotic Microcapsules

The process of *H. Seager; U.S. Patent 4,016,254; April 5, 1977; assigned to Beecham Group Limited, Great Britain* provides a powder comprising 0 to 95% of conventional pharmaceutical excipients and 5 to 100% of microcapsules which microcapsules have an average diameter of from 100 to 300 μ and which comprise 94 to 99.9% of a medicament coated by 0.1 to 6% of a coating agent.

The limits for the average diameter of the microcapsules are set at 100 μ and 300 μ because if the average diameter falls below this range the powder is likely to be dusty and if the average diameter is above this range the bioavailability of the medicament may be reduced. The lower limit of 0.1% for the quantity of coating agent in the microcapsules is chosen because if smaller quantities of coating agent are used the microcapsules tend to be of poor quality. The upper limit of 6% is chosen in order to keep the costs of the process low and to ensure acceptable biopharmaceutical properties.

When the medicament to be microencapsulated is of medium or high potency so that a diluent or like excipient is required in fairly high quantities one preferred powder comprises 10 to 95% of optionally microencapsulated excipient and 5 to 90% of microencapsulated medicament wherein the microcapsules have an average diameter of at least 100 μ and 90% of which microcapsules have diameters in the range 75 to 450 μ.

In such powders the microencapsulated excipient generally comprises 94 to 99.9% of excipient and 0.1 to 6% of coating agent and the microencapsulated medicament generally comprises 94 to 99.9% of medicament and 0.1 to 6% of coating agent. Normally the excipient is some conventional diluent. Preferably in such mixed powders, the microcapsules containing the medicament comprise 98% to 99.8% of medicament and 0.2 to 2% of coating agent. Preferably, the coating agent in both sorts of microcapsules, if microencapsulated excipient is used, is the same.

A very wide range of medicaments are suitable for inclusion in the microcapsules. Such medicaments include antibiotics and other antibacterial agents, analgesics, anti-inflammatory agents, antihypertensive agents, hypnotics, sedatives, tranquilizers, alkaloids, diuretics and vitamins or most other medicaments frequently used in oral dosage forms.

The powders of the process are especially useful when the microencapsulated medicament is one to which humans may become sensitized on repeated contact as the risk of such sensitization to process operatives is removed or greatly reduced when the medicament is covered with a coating agent. One class of medicaments to which humans may become sensitized are the β-lactam antibiotics. β-lactam antibiotics are therefore included among the medicaments which can benefit greatly from presentation as powder of the process. Such compounds may be in the form of their salts, hydrates, esters, or the like.

Such highly suitable powders consist essentially of microcapsules comprising 97.5 to 99.9% β-lactam antibiotic and 0.1 to 2.5% coating agent which microcapsules have an average diameter between 150 μ and 250 μ, 95% have diameters between 75 μ and 450 μ and 80% of which have diameters between 100 μ and 300 μ. Preferred powders consist essentially of microcapsules containing 98 to 99.8% of one of the β-lactam antibiotics and 0.2 to 2.0% of coating agent which microcapsules have an average diameter between 150 μ and 250 μ. The microcapsules in such powders may frequently contain less than 1% of coating agent.

The process comprises the formation of a slurry of a medicament in a solution of coating agent which slurry may contain up to 5% of conventional pharmaceutical excipients, dispersing the slurry as droplets substantially all of which have diameters of from 100 μ to 1,000 μ into a spray drying cavity and collecting the resulting microcapsules in conventional manner and thereafter, if desired processing the microcapsules into standard dosage forms.

For reasons of economy, the amount of suspended solids is normally kept as high as compatible with the spray drying apparatus. Thus the suspended solids usually comprise 15 to 66% of the slurry. About 33 to 60% often provides a satisfactory range, 40 to 55% is generally a particularly suitable range while frequently the best results may be achieved by using an approximately 45 to 50% suspension.

If required, small amounts of antifoaming agents such as octanol or deflocculants such as polyoxyethylene sorbitan monooleate (Tween 20) may be added to the slurry. The spray drying process is unusual in that the slurry to be spray dried contains only small quantities of dissolved coating agent, e.g., if total suspended solids plus total coating agent amount to 100% then the coating agent present will normally be only about 0.1 to 6%.

The slurry to be spray dried may be made in any suitable solvent such as water, ethanol, propanol, chloroform, methylene chloride, acetone, methyl ethyl ketone, methyl acetate, ethyl acetate, methanol, trichloroethylene, tetrachloroethylene, carbon tetrachloride or like solvents or homogeneous mixtures of such solvents. Obviously, since it is necessary to spray dry a slurry of the medicament, the choice of solvents is limited to those in which the medicament has low solubility and preferably to those in which the medicament is insoluble or substantially insoluble. Normally, the solubility of the medicament is less than 15% and preferably less than 10%, e.g., below 5% at the temperatures used.

If it is desired to use a particular coating agent then the choice of solvent is further limited to those which dissolve the desired coating agent. The solvent should be one in which the coating agent is at least 10% soluble at the temperature of forming, storing and spraying the suspension to be spray dried and preferably at least 20% soluble at that temperature. Microcapsules of good quality are generally most easily prepared if the coating agent is at least 30% soluble in the solvent used.

The medicament and any excipient present in the slurry may already be finely divided. However, if this is not the case, it will be necessary to include a wet milling operation to reduce the particle size of the suspension before the slurry is spray dried. Any convenient conventional method may be used for this purpose. Before the slurry is spray dried it is normally beneficial to homogenize it in conventional manner.

The process may take place in any conventional large spray drier but the best results are often obtained from the kind of conventional spray drying equipment shown in Figure 4.2. Although large spray driers of this kind are not generally used in the pharmaceutical industry they are well known in other industries where large-scale drying apparatus is used. The spray drier may be operated in a conventional manner wherein the various operating parameters such as inlet and outlet temperatures, pumping pressures, liquid flow rate, gas flow rate, atomizer design and the like affect the nature of the product in conventional manner.

When using an open cycle drying system of the sort shown in the figure, the homogenized slurry **1**, is stored in a tank **2** in which it is agitated by the homogenizer **3**, until it is pumped by the high pressure pump **4** to the atomizer **5** at the top of the spray drier. The atomizer **5** is generally of the nozzle type although spinning disc atomizers may be used on wide spray driers. The nozzle atomizer **5**, sprays droplets into the drying cavity **6** where the droplets dry in and with a cocurrent air-flow which originates at the outlet **7**. This drying air has been heated to the desired temperature in an air heater **8** before being pumped to the outlet **7**. After leaving the outlet **7**, the heated air descends through the drying cavity **6** into the bustle **9** where it turns upwards and leaves through the vents **10** from where it passes via a cyclone **11** to the exterior **12**.

Figure 4.2: Open Cycle Drying System

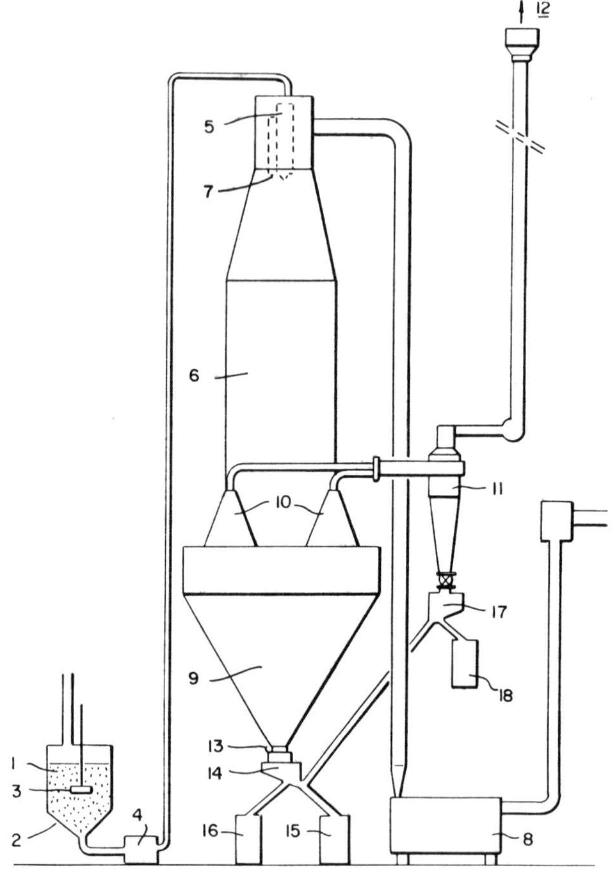

Source: U.S. Patent 4,016,254

As the air descends inside the dryer, the liquid present in the droplets evaporates to leave microcapsules; this process is completed by the time the air and the materials suspended in it reach the bustle **9**. As the air turns upward in the bustle, it precipitates most of the microcapsules which fall through the opening **13** at the bottom of the bustle **9** into a screen system **14** which separates the microcapsules in the desired size range from the fines.

The desired microcapsules and fines are respectively deposited in the collection vessels **15** and **16**. Any microcapsules present in the air leaving via the cyclone **11** are precipitated and separated into microcapsules of the desired size range and fines by a screen system **17**. The desired microcapsules and the fines are respectively deposited in the collection vessels **15** and **18**. The fines generally represent 5 to 10% of the spray dried product and may be added to the initial slurry for recycling thereby minimizing losses.

If it is desired to use a solvent which is to be recollected after passing through the apparatus, a condenser system may be included in the apparatus at some point after the cyclone **11**. In such conventional closed-cycle spray drier, the heated air is normally replaced by heated solvent vapor.

Both open-cycle and closed-cycle spray driers are equilibrated and operated in conventional manner. Suitable parameters for an open-cycle spray drier are generally (water as solvent):

Spray drier height	6-20 m
Spray drier chamber diameter	1-3 m
Feed rate of suspension	25-200 l/hr
Atomizer nozzle diameter	0.5-1.5 mm
Atomizer nozzle pressure	5-15 kg/cm^2
Rate of air flow	750-1,200 kg/hr
Inlet temperature	150°-250°C
Outlet temperature	50°-120°C

Example 1: Preparation of Microencapsulated Ampicillin Trihydrate – Formation of Slurry: Ampicillin trihydrate (27 kg) obtained from a wet cake of the material taken from a standard commercial production batch was added to a solution of sodium carboxymethylcellulose (K), (0.27 kg); i e., 1% of medicament weight in demineralized water (30 kg). The mixture was stirred during addition. This produced a slurry containing about 47.6% solids in suspension. Some foaming occurred during the continuing agitation but was reduced by the addition of a small quantity of octanol. The suspension was sieved through a 0.3 mm vibrating screen to remove clumps of medicament particles which had not disintegrated during stirring. The sieving stage increased the foam present. The suspension was transferred to a feed tank where it was kept stirred in order to maintain an even distribution of medicament particles.

Tower Operation: The suspension from the feed tank was pumped through a nozzle atomizer at about 33 kg/hr. The nozzle orifice diameter was set at 1.0 mm, the spray angle of the nozzle was set at 80° and the nozzle pressure at 11 kg/cm^2. A concurrent air flow was pumped through the spray drier at 925 kg/hr, and the temperature of the air adjusted to give an inlet temperature of 160°C and an outlet temperature of 81° to 87°C.

The encapsulated powder was collected from the bottom of the tower in a discharge hopper and a cyclone separator. In general, 20 to 25% of the products were recovered in the cyclones and 75 to 80% were collected from the chamber. There was no observable powder present in the exhaust gas leaving the stack. The product was screened in the apparatus prior to collection to remove particles below 75 μ (5 to 10%) and the encapsulated powders were stored for evaluation and pharmaceutical processing. The spray dried powders consisted of particles composed of an outer porous shell of polymer with an inner core of fine antibiotic powder. The core contained small quantities of air and interspersed strands of polymer. The coats appeared to contain blow holes.

Example 2: In order to reduce the quantity of foam, the medicament suspension was prepared as follows. The coating agent solution was prepared in one vessel using a Silverson LZR mixer with standard emulser head attachment. The ampicillin trihydrate suspension was prepared in a second vessel using a Silverson mixer and a turbo-stirrer. The coating agent solution was added to the medicament suspension, mixed and then defoamed with a small quantity of octanol. The suspension was then pumped to a feed tank via a 0.3 mm screen. The suspension was kept stirred in the feed tank to ensure an even distribution of particles. Slurries containing 22 kg of ampicillin trihydrate were made up as described containing the following constituents:

Run No.	Coating Agent*	Wt of Coating Agent (kg)	Water (kg)	Solids in Suspension (%)
1	K	0.054	33	45
2	K	0.081	33	45
3	K	0.108	33	45
4	I	0.11	27	45
5	L	0.11	27	45
6	N	0.11	30	42.5
7	A	0.11	27	45
8	P	0.11	27	45
9	N	0.11	27	45

*Coating agents are described below.

The tower was operated as described in Example 1 using a 45° angle nozzle and the following conditions:

Run No.	Nozzle Orifice (mm)	Nozzle Pressure (kg/cm^2)	Approx Throughput (kg/hr)	Inlet Temp (°C)	Outlet Temp (°C)	Air Flow (kg/hr)
1	0.9	9	24	162	78-79	800
2	0.9	12-9	23	143-160	64-72	800
3	0.9	9	21	105-140	61-71	800
4	0.9	9	18	140	68-70	800
5	1.0	9	21	150	72-73	925
6	1.0	9	32	150	71-73	800-925
7	1.0	9	29	150	70	925
8	1.0	9	33	150	68-71	800-900
9	1.0	10	28	190-200	81-83	750

The microcapsules produced in Runs 4 through 9 appeared to have continuous coats free of blow holes.

A Niro tower spray drier was used. The drier is similar to that shown schematically in Figure 4.2 and is approximately 12 m high and 1.75 m in diameter. Such apparatus is of an industrially used dosage. The coating agents of the examples are as follows:

Coating Agent	Trade Name (Supplier)
A Hydroxypropylmethylcellulose	Methocel HG60 (Dow)
I Polyvinylpyrrolidone	Plesdone K29-32 (G.A.F.)
K Sodium carboxymethylcellulose	Coulose P8 (British Celanese)
L Gelatin	Protein S (Coroda)

(continued)

Coating Agent	Trade Name (Supplier)
N Polyvinyl alcohol	Gelvatol 40-20 (Monsanto)
P Hydroxypropyl cellulose	Celacol He25 (British Celanese)

Encapsulated Chemotherapeutic Agents

R.T. Gordon; U.S. Patent 4,106,488; August 15, 1978 describes a treatment of cancer by the application of external electromagnetic energy capable of the generation of heat in intracellular particles to induce selective thermal death of cancer cells in living tissue. This process allows for the selective treatment of cancer cells in living tissue without damaging the normal cells.

The process comprises introducing minute particles into the interior of the cells of living tissue. These particles are injected intravenously while suspended in an appropriate solution and are of a size generally with a diameter of approximately one micron or less and are of a material with properties, such as ferromagnetic, paramagnetic, or diamagnetic, so as to be inductively heated when subjected to a high frequency alternating electromagnetic field.

After introduction of the particles as described, the patient is subjected to an alternating electromagnetic field to inductively heat the particles sufficiently to raise the temperature of the cells by an increment of 8.0° to 9.5°C, thus killing the cancer cells without harming the normal cells. Further selectivity and increased affinity of the cancer cells for these particles may be achieved by incorporating specific radioisotopes or tumor specific antibodies bound to these particles.

These particles introduced intracellularly as described may be used as a method of delivering a chemotherapeutic agent primarily to the interior of the cancer cells by having the chemotherapeutic agent encapsulated within the particles and released at the proper time by application of the high frequency alternating electromagnetic field or by solubilizing the particles within the cells.

Example 1: In the simplest form of the process, ferric hydroxide particles of 0.7 micron size are suspended in a 5% dextrose aqueous solution in an amount of about 50 mg of the particles per cc. Dosages in the amount of 30 mg/kg of body weight of each of the particles should be made twice, by intravenous injections, each being 24 hours apart. The patient is then ready for the electromagnetic treatment by insertion entirely within an inductive coil 3 ft in diameter. The coil is connected to an alternating current generator, producing a frequency of 3 MHz and a field of 600 oersteds.

The patient is to be subjected to the electromagnetic treatments about 12 hours after the last injection. The inductive heating of the particles within the cancer cells is between 8 and 10 minutes, during which time the temperature within the cell will have been increased 8.5°C. At this temperature, the cancerous cells in the living tissue will have been killed while the normal cells will recover normal cellular functions.

Example 2: (A) The following is an example of the method of coating 5-fluorouracil with a ferromagnetic material: 5-fluorouracil, a known acknowledged effective chemotherapeutic agent against cancer, is taken in its solid state and pulverized into particles 0.5 micron in size. These particles, in turn, are then coated with ferric hydroxide to approximately 0.1 micron in thickness, in accordance with any of the conventional methods of coating submicron particles as described in U.S. Patent 3,294,686.

These particles are then colloidally suspended in a 6 wt % aqueous dextran solution. This solution is introduced intravenously to the patient with the result that due to the phagocytic characteristics of the cancer cells, most of these particles will be deposited in the cytoplasm inside the cancer cells. This would take place about 4 to 8 hours after the intravenous injection. After the particles' deposition into the cytoplasm, the ferric hydroxide is acted upon by the cytoplasm and is converted to an organic iron complex (ferritin) which is then absorbed.

After approximately 24 hours, the ferric hydroxide coating is thus solubilized and the chemotherapeutic agent 5-fluorouracil is released within the cancer cell where it can effectively kill the cell. Time is not critical, and may vary from 1 to 48 hours or more. The other tumor specific cancer agents may be similarly utilized.

(B) The chemotherapeutic agent encapsulated in a ferromagnetic material, as described in (A), may be injected in precisely the same manner and alternatively subjected to the high frequency alternating electromagnetic field of Example 1 which then is capable of breaking up the microsphere of the magnetic material by a vibrational frequency produced by the electromagnetic field at which the outer surface resonates and its integrity is destroyed. Upon breakup of the microspheres the chemotherapeutic agent is released intracellularly and selectively within the cancer cells. The same example may be applied in the same manner to the other tumor specific cancer agents.

(C) The encapsulating material may also contain a low melting solid such as wax having a melting point higher than the temperature of the cells but below the death temperature of the normal cell. This temperature range may be therefore between about 37° and 46.5°C. This wax is in combination with the ferromagnetic material and applied as in (A).

Encapsulated Chelating Agents for Removing Metal Toxins in Tissue

In accordance with the process of *Y.E. Rahman; U.S. Patent 4,016,290; April 5, 1977; assigned to United States Energy Research and Development Administration* a chelating agent is encapsulated within liposomes to enable transfer of the chelating agent across a cellular membrane. Since toxic heavy metals are known to deposit intracellularly as well as extracellularly, a method for transferring the toxic heavy metal from the interior of the cell is necessary to insure complete removal of toxic heavy metals from the body. While chelating agents are known to be useful in removing extracellularly deposited toxic heavy metals, chelating agents have not heretofore been demonstrated to be efficient in removing intracellularly deposited toxic heavy metals.

It is believed that the large negative charge on the chelating ion prevents transfer of the chelating agent across the cellular membrane to the interior of the cell and, therefore, the chelating agent has no effect on intracellularly deposited toxic heavy metals.

One of the reasons toxic heavy metal poisoning, in particular radioactive toxic heavy metals, are of such concern is the fact that these metals concentrate selectively in vital organs, such as the liver and spleen. It has been found that the metal, such as colloidal plutonium in the liver, is associated mainly, if not solely, with lysosomes. The lysosomes are the usual location for matters foreign to the organism ingested by cells including the heavy metals.

Liposomes injected into the body also will be directed to and later found in the lysosomes. The term "liposomes" as used herein refers to artificial spherules formed by thin layers of phospholipid in the presence of any electrolyte. Phospholipids when placed in an electrolytic solution form concentric bimolecular lipid layers separated by the entrapped aqueous compartments. It can be seen then that the liposomes are composed of concentric bimolecular layers of lipid alternating with aqueous layers.

It has been found that polyaminopolycarboxylic acid chelating agents, EDTA and DTPA in particular, can be encapsulated in liposomes. A lipid mixture is dried to form a thin film on the walls of a flask. A solution of the electrolyte is introduced into the flask and the thin film of the lipid is wetted with the solution. The contents of the flask are then shaken, whereby small spherules will be formed. The small spherules are composed of lipid layers separated by entrapped aqueous layers, and are herein referred to as liposomes. The liposomes thus formed will have encapsulated layers of the electrolyte, in this process the electrolyte being a chelating agent.

Example: Liposomes were prepared from a 3 to 1 mixture of phosphatidylcholine, egg lecithin, and cholesterol dissolved in chloroform. In the process, 4.5 mg egg lecithin and 1.5 mg cholesterol were used. This mixture was dried in a round-bottom flask in a rotary evaporator. The flask was then placed in a 37°C water bath and 1 ml of a 25% trisodium calcium DTPA solution was slowly added to the flask with immediate and constant stirring with a magnetic stirror.

The resultant suspension of liposomes containing DTPA was centrifuged at 2,000 rpm for 5 minutes. The supernatant was carefully pipetted off and the liposome pellet was resuspended in normal saline. The same centrifugation and resuspension procedure was repeated five times to insure the complete removal of nonencapsulated DTPA solution. The liposomes were finally resuspended in saline solution.

The formation of the liposomes was found to be affected by the purity of the phosphatidylcholine used and by the concentration of the electrolyte. Under ideal conditions, the liposomes were small, usually less than 10 microns, and usually spherical and well separated from each other. When liposomes were prepared with partially degraded phosphatidylcholine, fewer liposomes were formed, and clusters of liposomes instead of single, separate liposomes were observed. However, when the phosphatidylcholine was purified, as by thin layer chromatography, within a week before use, spherical, single, well-separated liposomes were consistently obtained. When the concentration of EDTA was higher than 10%, fewer liposomes were formed. Consequently, it is preferred that EDTA liposomes be prepared with highly purified, fresh phosphatidylcholine and EDTA solutions at concentrations between 5 and 10%. When partially degraded or impure phosphatidylcholine was used to make liposomes containing DTPA, some of these liposomes were as large as 80 microns in diameter, and large clusters of liposomes were observed. Successful liposome formation can be achieved with a 25% trisodium calcium DTPA.

The encapsulation of chelating agents by the liposomes, i.e., within the artificial lipid spherules, was verified by use of radioactive, tagged chelating agents. Using the abovedescribed preparation technique, ^{45}Ca-DTPA and ^{14}C-EDTA were used in place of the usual electrolyte. Following extensive washing of the liposomes produced in accordance with the technique, the labeled chelating agents were formed within the liposomes.

The uptake and retention by the body and cells of the liposome encapsulated chelating agent was studied by use of the radio-labeled chelating agents prepared in accordance with the technique described above. Distribution of injected ^{14}C-EDTA liposomes was studied in mice and compared with that of free ^{14}C-EDTA to determine the delivery of the chelating agent to the various organs and retention of the so-introduced chelating agent over a period of time.

It was found that the free ^{14}C-EDTA was swept from the body quite rapidly, whereas the liposome encapsulated EDTA remained in the body for a substantial period of time. This is indicative of the fact that the liposome encapsulated EDTA was taken up by the cells. A substantial amount of the liposomes deposited in the liver, the liver containing about 41% of the total injected liposome at 6 hours after injection. The labeled chelating agent subsequently transferred out of the liver, at 3 days there being less than 10% remaining, and at 17 days less than 1%.

Since injected liposomes in the liver have been found to be mostly associated with lysosomes, intracellular organelles responsible for the storage and digestion of incorporated foreign materials, and since colloidal plutonium is also specifically localized in liver lysosomes, the encapsulation of chelating agents provides a means for removing the intracellularly deposited plutonium. In accordance with the techniques, a chelating agent, in this case DTPA being used in view of the greater complexing ability of the DTPA with plutonium, was encapsulated in liposomes, and the liposome encapsulated DTPA suspended in a saline solution for injection.

The suspension can be introduced to the body through intravenous injection, whereby the liposomes will deposit in various organs and, in particular, will be directed toward the liver. The liposomes can transfer across cellular membranes in the liver, thereby gaining access to the interior of the cells. Once in the cells, the lysosomal enzymes will break down the liposomes, releasing the DTPA chelating agent to the interior of the cell. The chelating agent will complex toxic heavy metal, plutonium, and the complexed heavy metal, its ionic charge much lower in comparison with either the toxic metal or the chelating ion itself, can diffuse back across the cell membrane out of the cell. After transferring across the membrane from the cell, the complexed ion will be removed from the body by normal body processes.

Experiments were conducted on mice showing the removal of toxic heavy metals from the body by treatment with liposome encapsulated DTPA. Each mouse received 0.4 μCi of ^{239}Pu/kg of body weight. Separate groups of five mice were treated at 3 and 6 days after administration of the plutonium with one of the following: (1) saline solution, (2) nonencapsulated DTPA, (3) liposome encapsulated DTPA, or (4) both encapsulated and nonencapsulated DTPA. The mice were sacrificed on day 10 after plutonium injection, i.e., day 4 after the second therapy. The liposome encapsulated DTPA given alone consistently reduced the level of plutonium in the liver below that achieved by conventional nonencapsulated DTPA therapy.

Other experiments were conducted with ^{198}Au, the results of which showed increased excretion of the ^{198}Au with liposome encapsulated DTPA as compared with excretion by free DTPA or saline. It is further believed that other toxic heavy metals, such as mercury, lead, yttrium and cerium, which can be complexed by chelating agents will similarly be removed by liposome encapsulated chelating agents.

VITAMINS

Vitamin A Encapsulated in Corn Flour

In a process developed by *S. Katzen; U.S. Patent 3,962,416; June 8, 1976* an encapsulating agent and a nutrient are admixed, and then the encapsulating agent is gelatinized or polymerized under high temperature and pressure so as to encapsulate the nutrient. The encapsulation allows the nutrient to be kept in a dry stabilized state for a long period of time without the loss of potency. Further the encapsulation allows the nutrients to be released into the digestive tract after a predetermined amount of time. The digestive tract solubilizes or digests the encapsulating agent thereby freeing the nutrient.

Encapsulation is preferably conducted using a heated extruder or expander. The encapsulating agent may be a high protein vegetable composition, such as, wheat flour gluten, a grain flour or carbohydrate flour. The nutrients may be in particulate or liquid form and can be such things as vitamins, amino acids, lipids, enzymes, inorganic salts (minerals). Additives such as surfactants can be incorporated into the admixture before the extruding step.

Preferably, 100 parts by weight of the encapsulating agent are admixed with about 40 to 50 parts by weight of the nutrients. The encapsulating agent is normally gelatinized or polymerized at a temperature between 250° and 450°F, preferably at 350°F. The temperature utilized must be such that the potency of the nutrients and/or additives is not seriously impaired. The pressure utilized will be above atmospheric and will vary with the type of encapsulating agent, nutrients and additives and the operating temperature, but will generally range from about 200 to 2,500 psi, preferably about 1,000 psi. The time of product formation at those pressures and temperatures will vary from about 3 seconds to 3 minutes, preferably about 10 seconds.

Example: 1 kg of vitamin A palmitate, having a rating of 1.7 million I.U. per gram, was thoroughly admixed with 4 kg of corn flour. The encapsulating agent was the corn flour and the nutrient was vitamin A palmitate. The admixture was extruded in an extruder operated at a pressure of 1,000 psi and has a temperature of 240°F. The temperature used was sufficient to gelatinize the corn flour but yet was not of such a level as to decompose, deactivate or otherwise impair or destroy the potency or effectiveness of the vitamin A palmitate.

The gelatinized corn flour completely enclosed individual or groups of particles of vitamin A palmitate. The extruded material was dried, cooled and reduced in size by grinding to particles of an average diameter of about 0.1 mm (millimeter). The resultant product contained 340 million I.U. of vitamin A per kg, which is above the conventional market standard of 325,000 I.U. per gram. The resultant product which contained encapsulated dry, stabilized vitamin was stored for two months and was then consumed by a man and a rat. The gelatinized encompassing corn flour was solubilized in the digestive tract and the vitamin A material was released, thereby making the vitamin A activity available to the organism.

Nonsticky Granules of Vitamin E Acetate

In a process described by *M. Murakami, H. Kawada, T. Ohmura and H. Sugiura; U.S. Patent 4,013,773; March 22, 1977; assigned to Yamanouchi Pharmaceutical Co., Ltd., Japan* a liquid is converted into a stable solid composition using an excipient of a small specific volume in a relatively small amount with respect to the liquid.

As a result of a detailed study of the method for the solidification of nonaqueous liquid, it has been found that a single phase solid composition, obtained by mixing one part of one or a mixture of two or more nonaqueous liquids with 0.5 to 6 parts of calcium lactate hydrate having a small specific volume and heating the mixture, is very stable and the resulting product can be formed into various kinds of moldings by a very simple operation and applied to many uses. It is quite unexpected that the mixing and heating of the components provides a very stable solid composition.

As regards the nonaqueous liquids which can be used, there are included compounds other than water, which are liquid such as wax or materials which are viscous semifluids at ordinary temperature, such as, for example, vitamin A, vitamin E acetate, linoleic acid, liver oil, methyl linoleate, ethyl α-(p-chlorophenoxy)iso-butyrate (common name: clofibrate), dimethyl polysiloxane, castor oil, soybean oil, peppermint oil, cinnamon oil, camellia oil, olive oil, eucalyptus oil, maize oil, oleic acid, liquid paraffin, polyethylene glycol, propylene glycol, nonyl phenyl polyoxyethylene ether, dialkyl benzyl ammonium halide, dodecyl polyaminoethyl glycine, kerosene, flavor oil, glycerin, silicone oil, octyl decyl triglyceride, and the like.

As for the calcium lactate hydrate which can be used for the preparation of the solid composition, in general, calcium lactate pentahydrate is used. For the preparation of the solid composition, one part of a nonaqueous liquid and 0.5 to 6, preferably 1 to 3 parts of calcium lactate hydrate are mixed homogeneously and illustratively by means of a mortar, mixer, etc. and the resulting cream thus obtained is heated at above 40°C, preferably from 60° to 150°C for from 5 minutes to about 1 hour generally in a thermostatically controlled drier, etc.

The solid composition thus obtained is quite different from the cream before the heating and a solid composition in the form of mass. In the preparation of the solid composition according to this process, the nonaqueous liquid and calcium lactate hydrate are dissolved or suspended in water or a low-boiling solvent, which is volatilized on heating, such as acetone or alcohol by means of a homogenizer, etc., and then dried by heating to yield a glossy gypsumlike solid composition. The mass or gypsumlike solid composition which is obtained as mentioned above can be changed to the solid composition in the form of particles by grinding with a pulverizer, etc.

Further, in the preparation of the solid composition, when the nonaqueous liquid and calcium lactate hydrate are dissolved or suspended in water or a low-boiling solvent, which is volatilized on heating, such as acetone or alcohol by means of a homogenizer, etc., and then heated and spray dried, the solid composition in the form of particles is obtained at once.

In the mixing of the nonaqueous liquid with calcium lactate hydrate, additives such as a coloring agent, tasting agent, perfuming agent, diluent, etc., may be added, if desired, and a mixture of more than two kinds of liquids may be used for the preparation of the solid composition.

Example: 50 g of calcium lactate pentahydrate and 50 g of vitamin E acetate are mixed at room temperature to yield a sticky cream. The mixture is heated at 80° to 100°C for 30 minutes in a thermostatically controlled drier to yield a solid composition. The solid composition is ground to form nonsticky fluid granules.

Riboflavin Added to Heat-Softened Blank Microcapsules

L.D. Morse, W.G. Walker and P.A. Hammes; U.S. Patent 4,123,382; October 31, 1978; assigned to Merck & Co., Inc. found that excellent results are obtained when blank capsules are prepared and heat softened, followed by addition of the solid to be encapsulated. The mixture is then stirred until the solid is encapsulated in the blanks, after which the microcapsules are solidified and recovered. This is accomplished by (1) preparing "empty" microcapsules, softening them, and "filling" them, or (2) preparing microcapsules, complete with internal phase, softening them, and adding internal phase to "fill" the capsules further. The fundamental principle here is that the coating polymer can be phased out of solution before the internal phase is added to the system. If the internal phase is added while the coating polymer is plastic, the internal phase enters the polymer and is enrobed. Advantages of the process are improved control of microencapsulation size, improved bioavailability, and increased production of microencapsulated product.

As the encapsulating material, ethylcellulose, methylcellulose, hydroxypropylmethylcellulose, polyvinyl alcohol, cellulose acetate phthalate, gelatin, gum arabic, and carrageenan alginates can be used, the first three and gelatin being preferred. The solid core can be any food or medicament used in microcapsules.

The blank capsule can be prepared by known methods. The hardening of the filled capsule, in the process, can be carried out in any way known in microencapsulation. Since the softening process in many cases is thermal—the capsules are produced at elevated temperatures or softened by heating up a slurry—the hardening is achieved by cooling. In some cases, it can be effected by chemical reaction on the surface of the soft microcapsules.

Example 1: A dispersion of 216 g of ethylcellulose (47.5 wt % ethoxyl content, viscosity 45 cp at 25°C, as a 5 wt % solution in an 80:20 toluene:ethanol mixture) in 5 liters of cyclohexane is stirred using a downthrust turbine impeller and baffles operating at 310 rpm with heating. At 80°C the ethylcellulose dissolves in the cyclohexane and stirring is continued while the system is allowed to cool. As the temperature drops, solvated ethylcellulose develops as a separate phase due to its lowered solubility in the cyclohexane. As the temperature drops further, the ethylcellulose loses solvent and develops into semiplastic, dispersed, small masses. At 50°C the cooling is discontinued and 1,088 g of crystalline riboflavin is added.

Microscopic examination of the small masses of ethylcellulose shows that it is plastic enough for most of the riboflavin to enter the masses and be enveloped. The temperature is raised to 57°C and from a microscopic examination it is apparent that the riboflavin is enveloped. The mixture is then cooled to 10°C and filtered. The solids are washed twice with 1.5 liters of hexane and dried in a fluid bed dryer to afford free-flowing discrete microcapsules containing the riboflavin. These microcapsules have the following size distribution:

Mesh	Percent by Weight
On 12	0.1
-12+16	0.1
-16+20	0.4
-20+30	0.6
-30+40	0.8
-40+60	1.3
-60+80	18.6
-80+100	31.4
-100+140	14.4
-140+200	23.6
-200+325	5.6
-325	1.1

Example 2: Using the same quantities of ingredients as in Example 1, the process is repeated but in this case the riboflavin is dispersed in the cyclohexane along with the ethylcellulose from the start. Under these conditions, the system becomes very viscous and large aggregated masses of encapsulated product are obtained. Essentially, the system is uncontrollable in terms of fluidity.

Example 3: Using the process described in Example 2 but reducing the amount of ethylcellulose to 137 g and the amount of riboflavin to 827 g, it is found that these decreased amounts are necessary to achieve proper fluidity. The resulting microcapsules consist of enrobed single crystals of riboflavin or enrobed agglomerates containing from 2 to 5 crystals. These capsules are all below the 50 micron range.

Oleaginous Shell Former for Vitamin C

The method of *S. Kondo and H. Nakano; U.S. Patent 4,102,806; July 25, 1978; assigned to Takeda Chemical Industries, Ltd., Japan* for producing a microencapsulated product comprises (1) dissolving an oil-and-fat in an organic solvent by heating, the oil-and-fat being solid at room temperature, the organic solvent being hardly or not capable of dissolving a core material to be encapsulated but capable of dissolving the oil-and-fat when hot and capable of coacervating the oil-and-fat when cold, (2) dispersing the core material in the resultant solution, (3) cooling the dispersion with stirring to coacervate the oil-and-fat on the core material, and (4) separating and drying the resultant encapsulated particulate product. Oil-and-fat is mainly composed of glycerin esters of fatty acids.

The oil-and-fat usable in this process is solid at room temperature and has a melting point not lower than 30°C, preferably not lower than 50°C, and further preferably not lower than 60°C. Preferred are the solvents which, when hot, will dissolve not less than 1% (w/v), desirably not less than 5%, of the oil-and-fat and, when cold, will coacervate not less than 50% of the dissolved oil-and-fat. Some examples of the preferred combinations of oils-and-fats with solvents are shown:

Oil-and-Fat	Solvent
Hydrogenated castor oil	Methanol
	Ethanol
	n-Propanol
	Isopropanol
	n-Amyl alcohol
	Ethylene glycol monomethyl ether
	Ethyl acetate
	Acetone
	Benzene
	n-Hexane
	Trichloroethylene
	Ether
Hydrogenated beef tallow	Ethanol
Cacao butter	Ethanol
Glycerin monostearate	Ethanol
Mixture of hydrogenated castor oil and hydrogenated soybean oil	Ethanol

The particulate core material may be either a water-soluble or a water-insoluble material, all that is necessary being that it is solid at room temperature and is either slightly soluble or insoluble in the vehicle. The core material may have a diameter within the range of 0.1 micron to several millimeters (e.g., 3 mm) and, preferably, between 10 microns and 840 microns. Examples of the core materials are vitamins, minerals, amino acids, antibiotics, synthetic antibacterial or antiprotozoal agents, analgesic antipyretics, enzymes, dried viable microorganisms, feed or food materials, agricultural chemicals, etc. Among them, preferably, are vitamins, antibiotics and enzymes.

The dissolution of the oil-and-fat is effected by increasing the temperature of the organic solvent but not to a level as high as to decompose the core material. An advantageous range of the temperature is 50° to 100°C. The resultant solution has generally a viscosity lower than 100 cp, advantageously lower than 50 cp. The dispersion of the core material to the solution is effected at a temperature higher than the temperature at which the coacervation occurs. The range of the temperature is 30° to 100°C, and when the core material is changeable at a high temperature, for example, enzyme or dried viable microorganism, the preferred temperature is not higher than 40°C. The resultant dispersion is cooled to a temperature within the range from 0° to 60°C, advantageously from 20° to 45°C.

Generally, the coacervation of an oil-and-fat takes place at a temperature far below the temperature at which it was dissolved. By way of example, hydrogenated castor oil as dissolved in ethanol at 78°C would start undergoing coacervation in the neighborhood of 50°C and, as it has been discovered, this coacervation continues for a fairly long time even after the temperature of the system has dropped to room temperature, i.e., 25° to 30°C. Therefore, in order that the oil-and-fat dissolved in a solvent may be allowed to coacervate sufficiently from the solvent, it is necessary that the solution be maintained, under stirring, at the destination temperature of cooling for some time. While the appropriate duration of this time depends upon such variables as the shell-forming material, organic solvent, destination temperature, batch size, etc., it is generally within the range of 10 minutes to 2 hours, advantageously 30 minutes to 2 hours.

The ratio of organic solvent to core material is at least 3:1 v/w (not less than 3 ml/g), advantageously at least 5:1 v/w (not less than 5 ml/g) and a greater amount of the solvent is necessary where the solubility of the oil-and-fat in the solvent is low. Furthermore, the ratio of the oil-and-fat, which is the shell-forming component, to the core material in the solvent may be optional within the limits of 0.1:1 to 10:1, preferably within the limits of 0.3:1 to 5:1, further preferably within the limits of 0.75:1 to 2:1.

In this process, a polymer may be dissolved in the organic solvent together with the fat-and-oil. The polymer serves to support the oleocapsule in the encapsulated product under high temperature, e.g., a temperature when a feed pellet is formed, or to make the microcapsule possess a suitable property for sustained release or prolonged action. The polymer is generally dissolved in the organic solvent at a concentration not greater than 5 w/v %, advantageously at a concentration not greater than 2 w/v %. In this case, the viscosity of the resultant solution is lower than 100 cp, preferably lower than 50 cp in the presence of the oil-and-fat.

In the above concentration, the polymer itself does not coacervate or precipitate in the system, and, therefore, the polymer in the encapsulated products is based upon that dissolved in the solvent which was contained in the gel structure of the coacervated oleocapsule. Accordingly, the ratio of the polymer to the oil-and-fat in the resultant oleocapsule is generally not greater than 25 wt % basis, advantageously not greater than 10 wt % basis. The polymers are exemplified by cellulose derivatives and acrylic copolymers. When a polymer is employed, if necessary, a fine powder (e.g., cornstarch, lactose, magnesium stearate, talc and silicic acid anhydride) may be added to the solution after coacervation in order to prevent adherence among the resultant encapsulated products.

The method does not require a nonsolvent (a solvent which is otherwise employed to depress the solubility of shell-forming material in a system to cause a coacervation) and requires only a comparatively small amount of a solvent. Moreover, low-boiling alcohols, saturated hydrocarbons and other solvents that are easy to remove later can be successfully employed. Since nonaqueous solvents may also be employed, the method has the advantage that those kinds of core materials which are readily soluble in water or unstable in the presence of water can also be encapsulated without causing a loss of the ingredients.

Example 1: To 80 ml of ethanol was added 5.0 g of Castor Wax A (hydrogenated castor oil, MP 85°C) and, in a flask fitted with a reflux condenser, the mixture was boiled at 78°C. The resultant solution was transferred to a beaker of stainless steel, to which 5.0 g of calcium ascorbate (80 to 200 mesh) was added. Under agitation with a propeller stirrer, the mixture was allowed to cool under room temperature conditions whereby Castor Wax A was caused to coacervate on the calcium ascorbate by way of core material and, thereby, to produce an encapsulated particulate product. This system was centrifuged to remove the ethanol and dried under reduced pressure and at 40°C for 3 hours. By the above procedure was obtained 9.0 g of calcium ascorbate oleocapsules from 48 to 200 mesh in diameter.

Example 2: The procedure of Example 1 was repeated except that 5.0 g of dry iron sulfate not exceeding 200 mesh (The Pharmacopoeia of Japan) was used in lieu of calcium ascorbate. By this procedure was obtained 8.8 g of oleocapsules of dry iron sulfate from 32 to 100 mesh in diameter.

Example 3: The procedure of Example 1 was repeated except that 1.0 g of aluminum salicylate (average diameter about 5 μ) was used in lieu of calcium ascorbate to obtain 4.7 g of aluminum salicylate oleocapsules from 60 to 100 mesh in diameter.

HEALTH AND BEAUTY AIDS

Skin Cream with Encapsulated Active Base in Oil/Water Emulsion

G. Barnett, N. Gershaw and J.J. Mausner; U.S. Patent 4,087,555; May 2, 1978; assigned to Helena Rubinstein, Inc. describe a composition for use as a skin cream comprising an oil phase, a water phase and an encapsulated active base. The oil phase comprises an emulsifier, an emollient, a lubricant, a dispersing agent, and a nonionic surfactant. The water phase comprises hectorite clay, a peptizer for the clay, a humectant, milk protein, and water. The encapsulated active base comprises hectorite clay, a polar group affording compound, a peptizer for the clay, and water.

Because of uniformity in quality and analysis, the synthetic hectorite clays are preferred over the clay derived from natural hectorite clay mineral. It is preferred to use as the peptizer one or more of the water-soluble salts of a condensed phosphoric acid. Tetrasodium pyrophosphate and sodium hexametaphosphate are commonly used peptizers.

The polar group affording organic material is characterized by (1) the ability to form water-insoluble particles having a size above colloidal dimensions when added to an aqueous colloidal solution of synthetic hectorite clay and tetrasodium pyrophosphate peptizing agent, with commingling, and (2) having been selected from the group consisting of (a) simple organic compounds having at least one polar group and (b) organic hydrophilic colloids.

Example: Encapsulated Active Base – The encapsulated active base includes the following ingredients in percent by weight:

Cellosize WP-4400	0.5-2.50
Deionized water (A)	to make 100
Clay-Rheo-VIS	0.45-1.8
Sodium acid pyrophosphate (food grade)	0.05-2.00
Deionized water (B)	4.5-18.00
D&C Red 30	5-10
Casein, edible, 80 mesh	0.5-3.00
Tegosept M (methylparaben)	0.4

The deionized water (A) was transferred to a stainless steel kettle equipped with a Lightnin' Mixer. The Lightnin' Mixer was started to run at a fairly rapid speed and the Cellosize was sprinkled into the kettle. This was mixed until completely dissolved. The deionized water (B) was transferred to a separate stainless steel container equipped with a Lightnin' Mixer. The mixer was started and the sodium acid pyrophosphate was added. The clay was sprinkled into the container and the mixture was stirred well to allow the clay to hydrate fully.

When the clay was hydrated, the clay-peptizer-water mixture was added to the Cellosize solution and mixed well. The DC Red was added and stirred in well and then the casein and Tegosept were added and stirred well. The entire mixture was put through a homogenizer or colloid mill.

Oil Phase – The oil phase contains the following ingredients, in parts by weight: glyceryl monostearate, 1.5 to 3.5; cetyl alcohol, 1.25 to 2.5; Wickenol 155, 8.00 to 14.00; isostearic acid 875 D, 0.5 to 4.00; Myrj 52, 0.2 to 1.50; and Span 65, 0.1 to 0.4.

Water Phase – The water phase includes the following ingredients, in percent by weight: deionized water, to 100; clay Rheo-VIS, 1.80 to 3.96; sodium acid pyrophosphate (food grade), 0.20 to 0.44; propylene glycol, 2.00 to 5.00; Tegosept M (methylparaben), 0.40; triethanolamine, 1.00; and Lactolysate LS HR2, 1.25. Additionally, a perfume, Perfume 802, was included.

In the example, certain ingredients are shown by trademark, the compositions of these ingredients are as follows: Wickenol 155, 2-ethylhexyl palmitate; Myrj 52, polyoxyethylene stearate; Span 65, sorbitan tristearate; Lactolysate, milk protein; Cellosize WP 4400, hydroxyethylcellulose; and DC Red 30, 6,6'-dichloro-4,4'-dimethylthioindigo.

Mixing Procedure – The water of the water phase was transferred to a kettle equipped with a Silverson Mixer and a sweep anchor mixer. The Silverson Mixer was started and the sodium acid pyrophosphate was added and dispersed well. The clay was sprinkled in and stirred well until hydrated, approximately 10 minutes.

In a separate stainless steel container, the propylene glycol was weighed. The preservative and Tegosept were dissolved in the propylene glycol and then this solution was added to the kettle containing the clay and peptizer. The triethanolamine and the Lactolysate were then added.

All the ingredients of the oil phase were transferred to a stainless steel steam-jacketed kettle. Both the oil and water phases were heated to 167°F (75°C) and the Silverson Mixer was continued in the water phase during the heating. When both phases reached 167°F, the oil phase was strained through a cloth into the water phase. The mixture was allowed to stir for 10 minutes and then it was allowed to cool to 136°F (58°C). The perfume (0.20 part by weight) was added.

The Silverson Mixer was removed and replaced with an adequate Lightnin' Mixer. With the Lightnin' Mixer running at a moderately fast speed, but in a position which would not aerate the cream, 0.1 part by weight of the encapsulated active base was added. Stirring with the Lightnin' Mixer was continued until the particles broke up to the desired size. The composition was allowed to cool, with stirring, to 86°F (30°C) and then to room temperature. Stirring was stopped and the composition was tested. The cream spread easily unto the skin and was not sticky or oily. The skin cream composition is used as a conventional day or night cream. By applying conventional quantities to the face, neck or forehead in a rotating manner, and massaging in the usual way, the encapsulated particles will break down easily and smoothly.

This product was tested on 100 women and produced significant improvements with respect to softness and smoothness of the skin after only 20 days of use. The product is, therefore, a very effective softener and a smoothing and moisturizing agent.

It has been found that certain practical limits of the critical ingredients can be set. For example, the clay in the water phase of the emulsion should be present in an amount of up to about 3 to 5 wt %. The peptizer in the clay is used in an amount of about 0.2 to 1.0%. In the encapsulated active base, the limits are about 1 to 2 parts of clay to 2 to 3 parts cellulose. The preferred proportion is 2 parts clay to 3 parts cellulose on a dry basis.

Wet-Look Lipstick Containing Encapsulated Moisturizer

J.H. Murphy and G. Lieberman; U.S. Patent 3,947,571; March 30, 1976; assigned to Lanvin-Charles of the Ritz, Inc. are concerned with a lipstick which will impart a uniform long-lasting coloring to the lips, particularly a lipstick formulation containing low levels of pigment and dye and high levels of emollients, lubricants, and moisturizers so as to impart a "wet" or "moist" look to the lips and yet avoid a "creeping" or "feathering" effect.

This is achieved by including within the lipstick formulation water-soluble microcapsules containing an oil component functioning as an emollient, lubricant, or moisturizer. Thus, the lipstick contains a reservoir of ingredients which will impart a shiny wet or moist look to the lips. Sustained release of the encapsulated ingredient is effected by merely moistening the lips. It has also been found that the capsule shell material after releasing its contents forms a barrier which reduces creeping and minimizes mechanical removal.

The lipstick formulation comprises from about 2 to 20 wt % of water-soluble microcapsules containing a core of an oily material which functions as an emollient, lubricant or moisturizer dispersed in from about 98 to 80 wt % of an anhydrous base including waxes, oils, coloring agents, and minor amounts of other ingredients. It is preferred that the lipstick formulation comprise from about 10 to 15 wt % of microcapsules, with about 10% being most preferred. Sufficient anhydrous base must be employed so that the formulation is rigid enough to be moldable.

The microcapsules comprise an outer shell of water-soluble material and an inner core of one or more of the oily emollients, lubricants and moisturizers, with mineral oil being the preferred core material. The shell material is continuous and self-supporting and comprises from about 50 to 90 wt % of each microcapsule with about 70% being preferred. The core materials comprise from about 10 to 50 wt % of each microcapsule with about 30% being preferred. The microcapsules have an average particle size less than 77 microns and preferably less than 38 microns.

The water-soluble shell material is preferably selected from food grade polymeric materials such as starches, gum arabic, gum tragacanth, dextrin, derivatives of dextrin, etc., with dextrin being the most preferred. Methods of forming microcapsules from such materials are known (for example, U.S. Patent 3,159,585).

Example:

Ingredient	Percent by Weight
Candelilla wax	13.73
Oleyl alcohol	13.22
Castor oil	13.00
Super wool wax	10.00
Mineral oil	7.50
Synthetic cocoa butter	4.00
Cetyl alcohol	5.00
Liquid lanolin USP	4.50
Sesame oil	4.50
Petrolatum USP	4.50
Isopropyl lanolate	3.00
Lanolin USP	1.50
Squalane	1.00
Ozokerite	1.00
Propyl p-hydroxybenzoate	0.10
Butylated hydroxyanisole	0.02
D&C Red No. 9	1.66
D&C Red No. 27	0.78
Iron oxide	0.49
Fragrance oil	0.50
Encapsulate	10.00

The encapsulate consists of microcapsules having an average particle size of less than 77 microns. Each microcapsule consists of 30% mineral oil and 70% water-soluble dextrin with the oil encapsulated within the dextrin shell. The ingredients are combined according to the following procedure:

(1) All of the waxes are melted in a steam-jacketed kettle with Lightnin' Mixer agitation while maintaining the temperature at from 75° to 85°C. After the waxes are melted, the oil components except for the castor oil are added and agitation is continued.

(2) The dyes and pigment are added to the castor oil in a separate kettle and heated with agitation at 70°C. Agitation is continued until a proper dispersion is achieved. The dispersion of oil and coloring agents is passed through a three-roll mill.

(3) The encapsulated moisturizer is sifted through a 77 micron screen.

(4) The melted waxes from step (1) and the ground coloring agent from step (2) are mixed at 75°C with Lightnin' agitation. After the mixing is completed the sifted encapsulated moisturizer is added. The formulation is either stored or poured directly into molds and maintained at room temperature to form the lipstick.

Alternatively, the encapsulated moisturizer can be added directly to the ground dye slurry of step (2). This mixture is passed through a three-roll mill and then added to the melted waxes from step (1) at 75°C with Lightnin' agitation.

Towel Containing Encapsulated Makeup Remover

In accordance with the process developed by *R. Charlé, C. Zviak and G. Kalopissis; U.S. Patent 3,978,204; August 31, 1976; assigned to L'Oreal, France* cosmetic towels and cottons are prepared by a method characterized in that the microcapsules containing the cosmetic agent are introduced in the course of the preparation of the solid cosmetic support itself and that there is then directly effected the workup of the preparations thus obtained, the microcapsules remaining unaltered in the course of this treatment.

The compounds used for preparation of the synthetic resin films which contain microcapsules C are preferably selected from among the following: acetal homopolymers and copolymers, methyl polymethacrylate as well as copolymers thereof formed with styrene and α-methyl styrene, ethylcellulose, cellulose acetate, cellulose propionate, cellulose acetobutyrate, vinyl polymers and copolymers such as vinylidene chloride or polyvinyl dichloride, polystyrenes and copolymers of styrene-acrylonitrile, allyl resins, casein base resins, polyethylene, melamine-formaldehyde resin, phenol-formaldehyde resins, etc.

The manufacture of the towels and cosmetic cottons is accomplished as follows. The suspension or mixture of the initial liquid compounds that are to constitute the support of capsules C in the final product is prepared. The support is prepared, i.e., either blotting paper from paper paste or synthetic polymer from a monomer or liquid prepolymer which is thermosetting, or catalytically condensable products, the latter possibly yielding foams. Microcapsules C which have been prepared separately are introduced at an appropriate moment in this process, conditions particularly of temperature and pressure being appropriately adjusted.

Microcapsules C are introduced either directly into the mass at a moment in which its fluidity is still sufficient, the density of the microcapsules moreover being close to that of the liquid phase, or they are introduced by spraying when it is desired to incorporate them in a thin foil, before termination of the polymerization of the foil. At the end of the manufacturing process, there are thus obtained microcapsules C incorporated in the body of the support, the support being a blotting paper, a thin film, or a porous mass of suitable synthetic material.

Example: Towel Containing a Microencapsulated Makeup Remover Milk – The following makeup remover composition is prepared in parts by weight: "O.E." stearyl alcohol (oxyethylene), 4.0; ropy vaseline, 6.0; isopropyl myristate, 5.0; glycerol, 10.0; antiferment, 0.1; perfume, 0.3; and water to make up, 100.0.

The makeup remover milk is then microencapsulated by the known technique, using polypropylene, the microcapsules having an average dimension of 50 to 100 microns and preferably from 60 to 80. The microcapsules are dispersed in a blotting paper paste at the moment at which the density of the paste is such that the microcapsules are distributed in it with sufficient uniformity. The blotting paper is allowed to drain and it is dried on a form in thin layers, possibly with slight pressure, or the microcapsules are "flash" projected onto the surface of sheets of blotting paper preliminarily coated with an adhesive layer. The sheets are cut to the desired size and thus makeup remover towels ready for use are obtained. The microcapsules release the makeup remover milk by simple pressure that crushes the microcapsules.

Soaps Containing Encapsulated Oils

Soaps, such as salts of long chain fatty acids, usually obtained by the saponification of fats, and synthetic detergents, have defatting properties and as a result have a drying effect on the skin. *J.E. Jedzinak; U.S. Patent 4,124,521; Nov. 7, 1978; assigned to Revlon, Inc.* provides a soap bar having therein an oleophilic substance which soap will produce a noticeable lubricious softening effect on the skin and still have good cleansing properties.

The soap bar has substantially uniformly distributed therein a microencapsulated oleophilic substance in a concentration of from about 1 to 30 wt % of the soap composition. Any nontoxic, liquid oleophilic substance may be enclosed in the microcapsules. The encapsulating material may be any one of the standard materials used for forming the matrix of a microcapsule. The matrix material may be of either the pressure sensitive or water-soluble type. Preferably, the diameter of the microcapsule is about 40 to 50 microns. The microcapsules may be prepared in the usual fashion about a base of the oleophilic material. These microcapsules preferably contain about 5 to 40 wt % of the oleophilic material.

The preferred microencapsulated oleophilic material is mineral oil encapsulated in gum arabic. These microcapsules have a diameter of about 44 microns and have a mineral oil content of about 40 wt %. The preferred material soap base is soap chips obtained by the saponification of an 80/20 blend of tallow and coconut fat, or by the neutralization with alkali of a similar blend of fatty acids derived from these fats.

Example 1: 990 g of soap chips obtained by the saponification with sodium hydroxide of an 80/20 tallow/coconut fat were placed in a Sigma amalgamator and the mixer started. 10 g of microcapsules of mineral oil in a matrix of gum arabic (the microcapsules containing about 40 wt % of the mineral oil and having a diameter of about 44 microns) were then added and the mixing continued until the blend was substantially uniform. The blend was then transferred to a soap plodder and twice passed through a multiple orifice head attached to the plodder. The material was then returned to the plodder and passed through a heater head attached to the plodder and kept at a temperature of 45°C. The billet of soap formed after passage through the heater head was then cut into bars of soap of desired size.

Example 2: A soap formulation contains the following in parts by weight: soap chips as described in Example 1, 934.5; encapsulated mineral oil as described in Example 1, 40.0; lavender fragrance, 25.0; and 25% dispersion of D&C Violet #2 in propylene glycol, 0.5. The soap chips, encapsulated mineral oil and fragrance were blended til a uniform mix was obtained. The colorant was then added and the blending continued til the mix was uniform. The mixture was then transferred to the plodder and the procedure as described in Example 1 was followed.

As the soap bars prepared as described above are used, the microcapsules are ruptured in the process either by the pressure exerted on them or by the solution of the matrix in water, to release the free oleophilic substance in amounts which do not interfere with the lathering and cleansing properties of the soap. After these soaps were used in washing hands, it was demonstrated that the hands were covered with a layer of the oleophilic substance. The soap bars were hard and retained their hardness during their entire periods of use.

Dentifrices Containing Encapsulated Flavoring

J.E. Grimm, III; U.S. Patents 4,071,614; January 31, 1978 and 3,957,964; May 18, 1976; both assigned to Colgate-Palmolive Company describes a dentifrice which releases "bursts" of flavor during use and which includes a minor proportion of an encapsulated flavoring material in a dentifrice base. The encapsulated flavoring is maintained separate from the dentifrice base during storage but is released into it by breaking of the encapsulating shells or coatings when the dentifrice is used. Other dentifrice constituents which are more stable during storage when kept separate from the dentifrice base, and various other adjuvants, including colorants, which may give special effects during use, are also encapsulatable with the flavor. Also disclosed is a method for the manufacture of such dentifrices.

Example: A spearmint flavoring is encapsulated in substantially spearmint-impenetrable shells or coatings of a variety of encapsulating materials, including (1) polyvinyl chloride; (2) polyethylene; (3) phenol-formaldehyde; (4) paraffin; (5) carob bean gum; (6) shellac; and (7) hardened gelatin. The microcapsules are of sizes distributed over the range of 50 microns to one millimeter, distribution being substantially normal. In other cases, the distribution is controlled so that the particle sizes are in the 500 to 800 micron range.

Capsule wall thicknesses are assorted through the 1 to 100 micron range, averaging about 50 microns. The proportion of spearmint flavoring in the microcapsule is about 30% and present with the spearmint is about 10% of sweetener (sodium saccharin), 2% of green colorant (FD&C Green) of the water-soluble type, and 10% of a soluble fluorophosphate sodium salt. In some instances, wherein permeability of the flavor and color are to be minimized, the various "internal" ingredients of the microcapsules are mixed with paraffin wax (25% of the ingredients) before encapsulation.

After preparation of the microcapsules, they are degassed by subjection to a vacuum (40 mm Hg absolute pressure) for five minutes and then are blended with a dental cream of the following formula, made as described.

	Parts
Glycerin (99% CP)	7.0
Sorbitol (70% aqueous solution)	12.0
Sodium saccharin	0.1
Preservative	0.5
Gelling agent (Sodium carboxymethylcellulose)	1.0
Water (irradiated tap)	19.0
Tetrasodium pyrophosphate	0.5
Water (irradiated tap)	1.2
Dicalcium phosphate SM	38.0
Calcium carbonate (precipitated, dense)	10.0
Sodium N-lauroyl sarcosine solution (25% aqueous)	9.5
Spearmint flavor (essential oil of spearmint)	0.3

The solution of vehicles is made, subjected to the vacuum described for the encapsulated flavor and the mixture of flavor, preservative and gelling agent, in the 19 parts of irradiated tap water is prepared and subjected to degassing by the same technique. Subsequently, the pyrophosphate solution is made in 1.2 parts of the tap water and is blended with the previous aqueous suspension and the mixture of vehicles. The temperature is elevated to 45°C, while the mixture is being degassed at about 40 mm Hg absolute pressure over 10 minutes. Then, the polishing agent and detergent solution are added, after preliminary degassing. The temperature is maintained at about 45°C and 2.5 parts of the encapsulated flavoring (and other ingredients) are mixed in, taking care not to have the viscosity over about 40,000 cp and making sure that the mixer (Dopp) clearances are such that the microcapsules are not broken.

After about 10 minutes mixing, with application of vacuum and maintenance of elevated temperature, the dentifrice preparation is considered to be complete and it is packed into tubes in conventional manner. The tubes are then sent to storage and cooled to ambient temperature, at which the viscosity of the product increases to about 10,000 cp. The product analyzes about 8% glycerin, 8.4% sorbitol, 2% sodium N-lauroyl sarcosine, 35% moisture and 48% alcohol insolubles. Its apparent specific gravity is about 1.52 and its pH is about 7.7.

Upon subsequent use, when the product is squeezed from the tube and placed on a toothbrush, there is a distinct fresh spearmint fragrance apparently resulting from fracturing of some of the microcapsules. Also, on use, the spearmint flavor is released from the microcapsules, as is the coloring, by contact with the toothbrush, teeth and mouth, to reinforce both the flavoring and coloring of the product. Some of the coloring, a small proportion thereof, leaches through the capsule walls on storage and lightly colors the product but the subsequent coloring from the ruptured microcapsules and the increase in flavor resulting when the user fractures the capsule walls by brushing the teeth with the dentifrice are significantly noticeable as bursts of flavor and color and indicate to the user by taste and appearance when brushing has been vigorous enough and may be terminated.

In variations of the formula, in which the various encapsulating materials mentioned herein are employed with the basic formula, the same results are noted. The capsules are small enough so that they are not of objectionable size or feel during use of the dentifrice. Because the dentifrice is not swallowed, and because the encapsulating material is employed in small quantities, the use thereof is found to be harmless.

In other experiments modeled after that reported above, when special efforts are not made to prevent crushing of the capsules during mixing there is a noticeable decrease in the effectiveness of the flavor release from the capsules during use of the dentifrice. However, when such procedures are followed and when various flavors and mixtures of flavors are employed, such as spearmint or peppermint in thicker walled capsules and cherry flavoring in thinner walled capsules, with the proportions thereof being about 50:50, both flavors are distinctly produced, the cherry during the earlier part of brushing and the spearmint or peppermint later on, signalling the end of the brushing operation.

In other experiments the capsules made are suspended in clear gel dentifrices, wherein the coloring materials are apparent, giving the clear gel a distinctive colored appearance. Instead of utilizing clear gels with suspended polishing agents in them, the capsules are also suspended in thickened liquid detergents, based on sodium lauryl sulfate and sodium carboxymethylcellulose, wherein they serve to release coloring and flavoring until the cleaning operation is complete.

In other experiments, the flavor(s) in the capsules are changed to eucalyptus, anethole, menthol and carvone and the proportions are varied over the 0.5 to 5% range, with similar results. Generally, however, the total amount of flavoring employed will be from about 0.5 to 2% for best taste effects.

Hollow Antiperspirant Spheres Produced by Atomization Spray Drying

The process of *J.F. Kozischek; U.S. Patent 4,089,120; May 16, 1978; assigned to Armour Pharmaceutical Company* pertains to hollow, thick walled macrospherical particles intended for use primarily as antiperspirants. The macrospherical particles may also be used in pigments, resins, catalysts, etc. For the last 10 or 15 years, aerosol sprays have been a major application form for many products such as hair spray, paint, antiperspirant powders, and countless others. For the purposes of this process, "aerosol" means a suspension of fine solid particles in a gas. The gas need not be halohydrocarbons such as Freon which have been widely used as propellants, but may include air or any other gaseous propellants.

J.J. Sciarra et al (*J. Soc. Cosm. Chem.* 20, 385-394, May 27, 1969) reported that while most particles below 50 microns will remain suspended in air for relatively long periods of time, only those particles less than 10 microns are likely to pass into the respiratory tract. Most of the particles of this size will be retained in the upper portions of the respiratory tract, while particles in the range of 2 to 5 microns will be deposited in the area of terminal bronchi and alveoli.

Thus, it is apparent that certain particles suspended in an aerosol may be harmful to the respiratory system. The particles of this process are hollow macrospherical particles having a size predominantly between about 10 to 74 microns, and preferably between about 14 and 74 microns, in diameter and having a density greater than 1. These particles are of a large enough size and density to be substantially filtered out by the nose and to avoid deep respiratory tract penetration and deposition.

The process for producing the hollow macrospherical particles comprises providing a solution containing the materials from which the particles are made, diffusing the solution through small pores by centrifugal force such that the diameter of the particles is larger than the nominal diameter of the pores, and drying the solution in a stream of heated air after it leaves the pores. Approximately 85% of the particles diffused through the pores have diameters of between about 15 and 74 microns.

The apparatus for producing the dry, hollow macrospherical particles comprises a centrifugal atomizer having a filter ring made of porous sintered metal of substantially uniform pore size which is mounted in a spray drying chamber. The outer surface of the porous sintered metal filter is ground or polished and etched to provide a smooth surface with sharp pore exits to produce hollow, thick walled macrospheres having a diameter larger than the diameter of the pores.

Filters which are particularly useful are the porous sintered metal filters manufactured in accordance with the process of U.S. Patent 2,792,302 and U.S. Patent 3,313,621. Other methods of making porous sintered metal elements having uniform porosity are disclosed, for example, in U.S. Patents 2,157,596, 2,398,719, 3,052,967 and 3,700,419. Uniform porosity can be enhanced by using spherical powdered metal particles for sintering and forming a filter ring.

The filter ring must be thick enough not to break apart at rotational speeds; ⅜" is useful. The height should be a function of the feed rate of the liquid solution from which the hollow macrospherical particles are produced. A suitable feed rate is 0.5 to 2.5 lb/min/in^2 of the inner surface of the filter ring. A feed rate of 1.2 lb/min/in^2 is preferred when using a filter ring having an effective height of 1" and a diameter of 8". The nominal filter pore diameter is 15 to 30 μ. A filter having a nominal pore size of 20 μ will produce particles having an average diameter of 30 μ. The dried macrospherical particles are larger in size than the nominal pore size of the filter because the dried particles blow up as they become hollow. The walls of the hollow macrospherical particles increase in thickness during this process.

In operating the atomizer, first, the spray-drying apparatus is turned on. As the atomizer begins to spin at peripheral speeds of 2,100 to 5,100 in/sec, solutions from which the macrospherical particles are made are fed in through an inlet from the solution feed port. The feed rate is adjusted so that the solution diffuses promptly through the filter ring and there is very little, if any, solution buildup within the atomizer.

The stream of liquid diffusing through the filter is cut off into tiny droplets. As the droplets are propelled into the air currents of the spray dryer, they dry and expand into hollow, thick-walled macrospherical particles. The spray dryer inlet temperature is, e.g., 450° to 540°F and outlet temperature is, e.g., 195° to 250°F. The liquid stream should be a clear solution to prevent blinding of the filter pores.

Example: This example provides a comparison between conventional centrifugal atomization and porous metal atomization spray drying of a 50% solution of 5/6 basic aluminum chloride. Into a 500-gal reactor equipped with agitator and a heat exchanger was charged 2,950 lb of 24° Bé $AlCl_3$ and 1,720 lb of water. After preheating, 580 lb of aluminum powder was added in 10-lb increments maintaining an average reaction temperature of 85°C. After 6 hours, when nearly all of the aluminum had dissolved, an additional 35 lb of aluminum powder was added and the batch filtered. The composition assayed 12.6% Al and 8.5 Cl. Two batches of the solution were spray dried as follows:

	. . . . Type Atomization	
	Conventional Centrifugal	Porous Metal
Run conditions		
Feed rate, ml/min	100	100
Total wt feed, g	4,000	4,000
Run duration, min	30	30
Inlet temperature, °F	445	445
Outlet temperature, °F	195	200
Atomizer diameter, inch	2	1½
Atomizer speed, rpm	20,000	27,000
Atomizer peripheral speed, in/sec	2,094	2,120
Build-up in chamber	Heavy	Light
Al in feed solution, %	12.6	12.6
Al in dry powder, %	25.6	26.0
Theoretical yield based on Al, g	1,969	1,938
Actual yield (cyclone product), g	821	1,699
Percent recovery*	41.7	87.7
Wt chamber build-up, g	877	Slight
Particle size distribution of cyclone product (by wet sieve)**		
% +74 μ	2.2	0.3
% +44 μ	25.2	12.9
% +15 μ	94.4	91.4

*Percent recovery = actual yield/theoretical yield x 100
**Retained on sieves of the indicated size and those above it (i.e., cumulative distribution).

FOODS

VOLATILE FLAVORS

Encapsulation in CMC or Vegetable Gum

E. Palmer; U.S. Patent 3,989,852; November 2, 1976 has developed a process for the encapsulation of materials which tend to lose at least part of their original properties upon exposure to auto-oxidative, thermal, or humid conditions. The process which can be carried out at room temperature, comprises constituting the material to be encapsulated in or as a viscid medium and dispersing the medium as particulates into an atmosphere containing an agitated quantity of a powdered, sorbent, film-forming agent. The dispersed particulates must have a tacky surface. The powdered agent adheres to this tacky surface and absorbs sufficient liquid to gel the coated particulates and to form a continuous, substantially noncrackable and dry encapsulating film around each of the particulates.

A wide variety of liquids may be used in forming the viscid medium including mono- and polyhydric alcohols, mineral oils, edible oils, and the like. Among the fillers which may be used, either alone or in mixtures, are vegetable and/or organic substances such as protein-base materials, including vegetable and/or animal proteins, such as gelatin, casein, pectin, soy protein; non-protein-base materials including gums such as vegetable gum, Irish moss, corn syrup solids, modified starches such as Capsul, Purity Gum BE and National 46 (National Starch Co.), starch ethers, and cellulose including carboxymethylcellulose, hydroxyethylcellulose, hydroxypropylcellulose, ethylcellulose; polyvinyl acetate, polysaccharides, and dextran.

The film-forming agents may be any substance which will sorb the liquid from the tacky particulates and form an encapsulating film around these particulates. The film-forming agent which is selected will be determined by the intended use of the encapsulated product. However, it is vitally important that the films produced from this agent are noncrackable. Any of the substances previously described as fillers may be used as film-forming agents although among the preferred film-forming agents are non-protein-base materials, such as vegetable gum, for example, gum arabic, as well as low viscosity carboxymethylcellulose. A preferred particle size for the film-forming agent will be between 100 to 150 mesh.

Example: Encapsulation of Ethyl Vanillin to Produce a Nonbakeout Flavor – A good amount of flavoring ingredients are lost in the baking process due to the steam distillation of the volatile flavor ingredients at the baking temperature. These losses could be overcome if it were possible to keep the flavor oils from coming into contact with the water of the dough mix until the end and then only slowly. Also, where yeast fermentation is involved, the release of flavoring oils during the raising process has a detrimental effect on the taste of the final products. These problems are overcome by forming capsules according to this process as exemplified by the following.

40 g of benzyl alcohol, 50 g of propylene glycol, and 30 g of ethyl vanillin were mixed and dissolved, and then heated to 110°C. 10 g of ethylcellulose were added to this mixture and dissolved. A thick liquid was produced. This was then cooled to 60°C and 20 g of ethyl alcohol were added. This cooled and thinned out the liquid. The mix was further cooled to room temperature to produce a smooth, viscous and sticky paste. Then it was sprayed under pressure into a mixing vessel containing 1,350 g of pulverized ethylcellulose that had passed through a 100 mesh screen. It was well mixed and allowed to set for a few hours. A fine powdered product resulted. This was screened and a 12% ethyl vanillin content encapsulated flavor was produced.

Some of this powder was added to water and heated. No aroma of vanilla was evident until almost the boiling point of the water was reached. The aroma grew stronger on further heating. This flavor was being released slowly as would be the case in baking.

Solid Matrix of Mixture of Polysaccharides and Polyhydroxy Compounds

The polysaccharides employed in admixture with polyhydroxy compounds in the process developed by *J. Brenner, G.H. Henderson and R.W. Bergensten; U.S. Patent 3,971,852; July 27, 1976; assigned to Polak's Frutal Works, Inc.* are solids characterized by solubility in water and by at least partial solubility in, or capability of at least partially dissolving, the polyhydroxy compounds within the ranges of proportions used. They are primarily not the sweet, readily soluble saccharides like sugar, but higher polysaccharides that may be natural, such as gum arabic and similar vegetable gums, or synthetic, such as degradation and modified products of starch, which usually form colloidal solutions.

Among the polysaccharides that may be used are dextrins derived from ungelatinized starch-acid esters of substituted dicarboxylic acids represented diagrammatically by the formula:

$$\text{starch}-O-\overset{\overset{\displaystyle O}{\|}}{C}-\overset{\overset{\displaystyle R^1}{|}}{R}-COOH;$$

in which R is a radical selected from the class consisting of dimethylene and trimethylene and R^1 is a hydrocarbon substituent of R selected from the class consisting of alkyl, alkenyl, aralkyl and aralkenyl groups. These ungelatinized starch-acid esters are prepared by reacting an ungelatinized starch, in an alkaline medium, with a substituted cyclic dicarboxylic acid anhydride having the following formula:

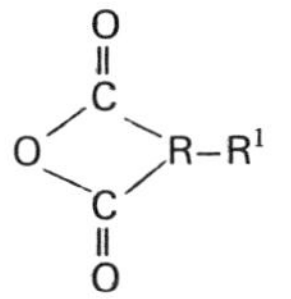

$$\begin{array}{c} O \\ \| \\ C \\ O \diagup \quad \diagdown R{-}R^1 \\ \diagdown \quad \diagup \\ C \\ \| \\ O \end{array}$$

in which R and R^1 represent the so designated substituent groups just defined. Examples of such anhydrides are the substituted succinic and glutaric acid anhydrides. Such a polysaccharide will be referred to hereinafter as polysaccharide X.

Other useful polysaccharides include products derived from dextrinized starch which will be referred to hereinafter as polysaccharide Y and hydrolyzed starch which will be referred to as polysaccharide Z. In general, these products contain minor proportions of lower saccharides such as dextrose and it is customary to classify them as to sweetness by a dextrose equivalent (DE) rating, number or range which for solids (as opposed to syrups) is in the approximate range of 10 to 25.

The polysaccharide should possess emulsifying properties either inherently or by reason of the presence of a minor proportion of a suitable emulsifying agent, such as sodium diisooctyl sulfosuccinate and sodium caseinate. If emulsifying agents are added, proportions in the range of 0.1 to 10% based on the weight of polysaccharide in the mixture are satisfactory. An important property of the polysaccharide or polysaccharide-emulsifier combination is that when dissolved in water with the polyhydroxy compound, the aqueous phase is capable of emulsifying oil to form the dispersed phase of an oil-in-water emulsion with the oil globules having diameters largely within but not limited to the range of about 0.5 to 5 microns and has sufficient stability not to invert or coalesce prior to moisture removal, e.g., by spray drying.

The polyhydroxy compounds employed in admixture with polysaccharide material are characterized by (a) solubility in water and at least partial solubility in the polysaccharide material or capability of at least partially dissolving such material, (b) forming with the polysaccharide material a liquid melt having a softening range at appropriate temperatures within the ranges of proportions used, (c) forming with the polysaccharide material a continuous aqueous phase in which oil is dispersible as a discontinuous phase to form a stable emulsion, (d) plasticity of the surface of the particle formed from the emulsion as water is removed through a drying operation, and (e) forming with the polysaccharide material a mixture that is in the solid state at the temperature of use.

The useful polyhydroxy compounds can be classified into three groups:

(1) Polyhydroxy alcohols, including glycerin, sorbitol, mannitol, erythritol and ribitol.

(2) Sugars from plant sources, including monosaccharides such as glucose, disaccharides such as maltose and sucrose, trisaccharides such as raffinose, and ketosaccharides such as fructose. These will be referred to as plant-type sugars whether actually derived from plants or produced synthetically.

(3) Polyhydroxy compounds containing other functional groups including glucuronolactone (lactone), sorbitan and mannitan (monoethers) and methylglucopyranoside (acetal).

In general, the proportion of polyhydroxy compounds is at least 20% of the matrix. The suitability of mixtures of these matrix-forming materials, e.g., polysaccharide material (referred to as A) and polyhydroxy compounds (referred to as B) for use in the process may be determined by the following test procedures.

Solubility Test:

(1) Dissolve A and B separately in water.

(2) Combine the two solutions in proper amounts to give various proportions of A:B on a solids basis over a sufficient range of proportions, in some cases varying the proportions from pure A to pure B, to determine if there are proportions that are useful.

(3) Evaporate water from the mixture, leaving a residue in solid state.

(4) Place some of the residue on the hot stage of a microscope and observe the melting behavior as it is heated. If the residue remains essentially homogeneous throughout the softening and molten range, it will be satisfactory for use, providing the criteria of the softening range test are met.

Softening Temperature Range Test:

(1) Determine the plastic or softening temperature range of each mixture of A and B, and use these data to construct a simple two-component melt diagram for each system which are typical melting behavior curves for mixtures used in the process.

(2) The softening, plastic or flowable state of A:B mixture must occur within the temperature range consistent with the drying technique used. It should be noted that the temperature range within which moisture removal occurs, e.g., the temperature of sprayed particles during drying of the emulsion, is not necessarily the same as or overlapping the range determined above, since the melt during moisture removal is a quaternary mixture of A, B, oil and diminishing proportions of water whereas on reheating it is a ternary mixture of A, B, and oil.

Example 1: A solution of an encapsulant comprising 32 parts glucuronolactone and 48 parts polysaccharide X is prepared by dissolving them in 250 parts of water with agitation at high speed in a household type Waring blender. Single fold orange oil containing 1% butylated hydroxy anisole as antioxidant is slowly added to the resulting solution until 120 parts are incorporated while continuing high speed agitation for 3 minutes, at which time an oil/water emulsion has formed with an average droplet diameter of 0.5 micron. The viscosity as determined with a Brookfield Model LVT Viscometer is 57.5 cp at 30°C.

The proportions are chosen to give an oil loading of 60% (120 parts oil and 80 parts encapsulant). The mixture is spray dried in a standard Anhydro laboratory drier, size No. 1, maintained at an air inlet temperature of 180°C and an air outlet temperature of 90°C at a feed rate of 3 lb/hr of emulsion. There is collected 170 parts of powdered product readily passing through a 140 mesh screen which upon analysis by standard steam distillation technique is shown to contain 66% by volume or 56% by weight of volatile oil based on the weight of the product. This represents an 85% weight recovery of product containing 93% of the theoretical load of orange oil initially employed to make the emulsion. This represents a total recovery of 79% of the original oil. The extractable oil of the product is 0.2% as determined by extraction as described above. The moisture content is 2.1% as determined by the Karl Fischer procedure. In general, the volatile oil content is determined by the standard steam distillation technique on product as produced. The volatile oil content as so determined includes the extractable oil.

Example 2: An emulsion is prepared from 32 parts of sorbitol, 48 parts of gum arabic, 120 parts of an orange oil, 2 parts of sodium diisooctyl sulfosuccinate and 300 parts of water. The resulting emulsion has an average oil particle size of 1.4 microns and a viscosity of 40 cp at 30°C. The spray dried powder obtained in a weight yield of 80.3% has 67.4% volatile oil [57.2% by weight, oil factor (total oil recovered:total oil input) 0.95] and 0.9% moisture. The product dissolves readily in cold water. Mannitol or sucrose gives comparable results.

Example 3: An emulsion was prepared from 60 parts sucrose, 24 parts sodium caseinate, 36 parts polysaccharide Z, 180 parts of cold pressed lemon oil, and 330 parts water. Prior to the addition of the oil, the pH of the emulsion was adjusted to 7, using 20% sodium hydroxide. An 83.8% by weight yield of product was obtained by spray drying and passing the product through a 60 mesh screen. The product has 3.6% extractable oil, and 53.8% by weight total oil.

Example 4: An emulsion is prepared from 60 parts of polysaccharide X, 30 parts of mannitol, 10 parts of polyvinyl alcohol 325 (Airco Chemicals), and 150 parts of an orange oil. The resulting emulsion has an oil particle size of 0.2 micron and a viscosity of 150 cp at 30°C, upon spray drying. The product obtained in 87.7% yield contains 65.8% volatile oil, 4.2% extractable oil and 1.2% moisture. This product illustrates the use of two polyhydroxy compounds instead of only one, as in the previous examples, and three or more polyhydroxy compounds may be used if desired.

The solubility rate of this product in water is lower than most of the above products, which is desirable for some applications, e.g., bath salts where a prolonged fragrance release is beneficial. The addition of a small proportion of glutaraldehyde to the abovedescribed emulsion gives an insoluble product.

Example 5: An emulsion was prepared from 40 parts of mannitol, 30 parts of polysaccharide X, 30 parts of polysaccharide Z, and 150 parts of an orange oil. The spray dried product obtained in 81% yield, has a volatile oil content of 63.3%. This product shows that two polysaccharides may be used instead of one, as in the previous examples. Comparable results are obtained by using three and more polysaccharides in suitable proportions.

Example 6: Additional polyhydroxy compounds (PHC) which may be employed in preparing emulsions with polysaccharide X (PSX), orange oil and water are listed in the table on the following page which gives suitable proportions and the percentage of volatile oil in the resulting products produced by spray drying in accordance with Example 1.

PHC, parts	PSX, pbw	Orange Oil, pbw	Percent Volatile Oil (v/w)
Mannitan 20	80	150	58
Sorbitan 20	60	120	62.5
Glucose 40	40	120	66.7
Maltose 60	40	150	54
Raffinose 70	30	150	58
Fructose 45	55	150	61
Glycerin 30	70	150	60
Erythritol 30	70	150	61
Methyl-alpha-glucopyranoside 40	40	120	63.3
Dulcitol 30	70	150	60

Lipophilic Modified Starch Derivatives

The use of volatile flavoring oils and perfumes in such applications as foods and cosmetics is often greatly hampered by the rapid evaporation and loss of the volatile component. The losses detract from the desirability as well as from the utility of the products concerned.

C.N. Richards and C.D. Bauer; U.S. Patent 4,035,235; July 12, 1977; assigned to Anheuser-Busch, Incorporated describe encapsulating agents which are water-dispersible and form films with the proper hydrophobic-hydrophilic balance upon drying to provide a gradual or controlled release of the substance entrapped by the encapsulating agent. This process produces a spray dried enzyme converted starch reaction product which may be used in the form of an aqueous dispersion with an oil to form a stable emulsion. The oil-in-water emulsion may be dried and later reconstituted to provide a stable emulsion. When resuspended in water, the spray dried product causes a cloud effect. The cloud effect is an opaqueness in the fluid which is used in certain types of drinks made from dried flavorings.

The method for producing a lipophilic derivative of starch to be used in encapsulating water-insoluble substances comprises:

(a) reacting in an alkaline aqueous medium granular waxy starch and a substituted cyclic dicarboxylic anhydride having the following formula:

```
      O
      ‖
      C
    /   \
   O     R–R'
    \   /
      C
      ‖
      O
```

wherein R is a radical from the class of dimethylene and trimethylene radicals and R' is the substituent group from the class consisting of an alkyl, alkenyl, aralkyl and aralkenyl to produce a granular starch reaction product which is the acid ester of the substituted dicarboxylic acid having a degree of substitution of about 2 to 3%,

(b) recovering the granular starch reaction product,

(c) washing the granular starch reaction product of step (b),

(d) treating the washed granular starch reaction product with an α-amylase enzyme treatment which gelatinized and depolymerized the granular starch reaction product to produce a dispersion of the lipophilic derivative of starch in water which derivative has the above degree of substitution and has a viscosity of 125 to 500 as measured by a Brookfield method at spindle 2 speed 20 rpm at 30% concentration and 25°C temperature.

The enzyme is inactivated by the addition of sodium hypochlorite and/or heat. The starch derivative is spray dried.

When using the α-amylase of the following examples, Rhozyme 86L, the following conditions are preferred. The temperature is raised to 90° to 100°C for 10 to 45 minutes. Preferably, the temperature is maintained from 90° to 94°C for 30 minutes. The amount of sodium hypochlorite added is from 0.01 to 0.25% by weight based on the weight of dry starch.

The modified starch is then spray dried using an inlet temperature of 175° to 700°F (preferably 500°F), and an outlet temperature of 150° to 350°F (preferably 225°F). Inlet and outlet conditions are selected so that desired drying is effected and no undesirable damage (browning, charring, etc.) occurs to the product. Any drying technique such as passing over heated drums may be used, but spray drying is a preferred method for waxy starch-n-octenyl succinate.

Example: 100 parts of waxy maize starch is slurried to a Baumé of 21.0. 3 parts of n-octenyl succinic anhydride is added to the starch slurry and the pH is kept between 7.0 and 8.0 with a basic solution (70 g NaOH, 150 g Na_2CO_3 per liter). The temperature is kept at 75°F. When the pH is stabilized, the starch is washed and filtered. The modified starch (10,000 parts) then is resuspended in water to a 35% solids suspension. 1.0 part of Rhozyme 86L is added to the suspension. The temperature is raised to 80°C until a Dudley viscosity of about 120 seconds at 80°C is achieved. Then 5.0 parts of sodium hypochlorite is added and the temperature is raised to 94°C for 30 minutes. The starch is then spray dried using an inlet temperature of 500°F and an outlet temperature of 225°F.

The product, when mixed with coconut oil in a 1:1:2 (starch:coconut oil:H_2O) ratio and emulsified, forms stable emulsions.

CONDIMENTS

Salt Seasoning Mixture Containing Encapsulated Citric Acid

There have been numerous formulations prepared as an aid to reducing or eliminating to a large degree the sodium intake. Some formulations completely eliminate sodium chloride; but seek to retain the salty taste associated with the sodium chloride since the taste appears to be a primary need and desire built into man throughout his evolution. These formulations, while eliminating sodium chloride from the diet from the seasoning standpoint, have been largely unsuccessful in satisfying the principal hunger man appears to have for the saline taste of salt.

Other formulations, to which class this process belongs, dilute sodium chloride with other additives. These additives are tailored to improve the processability of salt as well as enhance the salty taste derived from it.

A common additive or diluent is potassium chloride because of its acceptance in the body functions. Potassium chloride has a rather unpleasant, even bitter, aftertaste, however, and it has been found that other additives are needed to mask the unpleasant taste.

The process of *G.J. Moritz; U.S. Patent 4,068,006; January 10, 1978; assigned to Akzona Incorporated* is directed to a salt formulation having potassium chloride mixed with sodium chloride and containing citric acid as a bitterness suppressor for the potassium chloride taste. The action of the citric acid is augmented by delaying its effect on the taste buds of the mouth and tongue through the use of an encapsulating agent. The encapsulant also serves to prevent deliquescence of the citric acid and avoid caking of the mixture. Suitable encapsulants are hydrogenated vegetable oil, gelatin and a cellulose-wax mixture.

Example: (A) Control — A mixture of 55% sodium chloride and 44% potassium chloride and 1% citric acid was prepared by mixing the ingredients in a blending machine. Free flowing agents were added of 0.5 and 0.75% for KCl and NaCl, respectively. 100 g of the mixture were allowed to stand in a watch glass in ambient humidity conditions (40 to 50% humidity) for a period of one day. At the end of the day, the mixture was inspected and found to be encrusted and caked on the surface. The crust broke into large pieces when disturbed. The chunks were difficult to break.

(B) Use of Encapsulated Citric Acid — A mixture similar to (A) was prepared except that the citric acid was encapsulated with 15% by weight of hydrogenated vegetable oil. A sample mixture was placed in a watch glass in ambient humidity conditions (40 to 50%) for a period of 7 days. Some minor encrustation occurred, but the crust broke easily when disturbed.

(C) Evaluation — The mixture of (B) was tested to determine salty taste. Citric acid was found to be released by the encapsulation 1 to 3 seconds after placement in the mouth. One-eighth of one teaspoonful of the mixture was placed on 20-g servings of iceberg lettuce and served code marked to taste testing groups. Ratings of the mixture when compared with equal servings of lettuce sprinkled with sodium chloride were equal and the mixture was judged to have a good salty taste.

Sugar Encapsulated in Fat for Sweetened Coconut Products

L.A. Johnson and L.A. Walters; U.S. Patent 3,976,794; August 24, 1976; assigned to SCM Corporation are concerned with an edible coconut base particle coated with a mixture of powdered sugar particles and particles of sugar encapsulated in edible fat, the proportion of sugar in the encapsulated sugar particles constituting at least about 5% of the total sugar content of the coating mixture and not substantially in excess of that proportion which will impart a threshold textural difference to the product. The maximum particle size of the preponderance of the encapsulated sugar particles is restricted to about four times the maximum particle size of the powdered sugar particles.

The proportion of fat to sugar is from 0.67:1 to 2.33:1 or higher or lower, for example, from 100:1 to 0.1:1, the particles are from 20 to 60 mesh (U.S. Standard) average size, the fat has a capillary melting point of from 95° to 150°F. Fats for the process include triglycerides, fatty emulsifiers, and mixtures thereof, and especially those which are bland.

The fat encapsulated sugar particles comprising a portion of the coating mixture of the coconut of the process and the fat encapsulated sugar particles comprising a particulate sweetener replacement for straight powdered sugar in foods also can be made according to the process of condiment encapsulation by spray-chilling, of U.S. Patent 3,949,094. This represents an improved spray-chilling process for encapsulation of condiment with normally solid lipoidal material wherein a spray of the liquefied condiment (in this case sugar) or pumpable matrix of such condiment dispersed in lipoidal material is intercepted with a spray of lipoidal material in fluent state directed for enveloping the condiment-rich spray particles, the enveloped particles thereafter being passed through a chilling zone and therein congealing the lipids for handling.

Example 1: Encapsulated Sugar – Bland hydrogenated vegetable oil, capillary melting point specification of 124° to 130°F, was melted in a steam-jacketed tank. The liquid temperature was maintained at 140° to 152°F. Sufficient powdered 6xx sugar (about 60 mesh) was added to give a final concentration of 40% sugar and 60% fat. The resulting slurry was agitated for about one hour to assure a homogeneous mixture. The slurry was then sprayed into a conventional spray-chiller countercurrent to a stream of cold air. Solid particles of encapsulated sugar were collected from the bottom of the chiller. A series of runs gave particles of the following average analysis:

	Percent
Fat	58.5-59.4
Sugar	40.6-41.5
Sieve analysis	
Passes 20 mesh	91.63
Passes 40 mesh	56.55
Passes 50 mesh	8.75
Passes 80 mesh	1.34
Passes 150 mesh	0

Encapsulation appeared to be virtually complete. The encapsulated sugar particles were white, free-flowing spherical beads.

Example 2: Use in Coconut – Several batches of coconut were compounded in a rotating-drum tumble food mixer using as the sweetening coating various mixtures of the spray-chilled, fat-encapsulated sugar particles of Example 1 and 6xx powdered sugar (sucrose). In each run, the desiccated coconut was the same, namely shredded coconut. To it was added a mixture of 3 parts of propylene glycol and 17 parts water to obtain 20% water content in the final product. When this was sorbed, 0.5% salt was added, thus an edible coconut base particle was formed.

Finally, to the coconut base particle the straight powdered sugar and encapsulated sugar was added. All mixing was done in the rotating-drum tumble mixer at room temperature. In each batch the proportion of total sugar to the coconut base particle was the same, 27 parts of total sucrose per 73 parts of coconut base particle (the salted, humidified desiccated coconut), but in the first batch 5% of it was encapsulated, in the second batch 15%, in the third 25%. Coloring and flavoring, if desired, are added prior to coating the coconut particles with the straight powdered sugar/encapsulated sugar coating mixture.

In similar batch preparations, it was noted that like fat-encapsulated sugar substitutions for straight powdered sugar whitened off-color coconut substantially more than did a comparable straight powdered sugar coating.

Example 3: Evaluation – A consumer taste panel test (30 consumers) was conducted using samples of the sweetened coconut described in Example 2 to determine if the panelists could detect a textural or sweetness formulation change between sweetened coconut comprising only straight powdered sugar as the sweetening agent on the one hand and sweetened coconut of the compositions described in Example 2 on the other. Sample No. 1 (20% moisture content) was a control, sweetened only with straight powdered sugar 6xx. Samples 2, 3, and 4, were from the first, second, and third batches of sweetened coconut of Example 2, respectively.

The test results indicated that Samples 2, 3, and 4 (using various proportions of the fat-encapsulated sugar) were on the whole substantially more acceptable to the panel, with only statistically insignificant differences for the most part among the samples. The 25% substitution of fat-encapsulated sugar for the straight powdered sugar appeared to be about the threshold value, that is minimum textural perception reaction by the panel.

The other test results demonstrated that an edible sweetened coconut product comprising up to a 25% replacement of powdered sugar with fat-encapsulated sugar as the sweetening agent can be used with a carrier (white icing on cupcake) still maintaining excellent appearance, flavor, texture, and overall acceptance while substantially diminishing off-flavor in the coconut product.

Spray-Chilling Process for Encapsulation of Condiments in Fat

L.A. Johnson and E.J. Beyn; U.S. Patent 3,949,094; April 6, 1976; assigned to SCM Corporation describe a process for producing a lipid-coated condiment wherein spray-chilling is employed for congealing the lipid.

A condiment for purposes of this process can be a liquid, vapor, or solid phase seasoning, flavoring, salting, sweetening, souring, spicing, and/or coloring ingredient or ingredient mixture suitable for producing or enhancing a flavor, texture and/or color in an edible product.

The process for encapsulation of condiment with normally solid lipoidal material comprises liquefying the condiment; spraying the resulting liquefied condiment as a spray pattern of particles; intercepting the spray pattern with a spray of the lipoidal material in fluent state directed for enveloping condiment-rich spray particles; passing resulting enveloped particles into a chilling zone; and therein congealing at least their lipoidal exterior.

The resulting composite product of this process has a condiment-rich core and a congealed lipoidal-material-rich coating thereon. The distribution of particle sizes is characteristic of conventional spraying.

Final encapsulated particle sizes will range from about 5 microns or smaller to 150 microns or larger. The weight proportion of total lipid to condiment in the encapsulated particles ordinarily will range from about 100:1 to 0.1:1 depending upon the intended usage of the encapsulated particles. The size of and the condiment content in the encapsulated particles each can be varied over the above ranges to produce particles of the desired size and condiment content, and particles can be classifed as to size after production for particular use.

By a normally solid lipoidal material (including a mixture of lipoidal materials) is meant that such material at 90°F, advantageously at 95°F, and preferably at 115° to 180°F, is ostensibly dry to the touch, free-flowing in small (e.g., 60 to 100 mesh) beaded form, and such beads do not tend to agglomerate strongly or appreciably or to deform appreciably even when standing unpacked to a depth of 6 inches high in a one-inch diameter cylinder for 24 hours at 75° to 80°F.

In practicing this process, the first step is to liquefy the condiment which is to be encapsulated. An already normally liquid condiment can be sprayed (atomized) in its liquid form for purposes of this step. A vaporous condiment to be encapsulated is best dissolved or sorbed into a fluent high-boiling matrix, particularly a congealable hard fat, like that used to envelop the core spray particles. Alternatively such condiment can be sorbed on an edible solid and handled like a solid condiment. Certain solid condiments being encapsulated can be melted in order to spray the condiment provided that the desired organoleptic characteristics of such condiment are not grossly damaged by the melting.

Alternatively and preferably, however, solid and most liquid condiments to be encapsulated can be liquefied by dispersing them in finely divided state or dissolving them in a sprayable lipoidal matrix that is congealable in the chilling operation, for example, a molten normally hard fat for efficiency and economy.

Liquefaction means then converting (by melting, sorbing, dissolving or suspending) the condiment in such form that it can be atomized by conventional means, for example, airless spray, gas-assisted spray, spinning disc, or the like. The process is described with reference to Figure 5.1.

Figure 5.1: Spray-Chilling Process for Encapsulation of Condiments in Fats

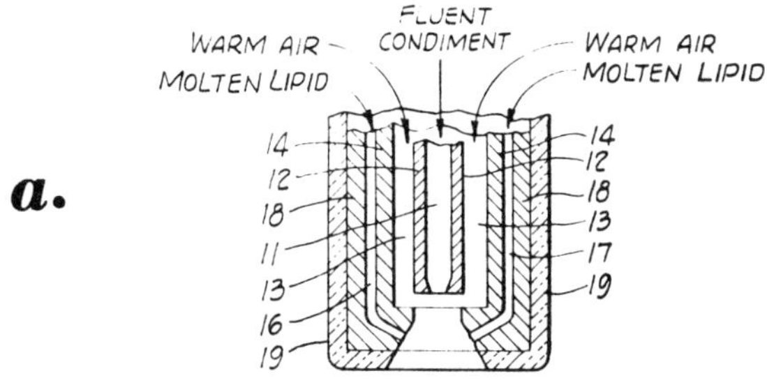

(continued)

Figure 5.1: (continued)

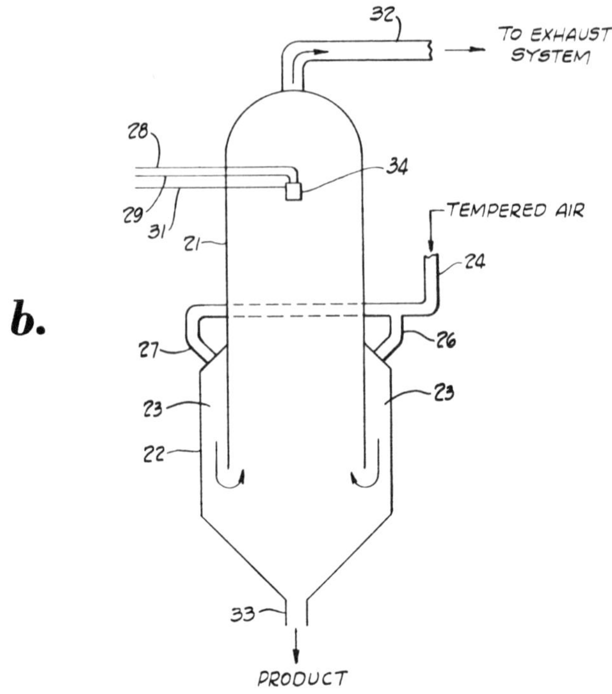

(a) Nozzle tip assembly in cross-sectional elevation
(b) Spray chiller, vertical cross-sectional elevation

Source: U.S. Patent 3,949,094

Figure 5.1a shows a useful nozzle tip assembly in cross-sectional elevation. The fluent condiment flows through passage **11**, which passage is defined by tube wall **12**. Annular to tube wall **12** is passage **13** conveying warm air transverse to the jet of fluent condiment exiting from passage **11** and atomizing this jet. Annular passage **13** is defined by tube wall **12** and the inner wall of interior casing **14**.

A pair of peripheral passages **16** and **17** (180° opposed and small in diameter) convey the molten lipid through exterior casing **18** and discharge it as a spray into the zone of atomized condiment. There can be additional such peripheral passages, generally opposed to each other and tending to intersect if unimpeded into a conical pattern looking down, but when the nozzle is in full operation, the molten enveloping lipid is atomized quite thoroughly and additional such streams of molten lipid tend to make more perfect lipid coatings on the core particle rich in condiment. Lagging **19** insulates the nozzle assembly from substantial heat loss. Obviously, more than one kind of lipoidal material can be used for the coating spray, each projected from a different spraying outlet.

Figure 5.1b shows a typical spray chiller schematically in vertical cross-sectional elevation. Shell **21** (the chilling zone) is a vertical cylindrical body extending into base **22**. Tempered air (typically 40°F and 40 to 80% relative humidity) enters line **24**, is manifolded to inlets **26** and **27**, and flows into annulus **23** formed by the downward extension of shell **21** and the wall of base **22**. Liquefied condiment enters the apparatus through line **28** along with a flow of warm air through line **29** and molten enveloping lipid through line **31.** These are discharged downwardly into shell **21** through nozzle **34**, typically a nozzle like that shown in Figure 5.1a.

The spray of lipid-coated condiment congeals as it falls countercurrently through the rising flow of cool air. Finished particles of the encapsulated condiment product are discharged through outlet **33** in base **22** and fall into a lock hopper (not shown). Spent air and entrained fines pass through overhead discharge line **32** to an exhaust system (not shown). Such exhaust system generally comprises a cyclone separator for a collection of particulates and even can be followed by a bag filter or like solid separation collector for additional recovery of undersized values. Additionally, the finished particles can be cooled further by cold gas fluidization.

Example: Referring to Figure 5.1b, a molten blend of 10% five-fold orange oil and 90% of triglyceride fat (specification melting point of 124° to 130°F) is introduced through line **28** at the rate of 100 ml/min and temperature of 145°F. 3 scfm (measured at 760 mm Hg and 70°F) of air at 145°F passes through line **29**. Molten triglyceride fat at 170°F (of the same type as fed into line **28**) passes through line **31** at the rate of 40 ml/min as the coating lipid. These liquid flows are atomized in nozzle **34**, the nozzle having a tip like that described in connection with Figure 5.1a, but having four peripheral jets for the coating lipid.

The net spray is directed downwardly and countercurrently to a flow of tempered air (18 scfm at essentially atmospheric pressure, 40°F and 80% relative humidity), entering line **24**, passing through lines **26** and **27**, annulus **23**, and eventually shell **21** which is at about atmospheric pressure. Chilled, congealed product, about 80 mesh average particle size, collects in the bottom of base **22** and is withdrawn through outlet **33**. It is appreciably coated with congealed triglyceride fat enrobing a core rich in orange oil. An exhaust of the spent air containing any ultrafine particles is withdrawn from shell **21** through line **32** and discharged to a particle-collecting exhaust system comprising a cyclone separator in series with a bag filter.

Spray Drying Process with Condiment Spray Coated with Edible Coating Spray

L.A. Johnson and E.J. Beyn; U.S. Patent 3,949,096; April 6, 1976; assigned to SCM Corporation describe a process for producing encapsulated condiment particles by spray drying wherein the spray dried particles are cooled while they are maintained in gas suspended condition in order to prevent them from agglomerating upon collection.

The process involves contacting a first spray of particles with cold air to assist in atomizing it; then spraying a second particle stream which contacts the first. The particle stream which is formed is then discharged through a heating zone, after which it is cooled while being maintained in a gas suspended condition. Finally, the resulting coated particles are separated from the gas.

The condiment can be a liquid, vapor, or solid phase seasoning, flavoring, salting, sweetening, souring, spicing, proteinaceous material, and/or coloring ingredient or ingredient mixture suitable for producing or enhancing a texture, flavor and/or color in an edible product.

The edible surface coating dispersion comprises an edible coating material dispersed in a fugitive carrier or solvent, e.g., water or ethanol, wherein the carrier or solvent can be volatized in the heating zone to leave a dry surface coating residue. Edible surface coatings include sacchariferous material, proteinaceous material, edible gums, colorants, normally solid lipoidal material (including a mixture of lipoidal materials), edible waxes, edible resins or like edible materials suitable for spray coating core particles and mixtures thereof.

Final coated particle sizes can range from about 5 microns or smaller to 150 microns or larger. The weight proportion of condiment to surface coating material in the dry coated particles ordinarily will range from about 0.11:1 to 100:1 depending upon the intended usage of the coated particles.

The first step is to form and spray a dispersion containing the condiment. An already normally liquid condiment can be sprayed (atomized) in its liquid form for purposes of this step. A vaporous condiment to be coated is best dissolved or sorbed into a fluent, normally hard lipoidal material. Alternatively, such condiment can be sorbed on an edible solid and handled like a solid condiment. Certain solid condiments being coated can be melted in order to spray the condiment, provided that the desired organoleptic characteristics of such condiment are not grossly damaged by the melting. Alternatively and preferably, however, solid and most liquid condiments can be coated by dispersing them in finely divided state or dissolving them in a sprayable lipoidal matrix for efficiency and economy.

Condiments which tend to swell upon exposure to moisture (for example, wheat flour) and those which are chemically activated by exposure to moisture (for example, moderate heat-resisting baking powder) are dispersed in finely divided state or dissolved in the sprayable lipoidal matrix so that any moisture content of the surface coating dispersion does not so adversely affect or prematurely decompose them.

Forming a condiment-containing dispersion for the process means then converting (by melting, sorbing, dissolving or suspending) the condiment in such form that it can be atomized by conventional means, for example, airless spray, gas-assisted spray, spinning disc, or the like. Average particle size (diameter) for spraying can be as low as a few microns on up to 100 microns or even larger. While certain product particles, preferably are at about 5 microns (average), many condiment products in the resulting spray dried coated forms are advantageously of about 80 to 90 microns average diameter. Thus, the atomizing device, e.g., nozzle, used is made to produce such size, and solids sprayed are, of course, fine enough to preclude nozzle stoppage.

The spray containing the condiment is intercepted with a further spray of edible surface coating dispersion convertible by spray drying into a dry surface coating. The multispray pattern usually is formed by use of a multicomponent spray nozzle. The resulting composite particles thereupon pass into a heating zone, therein drying the condiment core and coating simultaneously if both are dryable, otherwise, drying only the dryable dispersions. Such drying is accomplished by vaporization of volatile matter from the particles by hot gas, preferably hot air for efficiency and economy. The hot air preferably passes cocurrently with the coated particles in the heating zone for efficiency and economy. However, when the final particle size (effective diameter) becomes as large as 80 to 100 microns or larger, a countercurrent or cross-flow heating gas stream can be employed appropriately. Thus, a heating gas stream can be countercurrent, cocurrent, or crosscurrent to the spray particles as is necessary or desirable (for example, to resist or promote classification).

The dry coated particles suspended in the current of hot air are discharged from the heating zone and mixed with a flow of cold gas (preferably cold air for efficiency and economy) in a chilling zone. The discharged current is generally at about 100° to 200°F and at such temperatures many coating materials can be somewhat tacky or sticky in this environment. The cooling of the particles is done while same are maintained in gas-suspended condition in order to minimize any such subsequent caking or blocking.

Accordingly, a sufficient flow of cold gas at a suitable temperature calculated to substantially cool the suspended particles is mixed with the discharged current from the heating zone in the chilling zone while the particles remain in such gas-suspended condition. Substantial cooling is achieved when, upon collection of product particles and at the collection temperature, such product particles will resist appreciable blocking, caking and agglomeration, even when standing unpacked to a depth of 6 inches high in a 1-inch diameter cylinder for 24 hours. They will tend to be free-flowing. The process is described with reference to Figure 5.2.

Figure 5.2a shows a useful nozzle tip assembly in cross-sectional elevation. The condiment-containing dispersion flows through passage 11, which passage is defined by tube wall **12**. Annular to tube wall **12** is passage **13** conveying cold air transverse to the jet of condiment-containing dispersion exiting from passage **11** and atomizing this jet. Annular passage **13** is defined by tube wall **12** and the inner wall of interior casing **14**.

Figure 5.2: Spray Drying Process

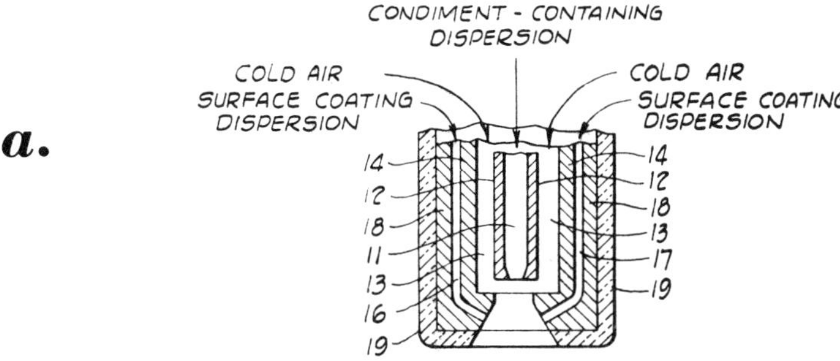

(continued)

Figure 5.2: (continued)

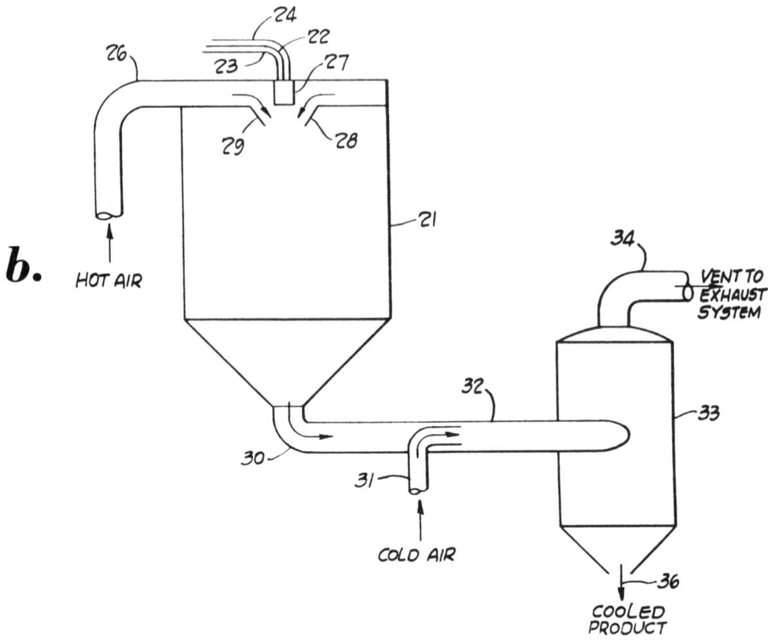

(a) Cross section nozzle tip assembly
(b) Vertical cross section of spray dryer

Source: U.S. Patent 3,949,096

A pair of peripheral passages **16** and **17** (180° opposed and small in diameter) convey the surface coating dispersion through exterior casing **18** and discharge it as a spray into the zone of atomized condiment-containing dispersion. There can be additional such peripheral passages, generally opposed to each other and tending to intersect if unimpeded into a conical pattern looking down, but when the nozzle is in full operation, the surface coating dispersion is atomized quite thoroughly and additional such streams of surface coating dispersion tend to make more perfect coatings on the core particles rich in condiment. Lagging **19** insulates the nozzle assembly from substantial heat loss. Obviously, more than one kind of surface coating dispersion can be used for the coating spray, each projected from a different spraying outlet.

Figure 5.2b shows a typical spray dryer for this process schematically in vertical cross-sectional elevation. Shell **21** (the heating zone) is composed of a vertical cylindrical body with a tapered base. Hot air is fed into line **26** and is at a suitable temperature and flow rate for drying at least the surface coating dispersion that coats the spray particles of condiment-containing dispersion. Typically, the hot air will range in temperature from about 200° to 400°F. Hot air from line **26** enters shell **21** through passages defined by louvers **28** and **29**, which louvers are positioned for causing the hot air and coated particles to swirl in and down through the heating zone **21**. Condiment-containing dispersion enters the apparatus through line **22** along with an atomizing flow of air through line **23** and surface coating dispersion through line **24**. These are discharged inwardly into shell **21** through nozzle **27**, typically a nozzle such as that shown in Figure 5.2a.

The surface coating dispersion dries as the particles flow cocurrently with the hot air in the heating zone. The current of suspended particles (typically at 100° to 200°F) is discharged through outlet **30** located at the tapered base of shell **21** and is mixed in chilling zone **32** with a flow of cold air which enters the chilling zone through inlet **31**. The spent gas and entrained cooled particles pass from chilling zone **32** into cyclone separator **33** wherein the cooled product is seprated from the spent gas. Cooled product is discharged through outlet **36** located at the base of the separator and collected. Spent gas is withdrawn through vent outlet **34** located at the top of the separator and passed to a conventional exhaust system (not shown).

Additionally the product can be dried further and/or cooled by gas fluidization. The spray dryer can be operated under superatmospheric or subatmospheric pressure, although atmospheric pressure whenever feasible is preferred for efficiency and economy.

Example: Referring to Figure 5.2b, a molten blend of 10% five-fold orange oil and 90% of a 50% sucrose solution in water is introduced through line **22** at the rate of 100 ml/min and temperature of 145°F. 3 scfm (measured at 760 mm Hg and 70°F) of air at 70°F passes through line **23**. Edible shellac solution (10% in ethanol) passes through line **24** at the rate of 400 ml/min. These liquid flows are atomized in nozzle **27**, the nozzle having a tip such as that described in connection with Figure 5.2a. The net spray is directed downwardly and cocurrently into a flow of hot air (350°F) entering shell **21** through louvers **28** and **29** at a rate of about 67 scfm.

This rate is adjusted in response to maintaining temperature of 200°F sensed by a thermocouple positioned on the central axis of the shell **21** inches below the nozzle tip. The current of suspended particles is discharged through outlet **30** at temperature of about 100°F and is mixed in chilling zone **32** with a flow of cold air (135 scfm) at essentially atmospheric pressure, 40°F and 10% relative humidity, which enters the chilling zone through inlet **31**. The spent air and entrained cooled particles, essentially at 80°F, pass from chilling zone **32** into cyclone separator **33** wherein the cooled product is separated from the spent air.

The cooled, dry product, about 20 micron average particle size, is discharged through outlet **36** located at the base of the separator and collected. The spent gas is withdrawn through vent outlet **34** located at the top of the separator and passed to an exhaust system. The product is appreciably coated with sucrose enrobing a core rich in orange oil.

OTHER FOOD PRODUCTS

Chewing Gum with Surface Impregnated Microencapsulated Flavor Particles

F. Witzel; U.S. Patent 3,962,463; June 8, 1976; assigned to Life Savers, Inc. found that chewing gum having an immediate, high level of flavor with a substantially lessened amount of flavoring ingredient is obtained by impregnating or depositing solid flavor particles, preferably microencapsulated flavor particles or flavors sorbed on an edible substrate on the surface of the gum. The interior of the gum which will preferably be in the form of a stick, is substantially free of flavor particles, although, if desired, the interior of the gum may include flavoring as well.

The solid flavor particles are deposited or impregnated on the surface of the gum which will ordinarily have a thickness ranging from 1,250 to 2,300 microns and usually 1,750 to 1,800 microns in such a manner that the solid particles penetrate the gum surface to a depth of at most within the range of from 35 to 230 microns or a penetration of at most about 10%, and preferably from 36 to 42 microns. Accordingly, it is apparent that the flavor particles do not penetrate the surface of the gum stick to any substantial degree and thus the interior of the gum can be substantially free of flavor particles.

The solid flavor particles will be applied to the surface of the gum stick so as to provide an amount of flavor of from 0.14 to 0.54% (preferably from 0.14 to 0.45% by weight) of the gum stick. In this manner, the gum will have a pleasing initial burst of flavor which will last a substantial period of time. Chewing gum sticks are normally flavored at a level of about 0.9% by weight.

Thus, the amount of flavoring employed in the gum in accordance with the process will be anywhere from 40 to 85% less than that employed in prior gum to produce the same level of taste for the same period of time.

The flavoring ingredient is microencapsulated in gelatin, waxes, polyethylene and the like, and printed on the surface of the gum as an aqueous slurry. The encapsulation is effected in conventional manner by blending the liquid flavoring with a concentrated aqueous solution of gelatin at a temperature below about 25°C whereby a very fine, stable emulsion is formed. The emulsion, preferably after treatment to impart moisture resistance, is spray dried while still cool, thereby producing a fine free-flowing powder each particle of which consists of a core of flavoring surrounded by a dry gelatin wall. The particles may vary in size from about 1 to 100 microns, preferably from 1 to 50 microns.

Example: A peppermint flavor chewing gum is prepared from the following ingredients: 21.6 parts by weight gum base, 18.0 parts by weight corn syrup (44°Bé), 60.4 parts by weight powdered sugar, and 0.2 part by weight lecithin.

The melted gum base (temperature 2502°F) is placed in a standard dough mixer equipped with sigma blades. The corn syrup and lecithin are added and mixed for 5 minutes. Powdered sugar is added and mixed another 5 minutes. The gum is discharged from the kettle, cut into 25-lb loaves and allowed to cool to 90° to 120°F. It is then rolled to a thickness of 0.178 cm on a standard Gimpel machine and scored into strips 7.26 cm wide and 41.9 cm long. After cooling 12 to 18 hours, the gum is ready for the printing operation.

The gum is then fed into a printing machine equipped with gravure cylinders and printed with an aqueous slurry of microencapsulated flavor particles on both top and bottom. The aqueous flavor slurry has an actual peppermint oil content of 15.6%. The printing operation is conducted on a modified breaking machine. The machine automatically discharges from a cartridge, slabs of gum 7.26 cm wide and 41.9 cm long at a speed of 270 slabs per minute. The gum is fed between two gravure printing cylinders set at approximately 0.127 cm for gum rolled to a thickness of 0.178 cm. Each cylinder has about 69 lines or cells/cm. The top cylinder has a cell depth of from 38 to 42 microns and a cell wall (distance between parallel cells) of 25 microns. The bottom cylinder has a cell depth of from 36 to 38 microns and a cell wall of 20 to 25 microns. The flavor capsules containing 80% flavor are thus impregnated onto the gum. After passing through the cylinders, the gum stick is about 0.142 cm in thickness and contains about 0.14% by weight flavor deposited on the surfaces thereon; the flavor capsules penetrate one surface to 38 to 42 microns and the other surface to 36 to 38 microns.

Frosted Coating of Encapsulated High Intensity Sweetener for Breakfast Cereal

High intensity sweeteners such as the dipeptide sweetener L-aspartyl-L-phenylalanine methyl ester, i.e., APM, and similar lower alkyl esters of aspartyl-phenylalanine have been proposed as sweetening compounds to be applied to the surface of ready-to-eat breakfast cereals and like comestibles.

Such dipeptide sweeteners as methyl ester (APM) have a sweetening power 150 to 200 times that of sucrose and therefore must be applied as a uniform dispersion in order to dilute sweetness impact. Uneven application of such dipeptide sweeteners can result in the oral sensation of hot spots of high sweetness intensity which may linger.

H.R. Schade, P.A. Baggerly and D.R. Woods; U.S. Patent 4,079,151; March 14, 1978; assigned to General Foods Corporation provide a coating method which readily produces a pseudo-crystalline frosted appearance on comestibles, the coating containing a high intensity sweetener as the primary source of sweetening.

This is accomplished by spraying a liquid coating of dextrin or like encapsulating solid and the high intensity sweetener in solution while causing the droplets thereof to undergo partial evaporation incident to the process of transfer from the spray source onto the cereal or other comestible base, which evaporation continues during a progression of successive applications of the spray droplets as discrete microcapsules. The moieties of coating solution thereby accumulate upon one another and result in the foamy coating which will eventually dry to provide a frosted appearance as well as a uniform sweetness application to a comestible base.

A typical application employs a heated coating reel wherein the comestible is tumbled, successive quantities of droplets of the coating composition being thereby successively applied either in a batch or in a continuous manner. Indeed, tumbling is thought to be a preferred means for maximizing a pseudo-crystalline appearance; tumbling of the foam coated particles abrades the drying surface of the foam, thereby increasing the irregular surface and scattering the reflected light.

The encapsulation carrier is ideally a starch hydrolyzate recovered by the acid or enzymatic hydrolysis of an amylaceous substance preferably having a low dextrose equivalency and providing oligosaccharides of elemental monosaccharides and di-, tri-, tetra-, penta- and hexasaccharides which may be of varying dextrose equivalency but commonly would have a DE less than 30 and more preferably less than 20 and of the order of 10 to 20, such as reduces the hygroscopicity of the dextrin carrier coating solid; indeed a dextrin as low as 1 or 2 DE can be used. Advantageously such dextrinous materials even the taste impact generated by the sweetening agent and any inbalance attributable to incomplete solution thereof or nonuniformity of its dispersion.

The coating solution preferably includes 1 to 15% of a vegetable oil or like triglyceride which controls uptake of milk and moisture generally whereby the base product will retain sweetness and crispness and have a limitation on the imbibition of water either incident to consumption or to packaging.

A coating solution is prepared containing 55.6% maltodextrin (Frodex 15 DE), 0.4% spray dried flavor, 10.0% vegetable oil, 0.7% APM dipeptide and 33.3% water. After dry blending the dextrin, flavor and APM, water is added and blended well at a low speed with a Hobart whip. This is followed by a high speed blend for two minutes to evenly distribute ingredients. Whip speed is reduced and the vegetable oil is added. The composition containing the vegetable oil is blended at high speed for an additional minute to evenly emulsify the oil and generate moderate overrun.

In a batch coating apparatus, approximately 5 lb of conventional gun-puffed ready-to-eat breakfast cereal dough particles that have been preheated to about 175°F, broadly 150° to 225°F, are inserted into the coating reel and 3 lb of the coating solution are sprayed (nozzle pressure 50 to 80 psig) thereon over a period of 12 to 15 minutes. With continued constant rotation, the foam structure is developed on the surface of the puffs.

After development of the foam structure, the coated product is then further dried at 170°F drying air temperature for 15 minutes to remove additional moisture from the product to a final moisture content of 1.5%, broadly 1 to 6%, preferably 4.5%. The finished dipeptide sweetened product yields a frosted appearance and a sweetness profile similar to sucrose-sweetened frosted ready-to-eat cereals.

Microcapsules produced by the high pressure spray system and deposited on the cereal puff as discrete moieties are caused to be more-or-less localized in place of the surface with minimum migration, if any, to the interior of the comestible. To effect this functionality, the concentration of the solvent for the coating solution will be a factor; it is estimated that in those coating solutions which are predominantly composed of dextrin that an aqueous solvent will be significantly evaporated incident to transfer from the point of origin of the droplets to the point of their application. Other solvents than water may be employed such as alcohols.

A practical upper limit for solvent temperature will be about 200°F; temperatures above 200°F are believed to involve a risk of degradation and loss of functionality and development of undesired by-product, i.e., the temperature of formation of the L-aspartic acid derivative itself.

Size of the spray coating droplet will play some part in ability to effectively evaporate the solvent for the coating solution. With finer microcapsules the opportunity for maximal evaporation will be afforded and, hence, a high pressure spray system is preferably employed.

In general, in the finished food the total sweetener solids will be a very minor weight percent of the coating solids and generally range from 0.1 to 1.5% by weight thereof, the range being dependent upon organoleptic considerations and not being critical.

Storage Stable Premixed Batter Containing Encapsulated Leavening Agent

According to *W.M. Selenke; U.S. Patent 4,022,917; May 10, 1977* storage stable aqueous batters are provided for use in the preparation of leavened culinary products. To the batter is added a quantity of powdered edible acid sufficient to maintain the pH at an acid level below about 5 to inhibit microbial growth.

Particles of alkaline leavening agent, encapsulated in a water-insoluble coating are also added to the batter. The alkaline leavening agent is capable of dispersing in the batter ingredients at a cooking temperature safely above the storage temperature to release the leavening agent into the acid batter mixture, thereby neutralizing the acid, and leavening the product. The batter premixture is storable with preservation against microbial growth, and the acid-base leavening system isolated to avoid prereaction prior to preparing a leavened product. The entire mixture is packaged in a pressurized watertight can.

The encapsulated microspheres of the leavening agent are illustrated in Figure 5.3a. The leavening agent itself is typically in the form of a powdered substance **21**, most commonly sodium bicarbonate. The leavening agent **21** is formed into small pellets **22**, preferably through the use of a bonding agent **23**. The bonded pellets **22** of the leavening agent **21** are then coated in a waterproof but meltable or heat-dispersible coating substance **24**. The coating **24** prevents reaction of leavening material with the ingredients of the batter until the material **24** is melted or dispersed upon the cooking of the batter so that the leavening agent **21** is then released into the batter.

The bonding agent **23** and the coating **24** may be of the same substance or may be of different substances. Preferably, at least one of these substances is composed of a fat which will contribute to one of the ordinarily required ingredients of the batter, that of the shortening or oil. Normally, however, the oil or shortening substance in a batter is of a melting point of approximately 50° to 110°F which is not sufficiently high to ensure that the coating will not melt or disperse during storage temperatures which may be encountered. Therefore, a higher melting point fat, such as FIX-X (Procter & Gamble) having a melting point of approximately 140°F, is preferred for the outer coating.

Whereas the bonding agent may also be composed of this substance, it may be suitable merely to pelletize the leavening agent under pressure or to bond it with a lower melting point fat. The latter is preferable in that it contributes to a quicker disbursement of the leavening agent into the batter upon cooking.

The reason that the entire microsphere is preferably not of the high melting point fat is that when such a high melting point fat substance is employed in a batter in high percentages, a noticeable aftertaste results in the product which it is desirable to avoid.

Figure 5.3b is a block diagram illustrating the method of preparation of the batter.

Figure 5.3: Storage Stable Premixed Batter Containing Encapsulated Leavening Agent

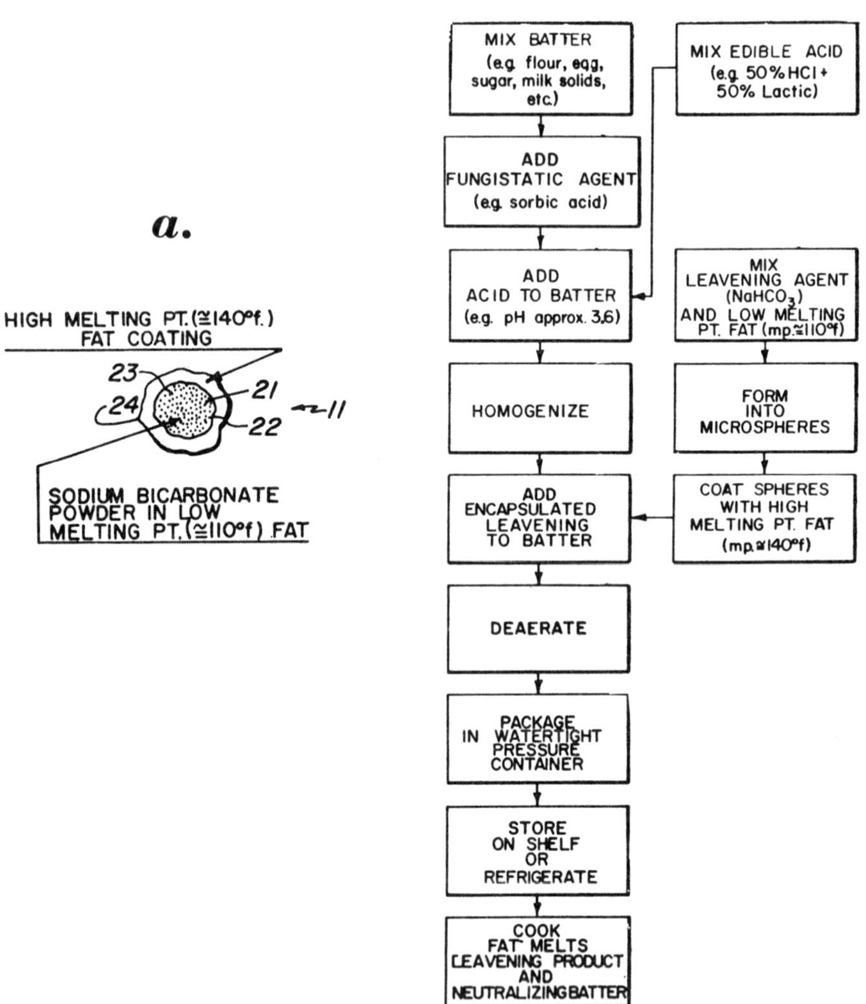

(a) Encapsulated microspheres of leavening agent
(b) Block diagram of process

Source: U.S. Patent 4,022,917

Example: The following ingredients were mixed in a conventional mixer to form a smooth batter having a 24 hour pH of about 3.8.

Flour	150 g
Sugar	8 g
Nonfat dry milk	14 g
Liquid vegetable oil	13 g
Water	190 g
Egg (1)	50 g
Vinegar (5% acidity)	4 g
Concentrated HCl (12 N)	1.2 cc
Sorbic acid	0.316 g
Lactic acid	1.2 g
Polyoxyethylene sorbitan monooleate	0.2 cc

Separately, a leavening agent of $NaHCO_3$ was encapsulated by first mixing 1 part by weight of the $NaHCO_3$ powder with 1 part by weight of Crisco to form a uniform suspension of powder in the Crisco. Then, the resulting mixture was broken up into small particles on the order of 1/16 to 1/8 inch. The particles were quickly dipped in a FIX-X fat bath heated at about 150°F to coat them with the fat, after which the coated particles were solidified by dipping in dilute aqueous solution of polyoxyethylene sorbitan monooleate. The resultant particles each representatively comprised about 1 part by weight each of the $NaHCO_3$, Crisco and FIX-X.

Upon blending the above batter with 9.4 g of the encapsulated leavening agent, the mixture exhibited room and refrigeration storage stability for 3 months. Furthermore, after frying the batter-leavening agent mix at a temperature in the order of about 400°F pancakes were prepared having a leavening comparable to freshly prepared batter and quite acceptable taste. Final pH of the prepared pancakes closely approximated 5.5 which was an entirely acceptable level similar to fresh pancakes. The pH of the cooked pancakes was determined by mixing the cooked pancakes with water to disperse the ingredients and measuring the aqueous mixture with a pH measuring apparatus.

ANIMAL FEED SUPPLEMENT

Containing Encapsulated Lipid

T.W. Scott and G.D.L. Hills; U.S. Patent 4,073,960; February 14, 1978; assigned to Commonwealth Scientific and Industrial Research Organization, Australia found that improved ruminant milk and meat products are formed by feeding ruminant animals prior to slaughter or milking a feed supplement comprising lipid encapsulated by a protein-aldehyde reaction product which protects the lipid from degradation in the rumen and allows the dietary lipid to digest in the abomasum and lower gut and become assimilated by the ruminant animal. When, the dietary lipid is unsaturated, e.g., polyunsaturated vegetable oil, the resulting meat and milk products are correspondingly high in unsaturated lipid content.

Example: (a) Acid precipitated casein (30% by weight) was dissolved in water, using a colloid mill as the mixer and with sufficient addition of NaOH to bring the pH to approximately 6.8. Safflower oil (to give a 1:1 lipid/protein ratio) and a dodecyl gallate emulsifying agent (0.1% by weight of oil) were mixed with the casein solution by a second passage through the colloid mill and emulsification completed in a two-stage homogenizer allowing air-entrainment. After heating to about 70°C, the emulsion was spray dried to form particles which were then sprayed down the inside of a column through a fine mist of formalin; the input of formalin was controlled to supply formaldehyde at the rate of 4 to 5% (on a protein basis), the product being collected from the base of the column. A second feed supplement was prepared in the same way using linseed oil instead of safflower oil.

The feed supplement particles produced in this way are hollow spheres (10 to 60 μ in diameter) the shell of which comprises a matrix of casein crosslinked with formaldehyde which completely encases discrete globules (0.1 to 4.0 μ in diameter) of safflower oil or linseed oil.

(b) As an in vitro test, samples of the products were incubated anerobically at 38°C with strained rumen fluid obtained from a sheep which had been fasted for at least 12 hours. The degree of hydrogenation of the polyunsaturated acids was determined by comparing the proportion of these acids present in the mixtures before and after incubation; separate incubations were carried out to provide samples for analysis at several time periods up to 20 hours from start of incubation. Control incubations using non-formaldehyde-treated particles were carried out to assess the hydrogenating capacity of the rumen fluid. The results of these tests indicate that in particles which would otherwise suffer substantially complete hydrogenation of polyunsaturated fatty acid content within 5 hours, the polyunsaturated fatty acids are not significantly hydrogenated after 20 hours when the particles have been treated with formaldehyde.

(c) Feeding tests show that the linoleic acid content of cow's milk can be raised from 2 to 25% when the animals are fed the safflower supplement. After the control period, the cows were fed the supplement at the rate of 500 g/day (as 5% of a basal diet of lucerne and oats) for 1 week and thereafter until 6½ weeks at 1,000 g/day (10% of basal diet). When the supplement was replaced by non-formaldehyde particles after 6½ weeks the linoleic acid content of the milk fat declined to about 5% within 1 week.

More dramatic results are obtained by feeding the supplement at higher rates, for example, when fed the feed supplement of (a) at a higher level of 15 to 20% of the basal diet the linoleic acid content of the milk fat of cows and goats was observed to rise to 35 to 38% within 48 hours from start of feeding. Not only is the polyunsaturated fatty acid content of milk fat increased by use of the feed supplements, but also there is a significant increase in milk fat production.

LAUNDRY PRODUCTS

BLEACHES

Encapsulated Granulated Laundry Bleaching Agent

L.R. Mazzola; U.S. Patent 4,126,717; November 21, 1978; U.S. Patent 4,078,099; March 7, 1978; and U.S. Patent 4,136,052; January 23, 1979; all assigned to Lever Brothers Company provides a method for preparing encapsulated chlorine granules having a delayed release providing high effective levels of chlorine at both high and low temperatures, and minimal fabric color damage.

When using an active chlorine bleach, the coating involves a first nonreactive coat which separates the active chlorine-containing compound from the second or time control coat. A second or time control coat, including the material having inverse solubility, is then applied over the protective or first coat. In this way materials which may react with the encapsulate can be utilized.

In addition to the second or time control coat, a third coating can be used to further improve the coherency of the coating, and to increase the amount of time necessary for the coating to release the active chlorine-containing agents. The first coating is a combination of a fatty acid and preferably a microcrystalline wax. The second coating is a combination of a fatty acid with material which exhibits inverse solubility with respect to temperature. This provides for a greater release of the encapsulate in cold water than in hot water.

By this means, sufficient delayed release is provided in hot water to prevent pinholing. These materials may be, for example, Pluronic surfactants (Wyandotte Chemical Co.), i.e., a condensation product of polyoxypropylene and polyoxyethylene. In addition to this, a wax can be used in the second coating. The third coating, if desired, can be a fatty acid in combination with a wax.

If a compound is used as the encapsulate which is substantially nonreactive as compared to chlorinating agents, then the first protective coat can be eliminated and the second or time release coat can be utilized directly covering the encapsulate. If in addition, color damage is of no concern, then a material which is simply soluble in water and miscible with the other coating components can be substituted for the materials possessing inverse solubility. This still provides a significant benefit in that release of the encapsulate is substantially temperature independent since the water-soluble material is leached from the coating causing coating breakdown followed by release of the encapsulate.

Substantially nonreactive materials which will benefit from the encapsulation are oxygen-releasing bleaches, such as, for example, sodium percarbonate, sodium perborate, as well as reducing bleaches such as sodium bisulfite. In addition, other materials which can benefit from controlled release may also be utilized.

Generally, the total coating will be 45 to 55% by weight of the total particle. The minimum that can be used is about 35%. The maximum, of course, is not critical except that the coating will be too costly if an excess is used. The amounts of the various layers considered as a percentage by weight of the total encapsulated particle are as follows.

Three Coat System: Layer One – About 5 to 15%, preferably about 8 to 12%. The components of layer one are present in the layer in the following amounts: fatty acid, about 82 to 98% by weight of layer one, preferably about 85 to 95% by weight; and microcyrstalline wax, about 2 to 18% by weight of layer one, preferably about 5 to 15% by weight.

Layer Two – About 25 to 40%, and preferably about 30 to 35%. The components of layer two are present in the layer in the following amounts: fatty acid, about 16 to 86% by weight of layer two, preferably about 45 to 76% by weight; microcrystalline wax, about 0.5 to 16% by weight of layer two, preferably about 3 to 12% by weight; and inverse solubility material, about 12 to 80% by weight of layer two, preferably about 20 to 47% by weight.

In layer two, the amount of the material having inverse solubility is about 5 to 20%, and preferably about 7 to 14% of the total encapsulate weight.

Layer Three – About 5 to 15%, and preferably about 8 to 12%. The components of layer three are present in the layer in the same relative amounts as in layer one above.

Two Coat System: Layer One – About 15 to 25%, preferably about 18 to 20%. The components of layer one are present in the layer in the same relative amounts as in layer one of the three coat system above.

Layer Two – About 30 to 40%, preferably about 32 to 38%. The components of layer two are present in the layer in the following amounts: fatty acid, about 27 to 86% by weight of layer two, preferably about 48 to 78% by weight; microcrystalline wax, about 0.5 to 16% by weight of layer two, preferably about 3 to 12% by weight; and inverse solubility material, about 12 to 67% by weight of layer two, preferably about 18 to 44% by weight.

In layer two, the amount of inverse solubility material is about 5 to 20%, preferably about 7 to 14% of the total encapsulate weight.

One Coat System: About 35 to 55%, preferably about 45 to 50%. This layer has about 5 to 20%, and preferably about 7 to 14% of the total encapsulate weight of the material exhibiting inverse solubility. The components of this layer are present in the layer in the following amounts: fatty acid, about 35 to 89% by weight, preferably 59 to 82% by weight; microcrystalline wax, about 1 to 16% by weight, preferably 3 to 13% by weight; and inverse solubility material about 9 to 57% by weight, preferably 14 to 31% by weight.

Among the chlorine-releasing or active chlorine-containing substances suitable as encapsulates, there may be mentioned those oxidants capable of having their chlorine liberated in the form of free elemental chlorine under conditions normally used for detergent bleaching purposes. Sodium dichloroisocyanurate, typical of the cyanurates suitable as core substances, is commercially available (Monsanto Chemical Company).

Encapsulated particles of chlorine-releasing agent prepared in accordance with the process find utility in mixture with particulate detergent compositions having therein anionic and/or anionic detergent species.

Example 1: Preparation – Encapsulated chlorine bleach was prepared with the following composition.

	Percent
Sodium dichloroisocyanurate dihydrate	47.0
Coat 1:	
Emersol 150*	7.5
Witco X-145A**	0.83
Coat 2:	
Emersol 150	22.17
Witco X-145A	2.5
Pluronic F-127***	10.0
Coat 3:	
Emersol 150	9.0
Witco X-145A	1.0

*Stearic acid, 83%; palmitic acid, 11%; myristic acid, 2%; margaric acid, 2%; pentadecanoic acid, 1%; and oleic acid, 1%

**A microcrystalline wax containing a blend of alkylated naphthenes, isoparaffins and normal paraffins having a MP of 145° to 155°F

***A block copolymer of 80% polyoxyethylene and 20% polyoxypropylene with an approximate MW of 13,330

The first step in preparing a batch of the encapsulated material is to load the batch weight of the sodium dichloroisocyanurate dihydrate into the mixer. The hot air blower is started and the air temperature in the mixer is slowly raised to about 135°F, at which point a portion of Coat 1 is added by a two fluid spray nozzle. With the temperature at or near the melting point of Coat 1, agglomeration of any fines present in the chlorocyanurate occurs. With the air temperature in the mixer lowered below the melting point of Coat 1, the remaining portion of Coat 1 is sprayed. This first coating is also intended to act as a barrier to separate the chlorocyanurate from the Pluronic F-127 in the second coat.

Following addition of Coat 1, the air temperature in the mixer is lowered to 105° to 110°F and Coat 2 is sprayed followed by Coat 3. After spraying Coat 3, the internal air temperature of the mixer is allowed to drop and heat is applied to the outer shell of the mixer to burnish the particles and improve the coherency of the coating.

Evaluation – There was no pinholing. The following chlorine release was observed in wash water after 12 minutes at temperatures indicated

Wash Water Temperature (°F)	Chlorine Release (%)
105	100.0
100	87.8
75	75.0

Storage tests in aluminum-foil-wrapped boxes for 3 months at high humidity indicated no chlorine loss as compared with an unencapsulated bleach-rinse combination, which showed a 24% chlorine loss.

Example 2: An encapsulated oxidizing bleach has the following composition.

	Percent
Sodium perborate	47.00
Coat 1:	
Emersol 150	16.50
Witco X-145A	1.83
Coat 2:	
Emersol 150	22.17
Witco X-145A	2.50
Pluronic F-108*	10.00

*A block copolymer of 80% polyoxyethylene and 20% polyoxypropylene having a molecular weight of approximately 16,250

Example 3: An encapsulated reducing bleach has the following composition.

	Percent
Sodium sulfite	75.0
Coat 1:	
Emersol 150	16.0
Witco X-145A	1.8
Pluronic F-108	7.2

Dual Coated Bleaches

D.S. Alterman and K.W. Chun; U.S. Patent 3,983,254; September 28, 1976 and U.S. Patent 4,124,734; November 7, 1978; both assigned to Lever Brothers Co. found that the problem of insuring complete encapsulation of a particulate material without agglomeration may be solved by applying a solution of a coating substance to a fluidized bed of the particulate material, the nozzle from which the coating substance is sprayed being at a critical height from the bed when in a static state.

The problem of pinholing can be solved or greatly alleviated by applying to the particles of the substance which can cause pinholing (i.e., a substance having at least one reactive chlorine atom in its molecular structure), a first coating of a solidifiable saturated fatty acid, and sequentially applying a second coating of soap by treating the first coating of fatty acid with a solution of a fixed alkali hydroxide selected from the group consisting of sodium hydroxide, potassium hydroxide, and calcium hydroxide.

A preferred product made by the process is encapsulated potassium dichloroisocyanurate in particulate form, the particles having thereon an inner and an outer coating, the inner coating comprising a fatty acid from 12 to 20 carbon atoms or mixtures thereof, and the outer coating comprising a sodium salt of the acid, or mixtures thereof, the particles of potassium dichloroisocyanurate having the inner coating being completely encapsulated by the sodium salt.

Most preferably, the encapsulated particles suitable for bleaching fabrics in an aqueous medium comprise: a core of potassium dichloroisocyanurate; a primary coating contiguous to the core of a fatty acid comprising about 55% palmitic acid and about 45% stearic acid; and an outer coating of the sodium salt of the fatty acid, the primary coating and the outer coating being substantially continuous.

The process for coating particles of an oxidizing material having at least one reactive chlorine atom in its molecular structure comprises the steps of:

(1) placing the particles in such a configuration as to define a layer thereof having a thickness between about ½ inch and 6 inches, on a perforated support;

(2) adjusting the height of a downwardly disposed spraying means capable of producing a spray of liquid droplets in a downwardly diverging pattern to a level such that the outermost droplets of the spray contact the layer of particles at the perimeter thereof as defined by the layer in static state;

(3) causing a gas to flow upward through the perforated support, thereby expanding the thickness of the layer and maintaining the particles in continuous motion to form a fluidized bed;

(4) spraying a solution of a solidifiable fatty acid on the fluidized bed until all particles in the bed are completely coated with the fatty acid;

(5) treating the coated particles with an aqueous solution of a fixed alkali hydroxide selected from the group consisting of sodium hydroxide, potassium hydroxide and calcium hydroxide, and mixtures thereof, thereby reacting the hydroxide with at least a portion of the fatty acid, and completely encapsulating the particles with the reaction product of the fatty acid and the hydroxide, the concentration of the fixed alkali hydroxide in the solution being about 3 to 15% when the fixed alkali is sodium hydroxide, about 10 to 15% when the fixed alkali is potassium hydroxide and about 0.1% when the fixed alkali is calcium hydroxide, by weight of the solution.

It is critical to control the spray pattern and to use supplemental tangential air so as to insure adequate movement and circulation of all the particles during fluidization and as a result to achieve a complete and continuous coating on all the particles. A suitable spray nozzle is a Sprayco No. 26 nozzle (Spraying Systems Co.). This nozzle contains six holes in the atomizing head.

Figure 6.1: Fluidized Bed Apparatus for First Coating

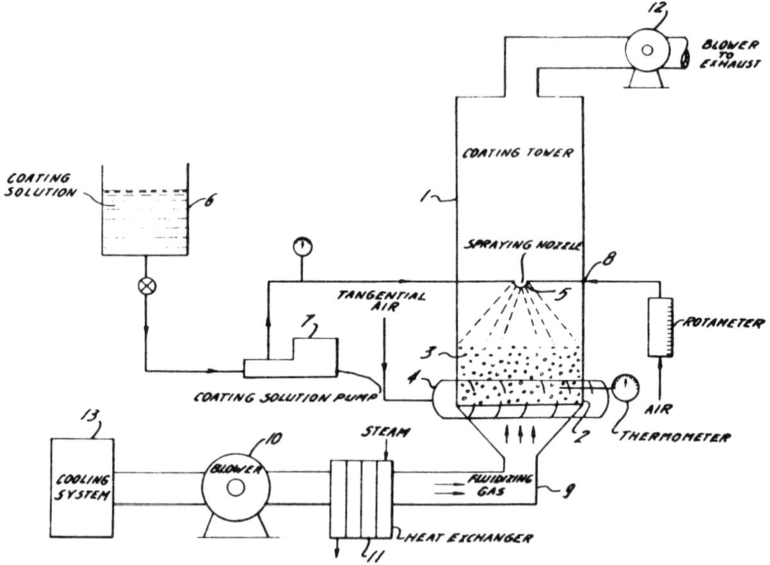

Source: U.S. Patent 3,983,254

Example 1: Dual Coating Process – (Described with reference to Figure 6.1) 13 pounds of extra coarse grade potassium dichloroisocyanurate are charged onto the perforated plate of the cylindrical coating tower **1**. The perforated plate is a 60-mesh stainless steel screen. The particles are fluidized and suspended by an upwardly moving air stream supplied by blower **10**. The superficial air velocity of the fluidizing air stream is 8.5 feet per second. The temperature of the air is maintained at 95° ± 2°F, by heat exchanger **11**.

The primary coating solution is prepared by dissolving triple-pressed stearic acid (about 45% stearic acid) in methylene chloride to form a 20% solution. A small amount of ultramarine blue is dissolved in the coating solution for subsequent use in observing the continuity of the primary coating.

The primary coating solution is sprayed on the fluidized particles **3**, through nozzle **5**, appropriately adjusted as to height. Nozzle **5** has six orifices disposed to provide the desired diverging spray pattern. An auxiliary stream of air is applied to the fluidized bed through nine nozzles horizontally disposed at the perforated support screen level with the tips of the nozzles placed close to the inner wall of the tower.

The air leaves these nozzles in a horizontal path substantially tangential to the wall of the tower. It is the function of this tangential air to assist in keeping in motion the particles at the outer periphery of the plate which do not obtain the full effect of the fluidizing air.

The coating solution is applied to the fluidized particles for a period of two hours. The weight of the coating is about equal to the weight of the original particles. The coated particles are of uniform blue color and size with substantially no agglomeration, and are dry and free-flowing. When some of the coated particles are left immersed for two days in an acidified potassium iodide solution, no color change is observed, indicating complete encapsulation of the particles.

The second coating is applied in the following manner. A 5.2% sodium hydroxide solution is prepared by diluting 60 g of 50% NaOH solution with 520 g of distilled water in a 2 liter beaker. The dilute solution is heated to 110°F in a water bath and 200 g of the particles coated as described above are placed in the NaOH solution and gently agitated for 30 minutes, maintaining the temperature of the solution between 105° and 110°F. The molar ratio of NaOH to fatty acid is 2:1.

After the 30 minute treatment, the solution is decanted through a 25-mesh stainless steel screen, and the particles on the screen are dried at room temperature for 24 hours. The particles are free-flowing and white, indicating complete covering of the blue-colored first coat. The single- and double-coated particles are tested for ease of chlorine release and for adverse effect on cloth in the following manner.

Six pounds of white cotton fabric are placed in a top-loading automatic washing machine. Three swatches of blue denim cloth and one swatch of black 65/35 Dacron/cotton cloth, each measuring 12" x 12" are placed on top of the cotton cloth in circular configuration. Next there is placed directly on the fabric 3.4 ounces of a detergent-bleach composition containing 8.0% of the encapsulated material prepared as above.

Water at a temperature of 132°±3°F is run directly on the detergent-bleach composition for about 150 seconds to a volume of 17.4 gallons. The wash solution is agitated for 10 minutes, and the fabrics are examined. The results are shown in the table below where (A) is about 45% stearic acid and 55% palmitic acid, MP 131° to 132°F; (B) is 95% palmitic, 4% stearic, 1% myristic acids, MP 138° to 144°F; and (C) is about 70% stearic acid and 30% palmitic acid, MP 138.5° to 143°F. The pinholing rating is as follows: 0 = none (excellent); 1 = minimal pinholing (acceptable); 2 = severe pinholing (unacceptable); and 3 = very severe pinholing (unacceptable).

From the data in the table, it may be seen that a single coating of fatty acid is inadequate to accomplish the dual purpose of providing a high chlorine release and at the same time avoid pinholing. It will be noted that fatty acid (A), having a melting point below the temperature of the wash water, melts to release all of the chlorine in the encapsulated material, but causes pinholing, due to contact of the encapsulated material with the fabric upon the melting of the fatty acid coating.

Fatty acids (B) and (C), having melting points above the temperature of the wash water, are unsatisfactory, since they do not allow a sufficient release of chlorine to be of any value as a bleach, although the low level of chlorine release prevents pinholing.

Bleach Composition KDC Coated with	Available Chlorine (%)	Pinholing (blue denim)	Chlorine Released (%)
Single coat of fatty acid			
Fatty acid (A)	35.0	3	97-100
Fatty acid (B)	37.5	0	20
Fatty acid (C)	39.0	1	41.5
Dual coat (second coating)*			
2.85% NaOH, 10 min	21.03	2	not determined
5.34% NaOH, 30 min	23.19	1	69.83
10.33% NaOH, 30 min	26.15	1	87.70

*First coating performed with fatty acid (A).

Referring to the above data, it will be observed that a dual coating applied in accordance with the process prevents pinholing to a substantial extent and additionally allows an adequate release of chlorine.

Encapsulated Diperisophthalic Acid

D.A. Stewart, B.D. Ricketts and C.H. Hoelscher; U.S. Patent 4,094,808; June 13, 1978; assigned to PPG Industries, Inc. are concerned with an organic peracid formulation in the form of an encapsulated core having a high rate of solution in aqueous media. The core comprises particles of a solid organic peracid in admixture with particles of a material substantially more water-soluble than the organic peracid as dispersing agent.

The core is essentially completely encapsulated with a water-dispersible encapsulating material capable, in the absence of free water, of preventing contact of the peracid with substances which cause its decompositions, e.g., alkalis. Water-dispersible encapsulating agents are those materials which distribute when placed in water either by dissolution or otherwise.

The core of the bleaching formulation has, as its essential ingredients organic peracid and dispersing agent. Organic peracids containing greater than 3 wt % active oxygen are preferred. Typically, perphthalic acids, such as mono- and diperphthalic, perisophthalic and perterephthalic acid are used with diperisophthalic acid being the preferred species. The diperisophthalic acid (DPI) may be either tabular habit or acicular habit. The formulation is especially useful when the peracid is only sparingly soluble in water, i.e., less than about 3% by weight. If desired, more than one organic peracid may be used, for example, a mixture of DPI and diperazelaic acid.

The dispersing agent may be one or a mixture of materials which are substantially more soluble in water than is the peracid. By substantially more soluble in water is meant having at least twice and preferably five times the solubility in water at 15°C. Those compositions which dissolve in water to the extent of at least 1 g/100 g of water at 15°C are useful as dispersing agents. Those agents soluble in water to the extent of 4 to 200 g/100 g of water at 15°C are preferred. The core particle containing the peracid and dispersing agent may contain from about 1 to 90% by weight of the dispersing agent. Typically, the core will contain from 2 to 75% dispersing agent with an amount of from 5 to 60% being preferred. A core composition is prepared by combining particles of the organic peracid with particles of dispersing agent. Preferably the organic peracid and dispersing agent are admixed in a manner such that they are evenly dispersed with each other. The mixing of organic peracid and dispersing agent is advantageously performed in an aqueous media.

The water-dispersible encapsulating layer surrounding the core is a substance which in the absence of free water prevents the core's contact with substances capable of causing decomposition of the contained peracid. Preferably the encapsulating layer contains a hydrated salt which retains water of hydration below 30°C, but gives up at least part of its water of hydration below the decomposition temperature of the peracid. Those hydrated salts which give up at least part of their water of hydration below 150°C and typically below 120°C are useful.

Hydratable inorganic salts in less than their maximum state of hydration (e.g., $MgSO_4 \cdot H_2O$) are preferred materials to form the encapsulating layer. When a nonhydrated salt is used as the encapsulating material, a binding agent capable of forming a gel when contacted with water is normally combined with the salt.

Use of a binding agent provides a more cohesive coating than would be obtained with the salt alone. Binding agents which may be mixed with encapsulating salt in order to provide a cohesive coating include magnesium aluminum silicate, polyvinyl alcohol, soluble starch, hydroxypropylcellulose, hydroxyethylcellulose, polyvinylpyrrolidone, casein, zein and agar.

Example: Diperisophthalic acid slurries containing less than 5% isophthalic acid were made by dissolving the salt to be used as dispersing agent in deionized water in an amount sufficient to yield the desired concentration of salt when the solution was slurried with a wet cake of diperisophthalic acid. The resulting slurries were homogenized in an electric blender, formed into thin layers between sheets of polyethylene, and quick frozen at dry ice temperatures.

The frozen sheets were broken up, ground, and screened to −18+70 mesh frozen cores. An encapsulating material was prepared by mixing Na_2SO_4 and $MgSO_4 \cdot H_2O$ in ratios of from 1:1 to 9:1. The frozen core particles were encapsulated by contacting them with the salt particles in a heated 3 inch diameter fluid bed. Heated air was used as the fluidizing gas to maintain the temperature at 40° to 45°C.

After a retention time of approximately 15 minutes, the bed contents were screened for 2 minutes on 8 inch diameter screens mounted on a Ro-tap sieve shaker at a loading of approximately 250 g. A product consisting of particles ranging in size from −14 to 30-60 mesh was collected. The samples prepared in this manner, as well as samples of encapsulated diperisophthalic acid containing no dispersing agent, were subjected to dissolution rate studies at 50°C and 20°C.

Dissolution rates were determined as follows. A simulated wash solution was prepared by dissolving 0.15% by weight of a household detergent in tap water. For each test, a 250 ml portion was placed in a 400 ml beaker on a temperature-adjusted stirring hot plate, or in a temperature-adjusted cooling bath, with

Comparison of Dissolution Rates of Encapsulated Diperisophthalic Acid With and Without Core Additives

Dispersing Agent Added to Core	Composition, Basis Encapsulated Product Weight (%): In Core*: Dispersing Agent (%)	In Core*: DPI**	In Core*: IPA***	In Coating: $MgSO_4$	In Coating: Na_2SO_4	In Coating: H_2O	Rate of Dissolution in 0.15% Detergent Solution: Solution Temperature (°C)	Percent of Added DPI Dissolved After Stirring: 15 Seconds	30 Seconds	60 Seconds	120 Seconds
None	0	26.9	1.5	45.2	0	26.3	20	–	13	13	20
							50	–	37	57	85
None	0	14.4	0.8	60.6	0	24.2	20	–	14	17	29
							50	–	46	66	90
Na_2SO_4	4.9	17.5	1.0	25.1	37.7	13.8	20	88	94	96	98
							50	98	99	99	100
Na_2SO_4 +	2.0										
$MgSO_4 \cdot 6H_2O$	1.9	9.8	0.5	22.8	53.2	9.7	20	95	96	98	98
							50	97	99	–	–
$Na_3C_6H_5O_7 \cdot 2H_2O$	3.2	9.0	0.5	24.7	49.2	13.4	20	74	81	97	98
							50	99	100	100	100
$NaH_2PO_4 \cdot H_2O$	3.0	8.5	0.5	24.4	52.8	10.8	20	80	95	98	98
							50	99	100	100	100
$NaHSO_4 \cdot H_2O$	3.2	9.3	0.5	24.4	49.5	13.1	20	87	92	96	100
							50	99	99	100	98
$KHSO_4$	2.8	9.1	0.5	24.5	50.7	12.4	20	87	94	97	98
							50	99	99	100	100
K_2SO_4	2.8	9.1	0.5	24.1	50.5	13.0	20	97	98	99	99
							50	99	99	100	100
Na_2SO_4 +	1.5										
$MgSO_4 \cdot 6H_2O$	2.8	9.7	0.5	24.2	49.8	11.4	20	94	97	98	99
							50	99	99	99	99
Na_2SO_4 +	1.0										
$MgSO_4 \cdot 6H_2O$	0.9	9.5	0.5	24.3	51.7	12.1	20	95	98	99	99
							50	98	99	99	100
Na_2SO_4 +	0.7										
$MgSO_4 \cdot 6H_2O$	1.3	9.0	0.5	24.3	53.0	11.2	20	94	98	98	98
							50	98	99	100	100
Na_2SO_4	7.9	12.8	0.7	25.3	41.3	12.0	20	94	97	98	99
							50	99	99	99	100
$MgSO_4 \cdot 6H_2O$	9.3	17.0	0.9	48.6	0	24.2	20	84	83	84	90
							50	96	99	100	100

*Assumes that all of the dispersing agent remained in the core and that no free water (only water of hydration) remained in the core after encapsulation.

**Diperisophthalic acid.

***Isophthalic acid.

a constant stirring rate provided by a magnetic stirring bar. A quantity of encapsulated diperisophthalic acid sufficient to yield a solution containing 60 parts per million active oxygen was added to the solution and stirred for a given length of time. At the end of the stirring period, the entire solution was quickly filtered through a Buchner funnel and into a flask containing approximately 250 ml of 4.3% H_2SO_4.

The wet filter paper and any residue were added to another flask containing equal amounts of isopropanol and 4.3% H_2SO_4 to dissolve any solids. Both solutions containing the filtrate and the solids were then analyzed for diperisophthalic acid by titration with a $Na_2S_2O_3$ solution. The procedure was repeated for each of several time periods at 50° and 20°C. The preceding table sets out the dissolution rates of encapsulated diperisophthalic acid with and without the presence of additives in the cores.

Encapsulated Calcium Hypochlorite Granules

J.P. Faust; U.S. Patent 3,953,354; April 27, 1976; assigned to Olin Corporation provides granular calcium hypochlorite compositions having materially lowered rates of propagation of decomposition and improved resistance to caking and loss of available chlorine compared with previously available compositions.

This is accomplished when particles of calcium hypochlorite containing less than about 5% by weight of water and at least about 65% by weight of calcium hypochlorite are mixed with an aqueous solution of a water-soluble salt which is nonreactive with and stable to calcium hypochlorite. The water-soluble salt is selected from the group consisting of alkali metal salts, alkaline earth metal salts and mixtures thereof.

When calcium hypochlorite particles of this type are contacted with the aqueous solution, a coating forms on the surface of the calcium hypochlorite particles which is comprised of a mixture of calcium hypochlorite dihydrate and the water-soluble salt. This coating which encapsulates the calcium hypochlorite particles generally ranges from about 5 to 60% by weight of each granule.

The proportion of water-soluble salt in the coating generally ranges from about 0.1 to 15% by weight of each granule. The resulting encapsulated calcium hypochlorite granules resist dusting, caking and decomposition of an exothermic nature. In addition, the calcium hypochlorite composition has improved retention of available chlorine on storage.

Example 1: A solution of 10 g of anhydrous $CaCl_2$ in 10 ml of water was prepared. Approximately 8 ml of this solution was sprayed on 100 g of commercial "HTH" spread out in a thin layer. The mixture was stirred while spraying to give a uniform coating of the granules and to break up any agglomerates. The final product was free-flowing. The coating on each granule was about 18.7%, the calcium hypochlorite dihydrate portion of the coating was about 14.7% and the calcium chloride was about 3.7%. Portions of this product were tested with lighted cigarettes and burning matches, but no self-sustaining reactions occurred.

Example 2: A solution of 10 g of $NaNO_3$ in 10 ml of water was prepared. Five ml of this solution was sprayed onto 95 g of commercial HTH containing

73.5% of available chlorine or about 74% of $Ca(OCl)_2$ spread out in a thin layer. The granules were stirred while spraying to obtain uniform distribution. The coating on each granule was about 11.7%, the calcium hypochlorite dihydrate portion of the coating was about 9.2% and the sodium nitrate was about 2.5%. Portions of this product were tested with lighted cigarettes and burning matches and no self-sustaining reactions took place.

Example 3: A slurry of 57 parts by weight of Microsized salt (NaCl) and 43 parts of water was sprayed on commercial granular HTH with stirring as in the preceding examples. The final product contained 67.5% available chlorine or 67.9% of $Ca(OCl)_2$ and 4.9% of water. For comparison, a sample of commercial granular calcium hypochlorite was sprayed with water to produce a hydrated product containing 9.8% water as described in U.S. Patent 3,544,267.

Neither of these products undergoes any self-sustaining decomposition reaction in contact with lighted cigarettes or burning matches. Both of these products were maintained at 100°C and ambient humidity for 2 hours. At the end of this time, the first product, sprayed with the salt slurry, contained 65.76% of available chlorine and the second product, sprayed with water, contained 60.14% of available chlorine. The latter product was badly caked, but the first product was not. Loss of available chlorine for the first product was 2.58% and for the second product was 14.92%.

FABRIC CONDITIONERS

Antistat/Softener plus Polyamide Encapsulated Melting Point Depressant

In the conventional home laundering process, soiled fabrics are subjected to cleaning with a detergent composition in the main wash cycle and rinsing with water in the final cycle. Optionally, during the rinsing cycle a fabric conditioning composition is added. Such compositions contain a fabric softener or fabric antistat material for imparting to the rinsed fabrics softening and antistat properties. The rinsed fabrics are oftentimes, thereafter, dried in an automatic clothes dryer.

A long-standing problem has been how to deliver the fabric conditioning agents during the rinse cycle and have the benefits retained after the drying operation. Another problem has been the attainment of satisfactory antistat properties on the dried fabrics. A static electric charge develops on fabrics during the tumbling of the fabrics in a clothes dryer. Such a charge is objectionable to the consumer because of difficulty it causes in sorting and folding of the dried fabrics. This is achieved by using an encapsulated fabric antistat/softener.

H.J. Pracht and S.H. Iding; U.S. Patent 4,018,688; April 19, 1977; assigned to The Procter & Gamble Company have developed a process for producing capsules having an outer wall of a polycondensation product formed from a first and a second monomer along an interface and containing as an inner core a fabric antistat/softener material and melting point depressant. Such capsules have a maximum particle dimension of less than 400 μ.

The process comprises the following steps:

(a) melting a fabric antistat/softener material and adding to it a melting point depressant, whereby the melting point depressant is a silicone oil or a nonaromatic alkyl or alkoxy ether free of functional groups which react with the first monomer and is capable of depressing the melting point of the fabric antistat/softener material by at least 5°C when added at a level below 50% based on the fabric antistat/softener material and has a boiling point greater than 30°C;

(b) forming a solution of the melted fabric antistat/softener material and melting point depressant of step (a) with the first monomer;

(c) forming an aqueous solution of the second monomer; and

(d) adding under agitation the solution of step (b) to the solution of step (c) to form the capsules along the interface of the two solutions wherein a degree of stirring is used such that the maximum particle dimension of the capsules so formed is less than 400 μ.

The wall constituent of the capsule is a synthetic resin selected from the polyurethanes, polyamides and polyesters. A polyamide wall constituent is preferred. The fabric antistat/softener material is selected from the group consisting of water-insoluble or water-dispersible quaternary ammonium compound, quaternary imidazolinium salt, diamine compound, sorbitan ester, fatty alcohol, fatty alcohol derivative or mixtures thereof.

The melting point depressant is selected from the group consisting of silicone oils, dimethyl and diethyl ethylene glycol, dimethyl and diethyl propylene glycol, bis(2-ethoxy ethyl)ether, 1,1-dimethoxy ethane, 1,2-dimethoxy ethane, dipropoxy methane and dicyclohexyl ether.

The aqueous solution of the second monomer contains from 0.1 to 10%, preferably 0.5 to 5% of the monomer. To this solution is added the solution of the fabric antistat/softener material, melting point depressant and first monomer. The solutions are added in amounts such that a ratio of the first monomer to the second monomer falls within the range of 2:1 to 1:1, preferably 1.1:1.0. The ratio of polycondensation product to fabric antistat/softener material is from 0.5:10 to 3:10, preferably 1:10 to 1.5:10.

The liquid fabric conditioning compositions consist essentially of about 0.1 to 15%, preferably 0.5 to 2.5% of the capsule component with the balance being water. Conventional liquid fabric conditioning composition components may be dissolved or dispersed in the composition. These conventional components include fabric softening agents, clay materials, emulsifiers, thickeners, opacifiers, coloring agents, brighteners, fluorescers, pH adjustment agents and perfume materials. Such optional materials generally comprise about 0.1 to 10% by weight of the composition.

Preferably the liquid fabric conditioning compositions comprise from 1 to 20% (preferably 3 to 7%) of cationic fabric antistat/softener materials as defined above which has not been encapsulated. It has been found that the addition of the unencapsulated fabric antistat/softener material aids in the deposition of the encapsulated material onto the fabrics. It is believed that the unencapsulated fabric antistat/softener material surrounds the capsules. Accordingly, the positively charged cationic fabric antistat/softener material is attracted to the negatively charged fabrics and carries with it the capsules of this process.

Use of the liquid fabric conditioning composition of the process results in the deposition of the capsules on the surfaces of the fabrics being rinsed. When the fabrics are dried in an automatic clothes dryer, the wall constituent of the capsules ruptures under the influence of heat and friction thereby releasing the fabric antistat/softener material. As a result of this release on the fabric surfaces, the dried fabrics have a very satisfactory antistat benefit imparted to them.

Example 1: The melting point of 128 g ditallowdimethyl ammonium methylsulfate (DTDMAMS) is depressed with 40 ml bis(2-ethoxy ethyl)ether to yield a fluid mixture of about 50°C whereas the DTDMAMS alone is normally fluid at about 60°C. To the fluid solution is added 31.3 g terephthalic acid dichloride.

A second solution of 14.4 g diethylenetriamine, 10.9 g sodium hydroxide and 1,450 ml water is prepared at room temperature. The solution of DTDMAMS is added to the aqueous solution under gentle stirring. Capsules containing the DTDMAMS and bis(2-ethoxy ethyl)ether as an inner core and an outer wall of a polyamide formed from the terephthalic acid dichloride and amine are produced. The capsules have a maximum particle dimension ranging from 20 to 60 μ. Liquid fabric conditioning compositions containing the abovedescribed capsules possess satisfactory antistat control.

Example 2: The capsules of Example 1 are tested for antistat control in the following manner. A 5½ lb test bundle of 53% all cotton, 12% 65/35 polyester/cotton blend, 17% nylon, and 18% Dacron is washed in a washing machine using a normal 38°C cycle. Forty-five grams of a fabric conditioning composition as indicated below is added in the rinse cycle. The test bundle is dried in a clothes dryer and the process repeated to ensure consistent results.

After the second drying, the test bundle is placed in a Faraday Cage connected with a volt meter. The bundle is taken out of the cage fabric by fabric and readings are taken at the beginning and after each fabric is removed. The increments are added up and compared versus values obtained from the compositions tested in the same manner as indicated below. Static readings closer to zero are more satisfactory. The formulations of compositions are shown below.

	Compositions, %			
Component	**A**	**B**	**C**	**D**
Water	100	94.6	93.4	94.6
Ditallowdimethyl ammonium chloride	–	5.2	5.2	–
Capsules of Example 1	–	–	1.2	5.2
Perfume and dye	balance			

The static readings (volts) are as follows: Composition A, 200; Composition B, 50; Composition C, 20; and Composition D, 30. The above results indicate that compositions of this process, i.e., Compositions C and D, possess satisfactory antistat control.

Polyamide Encapsulated Antistat/Softener

H.J. Pracht; U.S. Patent 4,081,384; March 28, 1978; assigned to The Procter & Gamble Company also provides another fabric conditioning composition intended for use in a home laundering operation where a fabric antistat/softener material can be effectively and efficiently applied to fibrous articles. The process produces capsules substantially free of organic solvent having an outer wall of a polycondensation product and containing as an inner core a fabric antistat/softener material. As used herein, substantially organic-solvent free, means that the capsules contain less than 25%, preferably less than 10%, organic solvent. The capsules have a maximum particle dimension of less than 400 μ. The method involves the following:

(a) forming a solution of fabric antistat/softener material and a first monomer capable of forming a polycondensation product along an interface with a second monomer where the first monomer is dissolved in the fabric antistat/softener material;

(b) forming an aqueous solution of the second monomer; and

(c) adding under agitation the solution of step (a) to the solution of step (b) to form the capsules along the interface of the two solutions where a degree of stirring is used such that the maximum particle dimension of the capsules so formed is less than 400 μ.

The preferred capsule wall and fabric antistat/softener material are those described above in U.S. Patent 4,018,688.

Example 1: 8 g of terephthalic acid dichloride are dissolved in 64 g of melted 1-methyl-1-tallowamidoethyl-2-tallowimidazolinium methylsulfate having a temperature of 50°C. The mixture is added slowly to an aqueous solution of 4 g diethylenetriamine and 4.3 g potassium hydroxide in 4,000 ml water under gentle stirring. The aqueous solution has a temperature of 70°C. Capsules having a maximum particle size ranging from 20 to 60 μ are formed instantaneously.

The capsules containing the imidazolinium fabric antistat/softener as an inner core and a polyamide outer wall as a result of polycondensation reaction between the terephthalic acid dichloride and polyvalent amine give satisfactory antistat control when used in a fabric conditioning composition.

Example 2: Capsules having an inner core of N-tallow-N,N',N'-trimethyl-1,3-propane diamine fabric antistat/softener material and a polyurethane outer wall are produced using the process. 0.6 g of hexamethylene diisocyanate are dissolved in 10 g of the melted diamine and added to a stirred aqueous solution of 200 ml water and 5 g bisphenol A. The resultant capsules have a maximum particle dimension ranging from 10 to 60 μ.

Example 3: The capsules of Example 1 are tested for antistat control in the following manner. A 5½ lb test bundle of 53% all cotton, 12% 65/35 polyester/cotton blend, 17% nylon, and 18% Dacron is washed in a washing machine using a normal 38°C cycle. 45 g of a fabric conditioning composition as indicated below is added in the rinse cycle. The test bundle is dried in a clothes dryer and the process repeated to ensure consistent results. After the second drying, the test bundle is placed in a Faraday Cage connected with a volt meter. The bundle is taken out of the cage fabric by fabric and readings are taken at the beginning and after each fabric is removed. The increments are added up and compared versus values obtained from the compositions tested in the same manner as indicated below. Static readings closer to zero are more satisfactory. The formulations of compositions are shown below.

	Compositions, %				
Component	A	B	C	D	E
Water	100	94.6	93.4	92.2	94.6
DTDMAC	–	5.2	5.2	5.2	–
Capsules of Example 1	–	–	1.2	2.4	5.2
Perfume and dye		balance			

The static readings (volts) are as follows: Composition A, 200; Composition B, 50; Composition C, 20; Composition D, 8; and Composition E, 25. The above results indicate that compositions of the process, i.e., Compositions C, D and E, possess satisfactory antistat control.

OTHER

Enzyme-Containing Beads for Use in Detergent

In accordance with the process of *M.H. Win, W.A. DiSalvo and E.J. Kenney; U.S. Patent 4,016,040; April 5, 1977; assigned to Colgate-Palmolive Company* an enzyme-containing preparation is blended with a molten normally solid nonionic detergent and the resulting blend is sprayed into a cool atmosphere to form tiny solidified droplets of the blend. These solidified droplets, or beads, are substantially spherical and despite the soft waxy nature of the nonionic detergent, they flow very easily.

Even when handled mechanically under severe conditions, e.g., when tumbled roughly with built detergent granules, they yield substantially no enzyme-containing dust and keep their identities. Mixtures of these enzyme-containing beads and detergent granules also flow well and have good stability and odor. Although such mixtures may form dust in the air under severe handling, the dust is found to be enzyme-free. The enzyme-containing beads dissolve very rapidly in water, releasing their enzyme content to the wash water quickly (e.g., in water at 40°C).

Preferably, the nonionic detergent is a waxy water-soluble material having a melting point up to about 60°C. In such preferred form, the melting point is at least 45°C, preferably at least 50°C and not above 60°C, and the nonionic detergent contains a hydrophilic polyethylene oxide chain attached to a hydrophobic radical. Particularly suitable types of materials are those which are ethylene oxide adducts of long chain alkanols (e.g., alkanols of about 12 to 20 carbon atoms) or long chain alkyl phenols (e.g., phenols having alkyl side chains of about 8 to 18 carbon atoms).

Preferred enzymes are subtilisin enzymes manufactured and cultivated from special strains of spore-forming bacteria, particularly *Bacillus subtilis*. The blend of nonionic detergent and enzyme concentrate from which the beads of this process are produced may contain an amount of enzyme concentrate such as to give beads containing about 0.1 to 5 Anson units or more per gram. There is substantially no loss of enzyme activity during the formation of the beads, particularly when the temperature of the blend is maintained below 65°C. The blend of molten nonionic detergent and enzyme concentrate may contain, for instance, in the range of about 5 to 50% of enzyme concentrate.

Example: 19 parts of a proteolytic enzyme concentrate (in the form of a dark brown salt-containing fine powder whose enzyme content is 4 Anson units per gram) are mixed with 81 parts of a molten nonionic detergent having a melting point of 48°C (Plurafac A-38) to form a free-flowing liquid slurry, which is then sprayed, at a temperature about 5°C above the melting point of the nonionic detergent and under pressure, through a single fluid nozzle (of standard type, having a small outlet orifice and having, just upstream of the orifice, a stationary four-vaned core which is arranged to impart a swirling motion to the liquid).

During spraying, most of the hot slurry is continuously recirculated from the nozzle to the heated storage vessel from which it is pumped continuously to the nozzle. The spray emerges continuously from the nozzle into a circular tower about 8 feet in diameter and about 40 feet high, to the bottom of which there is supplied a continuous stream of air at a temperature of about 13°C, so that the cool air flows upward into contact with the sprayed droplets, cooling and solidifying them within seconds after they leave the nozzle. The solid beads are collected at the base of the tower. The resulting free-flowing tan beads have the following screen analysis.

Screen Mesh	Opening, mm	Percent Remaining on Screen
10	2.0	0
20	0.84	trace
40	0.42	0.7
60	0.25	33.2
80	0.177	39.8
100	0.149	14.9
200	0.074	11.2
270	0.053	0
325	0.044	0
pan	0.044	0

The dust content of the beads is about 18 ppm. This dust content is determined in a standard manner by permitting a given quantity (50 g) of the beads to fall a predetermined distance (in an enclosed device) onto a base, then immediately putting a cover over the fallen beads and allowing any dust to settle for 10 minutes onto the cover.

To make a laundry detergent for use in the automatic machine washing of clothes, one part of the beads is blended with 99 parts of spray-dried hollow white granules of heavy duty built detergent composition having the following approximate screen analysis.

Screen size	10	20	40	60	80	100	-100
Percent retained	0.2	2.7	29.4	40.4	13.1	6.0	8.2

The enzyme-containing beads are not noticeable to the naked eye in the resulting mixture. The spray-dried granules of the heavy duty built detergent composition have the following approximate overall composition: 10% sodium linear tridecylbenzenesulfonate; 2% of the ethoxylation product made from ethylene oxide and primary alkanols of C_{14-15} chain length, the ethoxylation product containing 11 mols of oxyethylene per mol of alkanol; 2% of sodium soap of a mixture of 3 parts of tallow fatty acids and 1 part of coconut oil fatty acids; about 8.5% of total moisture; 34% of phosphate solids; 7% of sodium silicate solids ($Na_2O:SiO_2$ mol ratio 1:2.35); 0.5% of sodium carboxymethylcellulose; 0.2% of water-soluble polyvinyl alcohol; and the balance sodium sulfate together with small amounts of fluorescent brighteners.

The granules of built detergent composition are prepared by spray-drying a heated aqueous slurry containing the ingredients described and having a solids content of about 60% (i.e., the slurry has a total moisture content of about 40%). This aqueous slurry is prepared by vigorous agitation in a crutcher and is at a temperature of about 60°C; in making the aqueous slurry the phosphate (supplied as a powder of anhydrous pentasodium tripolyphosphate) is added last, just before spraying. Then the aqueous slurry is sprayed into a spray tower to which heated air, at a temperature well above the boiling point of water, is fed to evaporate off the water, in conventional manner.

PRESSURE-SENSITIVE COPYING SYSTEMS

One of the most widespread uses of microcapsules is in certain kinds of pressure-sensitive copying systems. In one such system, usually known as a transfer system, an upper sheet is coated on its lower surface with microcapsules containing a solution of colorless color former, and a lower sheet is coated on its upper surface with a color developing coreactant material, e.g., an acidic clay, a phenolic resin or certain organic salts. For most applications, a number of intermediate sheets are also provided, each of which is coated on its lower surface with microcapsules and on its upper surface with acidic material.

Pressure exerted on the sheets by writing or typing ruptures the microcapsules, thereby releasing the color former solution onto the acidic material on the next lower sheet and giving rise to a chemical reaction which develops the color of the color former. In another such system, usually known as a self-contained system, microcapsules and color developing coreactant material are coated onto the same surface of a sheet of paper, and writing or typing on a sheet placed above the coated sheet causes the capsules to rupture and release the color former, which then reacts with the coreactant material on the sheet to produce a color.

WALL FORMERS

Acrylamide Copolymer Crosslinked by Urea- and Melamine-Formaldehyde Precondensates

D.J. Hasler and T.A. McGhee; U.S. Patent 4,105,823; August 8, 1978; assigned to Wiggins Teape Limited, England provide a method of encapsulating finely divided particulate material to produce microcapsules in which the particulate material is surrounded by polymeric shells, comprising the steps of forming a dispersion of particulate material in an aqueous medium containing a water-soluble urea-formaldehyde precondensate, a water-soluble melamine-formaldehyde precondensate and a water-soluble polymer which is capable of being crosslinked by the precondensates, and condensing the precondensates by acid catalysis with resultant crosslinking of the polymer about the particulate material, forming shells.

The crosslinking action of the precondensates is primarily the result of the presence of methylol groups, but other groups may possibly be involved. The water-soluble polymer preferably contains alcohol, amine, amide, acid or acid derivative groups. Particularly preferred is an acrylamide/acrylic acid copolymer. Capsules made using such a copolymer have been found to be particularly resistant to aging. The urea-formaldehyde precondensate is preferably cationic, and the melamine-formaldehyde precondensate is preferably a methylated melamine-formaldehyde precondensate. Instead of a single precondensate, a mixture of two or more such materials may be used.

The process may be carried out in a number of ways. For example, the urea-formaldehyde precondensate, the melamine-formaldehyde precondensate and the water-soluble polymer may all be present in the aqueous medium before addition of the liquid to be encapsulated, and the acid catalyst may be added subsequently. Alternatively only the urea-formaldehyde precondensate and the water-soluble polymer may be present in the aqueous medium when the liquid to be encapsulated is added. The melamine-formaldehyde precondensate is then added subsequently.

The stage at which acid is added is not crucial. It is preferred that the acid is added once the material to be encapsulated has been added, either before or after addition of the melamine-formaldehyde precondensate. It is of course important that excessive condensation of the precondensates does not occur before the material is added, and that excessive condensation of the urea-formaldehyde precondensate does not occur before addition of the melamine-formaldehyde precondensate, if the latter is added after the acid. Conditions under which such excessive condensation is avoided, are readily determined by experiment.

The optimum pH for the condensation and crosslinking reactions depends to some extent on the precondensates and the water-soluble polymer used. For example, for the preferred acrylamide/acrylic acid copolymer a pH in the range 3.5 to 5.0 is preferred, more preferably 4.0 to 4.5, for example, 4.15. However, for a different polymer, vinyl methyl ether/maleic anhydride copolymer, a pH of 5.0 to 5.5 is preferred.

For minimizing coalescence, the dispersion may be chilled before addition of the melamine-formaldehyde precondensate and before addition of acid for bringing about condensation. Chilling is preferably to below 20° to 15°C. Chilling to any temperature below 30°C has however been found to have some effect.

Acidification may be followed by maintaining the mixture in a warm state, for example, at 55°C for 2 hours. If the melamine-formaldehyde precondensate is added after addition of the material to be encapsulated, without a chilling step, it is preferred to adjust the pH of the dispersion before addition of the melamine-formaldehyde precondensate and then to maintain the dispersion at 55°C for 2 hours after the addition of the melamine-formaldehyde precondensate. Adjustment may be in two stages, one before and the other after addition of melamine-formaldehyde precondensate.

Example: The following were first mixed:

(a) 95 g of BC 77 (British Industrial Plastics Limited), cationic urea-formaldehyde precondensate having a reactive resin content of approximately 45% and a solids content of approximately 35%;

(b) 60 g of BC 336 (British Industrial Plastics Limited), methylated melamine-formaldehyde precondensate having a reactive resin content of about 76% and a solids content of approximately 71%;

(c) 240 g of R1144 copolymer (Allied Colloids Limited), a 20% solution of an acrylamide/acrylic acid copolymer having a viscosity average MW of 400,000 and an acrylic acid content of 42%; and

(d) 850 g deionized water.

200 g of deionized water were then added to 800 g of the mixture described above, and the mixture was milled with 800 g of material to be encapsulated until a mean droplet size of 2 to 3 μ was reached.

The material to be encapsulated, (internal phase) was a color former solution. The solvent for the color former solution was a 4:1 w/w mixture of kerosene and HB40, the latter being a mixture of partially hydrogenated terphenyls (Monsanto Limited, HB40 is also known as Santasol 340). The color formers were crystal violet lactone and benzoyl leucomethylene blue, present in amounts of 1.7% w/w and 1.4% w/w respectively.

The remainder of the mixture was then added, followed by 1,405 g of deionized water as a diluent. The resulting composition was stirred for 30 min, after which its pH was lowered to 4.7 by adding acetic acid. Stirring was then carried out for a further 30 min. The temperature was then raised to 55°C using a water bath and the mixture stirred for 2 hours at that temperature, after which the composition was allowed to cool and left stirring overnight. Next morning capsules were seen to have formed and the pH was raised to 10.0. The capsules obtained were subsequently coated onto paper using a laboratory Meyer bar coater. When the sheet was placed on a color-developing sheet and written upon, a clear blue copy was developed on the color-developing sheet.

Interfacial Crosslinking of Polymeric Emulsifier by Isocyanate

A.E. Vassiliades and C.H. Chang; U.S. Patent 4,138,362; February 6, 1979; assigned to Champion International Corporation found that pressure-rupturable, oil-containing microcapsules having excellent thermal stability and friability may be provided by a system that avoids the somewhat complex process controls and multitude of ingredients normally required.

The process for forming microcapsules merely involves admixing a water-immiscible oily material containing an oil-soluble, nonpolymeric crosslinking agent in the form of a polyfunctional isocyanate and an aqueous solution of a water-soluble, polymeric emulsifying agent, which may be a natural or synthetic water-soluble nitrogen-containing polymer containing recurring $-NH_2$ or $=NH$ groups, or a natural gum containing recurring hydroxy groups.

The oily material and the aqueous solution are admixed under conditions that are effective to form an oil-in-water emulsion wherein the oily material containing the polyfunctional isocyanate is dispersed in the form of microscopic emulsion droplets in the aqueous continuous phase containing the emulsifying agent, which surrounds each of the droplets and is crosslinked by the isocyanate to form a solid, crosslinked capsule wall.

Preferably, a viscosity lowering agent is included in the emulsion when natural polymeric emulsifying agents are utilized in order to provide a microcapsular dispersion having a lower viscosity while having a relatively high solids content. It is vital from a commercial viewpoint to provide a microcapsular dispersion having as high a solids content as possible for coating purposes; however, at the same time it is necessary that the dispersion have a low enough viscosity to permit it to be coated onto a substrate, such as paper, in the case of carbonless copy paper production.

Suitable natural nitrogen-containing polymers include proteinaceous, hydrophilic materials, such as gelatin, chitosan, or the like $-NH_2$ or $=NH$ group-containing natural polymers. Suitable synthetic hydrophilic polymers containing recurring $-NH_2$ or $=NH$ groups include polymeric amines, such as polyethyleneimine; polyamides, such as water-soluble polyacrylamide; water-soluble copolymers of acrylamide and N-monoalkylacrylamide, wherein alkyl groups have 1 to 10 carbon atoms; amino-aldehyde resins, such as melamine-formaldehyde prepolymers; urea-aldehyde prepolymers, such as urea-formaldehyde prepolymer.

Suitable natural polyhydroxyl gums which may serve as both the emulsifying agent and the wall-forming material include water-soluble polyhydroxy-containing gum arabic, gum tragacanth, guar gum, carrageenan. Water immiscible oily materials include hydrophobic liquids which have been conventionally utilized in copy systems as the solvent for the chromogen, such as isopropyl naphthalenes, isopropyl biphenyls, etc.

Oil-soluble polyfunctional isocyanates that may be employed in the process include, e.g., diisocyanates, such as 2,6-toluenediisocyanate; 2,4-toluenediisocyanate; 4,4'-diphenylmethanediisocyanate; 1,4-naphthyldiisocyanate; hexamethylenediisocyanate; 1,4-cyclohexyldiisocyanate, and the like; triisocyanates, such as 4,4', 4''-triphenylmethanetriisocyanate; 2,4,6-toluenetriisocyanate, and the like; and isocyanate adducts, such as an adduct of hexamethylenediisocyanate with hexanetriol, an adduct of toluenediisocyanate with trimethylolpropane, and the like.

The microcapsular wall or shell is formed directly by the interaction between the polyisocyanate crosslinking agent and the emulsifying agent which may be, if desired, the sole coreactant for the isocyanate.

Viscosity-lowering agents include: alkali metal periodates, such as sodium or potassium periodate; or urea-aldehyde prepolymers, such as urea-formaldehyde prepolymer. Amounts of the viscosity-lowering agent are, preferably between 0.5 and 1.0% by weight of the alkali metal periodate and between 25 and 35% by weight of the urea-formaldehyde prepolymer based upon the dry weight of the emulsifying agent.

The ratio of polymeric emulsifying agent that is provided to the emulsion is at least one part by weight of emulsifying agent per part of crosslinking agent. Thus, suitable ratios of emulsifier to crosslinking agent include between 1 and 40 parts by weight of emulsifying agent per part of crosslinking agent, preferably between 2 and 10 parts by weight of emulsifying agent per part of crosslinking agent. Emulsification may be conducted at any suitable temperature, between ambient temperature up to 100°C. Subsequent to or concurrently with emulsification, the microcapsular dispersion may be heated to a temperature preferably between 50° and 70°C for a period between 1 and 4 hours in order to effect the crosslinking of the emulsifying agent by the polyfunctional isocyanate agent. The solids content of the resulting emulsion is preferably between 20 and 51% by weight.

In the preferred utility of this process, e.g., transfer sheet record material, the process may be used to encapsulate an oily printing ink, which may be used in smudge-proof typewriter ribbons or carbon papers. In such a use, it has been found expedient to encapsulate a colorless, water-insoluble dye intermediate dissolved in the oil. Typifying colorless dye intermediates are leuco dyes, such as crystal violet lactone, and derivatives of bis(p-dialkylaminoaryl)methane.

According to a modification of the process, a pigment, such as carbon black, is dispersed in the oily droplets, rather than a chromogen. The resulting capsules are coated onto paper to provide a copy sheet which produces a black image on an underlying copy sheet upon rupture of the capsules. Such products have significant advantages over conventional carbon paper products in that they minimize smudging during handling. Moreover, such microcapsules containing, e.g., carbon black particles may be incorporated into plastics, plastic films, rubber, etc. to improve the stability of the substrate towards ultraviolet light and thereby avoid deterioration of the physical and mechanical properties. Moreover, such capsules may be used in conventional printing methods, such as xerography, for elimination of the less desirable liquid toners.

Example 1: 3,300 g of 37% formaldehyde and 900 g of deionized water are mixed thoroughly in a flask. The pH of the solution is adjusted to 9.0 with sodium hydroxide. After the addition of 1,790 g of urea and 10 g of melamine, the resulting solution is heated at 65°C for one hour to provide a water-soluble urea-formaldehyde prepolymer having a solids content of 50.3% by weight.

A solution of 126 g of crystal violet lactone, 108 g of benzoyl leucomethylene blue, 240 g of dimethyl phthalate, 360 g of an adduct of toluenediisocyanate with trimethylolpropane in 5,490 g of an isopropyl naphthalene solvent is emulsified into a mixed solution of 6,300 g of 10% technical gelatin (No. 164, Hudson Industries Corporation) and 540 g of the water-soluble urea-formaldehyde prepolymer, a viscosity lowering agent, at 50°C. The resulting dispersion has an average particle size of about 5 μ and is diluted with 10,668 g of water and cured at 60°C for about 2 hours. The viscosity of the cured emulsion is only 10 cp at 20°C at 30% total solids.

Example 2: A solution of 2.1 g of crystal violet lactone, 1.8 g of benzoyl leucomethylene blue in 91.5 g of isopropyl naphthalene is admixed with 6 g of the isocyanate adduct of Example 1 and 2 g of tributyl phosphate. The solution is emulsified at ambient temperature into 660 g of a 2.3% chitosan solution containing 0.15 g of sodium periodate until particle size of about 5 μ is obtained. The emulsion is then heated at 60°C for about 2 hours to complete the microencapsulation. The resulting low viscosity (40 cp at 20°C) dispersion may be readily coated by conventional paper coating methods.

Example 3: Into a solution of 15 g of gum arabic in 135 g water is emulsified a solution of 100 g of an alkylated, partially hydrogenated naphthalene oil containing 2.1 g of crystal violet lactone, 0.9 g of benzoyl leucomethylene blue, and 4 g of toluenediisocyanate. Agitation is continued until a particle size of about 5 μ in diameter is obtained. The emulsion is heated under mild stirring at about 60°C for 2 hours. It is then coated on a paper to provide a pressure rupturable transfer sheet.

Example 4: In a mixture of 40 g of tricresyl phosphate and 10 g of tributyl phosphate is dispersed 25 g of carbon black (Continex F-1, Whitco Chemical Company). Then, 5 g of an adduct of toluenediisocyanate with trimethylolpropane is added and well stirred in this dispersion. The resulting mixture is emulsified into 250 g of a 3% by weight aqueous solution of chitosan in a Waring blender. Emulsification is continued until the average particle diameter of the droplets is about 5 μ. The microcapsular emulsion is cured at 60°C for 2 hours. The microcapsules are then coated onto a paper to provide a transfer copy sheet which produces a black image on paper upon rupturing the capsules.

Example 5: A solution of 2.1 g of crystal violet lactone and 0.9 g of benzoyl leucomethylene blue in 91.5 g of propylated naphthalene is dissolved into an adduct of toluenediisocyanate and trimethylolpropane. The solution is emulsified into a solution of 30 g of urea-formaldehyde resin (RP 703-78 Casco-Resin, Borden Chemical Company) in 120 g of water until an average particle size of 5 μ is obtained. The emulsion is cured at 60°C for 2 hours while under agitation to complete the microencapsulation. 70 g of a 7% polyvinyl alcohol solution (Vinol 540, 87 to 89% hydrolyzed, Air Products and Chemicals) is added to the emulsion.

Polyisocyanate Adduct plus Polyamine Adduct as Polymerization Promotor

M. Kiritani, H. Matsukawa, A. Watanabe and H. Imamiya; U. S. Patent 4,021,595; May 3, 1977; assigned to Fuji Photo Film Co., Ltd., Japan have developed a process for producing fine oil droplets in capsules having strong protective shells and more particularly it relates to a process for producing fine oil droplets or oil-containing microcapsules having strong protective outer shells by dispersing or emulsifying in a polar solvent a polyisocyanate adduct having a free isocyanate group and adding to the dispersion or emulsion a polyamine or a polyamine adduct having a free amino group as a polymerization promotor, whereby the polymerization of the polyisocyanate adduct is caused from the outer side of each oil droplet to insolubilize the polyisocyanate adduct.

The size of the capsules can be controlled easily and the oil-containing microcapsules have strong outer shells with quite a low permeability. The oil-containing microcapsules produced may be used for the preparation of pressure-sensitive copying sheets as well as for the purpose of generally protecting dyes, inks, perfumes, adhesives, and medicaments.

The polyisocyanate adduct having a free isocyanate group employed in the process are prepared by adding oleophilic polyisocyanates to hydrophilic group-containing compounds such as polyamines, polycarboxylic acids, polythiols, polyhydroxy compounds, epoxy compounds, etc. The term polyisocyanate includes polyisocyanates and polyisothiocyanates.

Suitable polyisocyanate adduct are an adduct of hexamethylene diisocyanate and trimethylolpropane, an adduct of tolylenediisocyanate and trimethylolpropane or a xylylenediisocyanate adduct.

The polyamines which can be used as the polymerization promotor for promoting the polymerization of the polyisocyanate adduct having a free isocyanate group, include aromatic polyamines such as o-phenylenediamine, p-phenylenediamine, diaminonaphthalene, etc.; aliphatic polyamines such as 1,3-propylenediamine, hexamethylenediamine, etc.; and the adducts of those aromatic or aliphatic polyamines and epoxy compounds. Also, a compound having many amino groups in the molecule such as a free amino group having adduct of polyamine and epoxy compound, thiourea-formalin resin and gelatin may be used. That is to say, any compound having more than two amino groups in the molecule may be used as the polymerization promotor.

The oily liquid to be encapsulated is an organic solvent immiscible with water, e.g., natural oils, synthetic oils, and solvents. The polar liquid used for forming the continuous phase can be a liquid immiscible with the oily liquid. Generally water but other polar liquids (immiscible with an oily liquid to be capsulated, e.g., alcohols etc.) may also be used simply or in a mixture with water.

The oily liquid to be encapsulated may be dispersed or emulsified in the polar liquid by using a protective colloid or a surface active agent. Suitable protective colloids are, gelatin, gum arabic, casein, carboxymethylcellulose, starch, polyvinyl alcohol. Suitable surface active agents are, anionic surface active agents, e.g., an alkylbenzene sulfonate, alkylnaphthalenesulfonate, a polyoxyethylene sulfate, Turkey red oil etc., and nonionic surface active agents, e.g., polyoxyethylene alkyl ether, polyoxyethylene alkylphenol ether, sorbitan fatty acid esters, etc. The sizes of the microcapsules are from 1 μ to 1 mm and, generally 2 to 500 μ.

Example 1: In 30 g of dipropylnaphthalene (oily liquid) containing 0.6 g of crystal violet lactone and 0.5 g of benzoyl leucomethylene blue as color formers for pressure sensitive copying sheets was dissolved 6 g of Coronate HL (a trimethylolpropane adduct of hexamethylene diisocyanate having a free isocyanate group) as a wall-forming material.

The oily liquid thus prepared was added to 55 g of water at 20°C having dissolved therein 3 g of carboxymethylcellulose and 3 g of polyvinyl alcohol with vigorous stirring to form oil droplets having diameters of 4 to 10 μ and thereafter the dispersion was diluted by adding 100 g of water. Then, 40 g of water containing 6 g of Epikure U (amino group-containing adduct of aliphatic polyamine and glycidyl ether; viscosity of from 60 to 120 poises, at 25°C), was added to the diluted dispersion. During the above procedure, the temperature of the system was maintained below 25°C.

For promoting the hardening of the abovedescribed polyisocyanate adduct, the temperature of the system was increased to 60°C by heating to finish the formation of the capsules, whereby the polyisocyanate initial addition product was hardened around the oil droplets containing crystal violet lactone and benzoyl leucomethylene blue, and quite strong and less permeable shells were formed thereby.

The capsule-containing composition was applied to a paper and dried to give a microcapsule sheet for pressure sensitive copying sheets. When the capsule sheet thus prepared was heated to 100°C for 10 hours, none of the contents exuded from the microcapsules and no reduction in the coloring ability of the capsule sheet with a developer sheet was observed.

Furthermore, a developer composition consisting of 300 parts of water, 100 parts of acid clay, and 20 parts of a styrene-butadiene rubber latex was applied to the microcapsules to form a self-recordable pressure sensitive copying sheet. No color stains or fogs were observed in the pressure sensitive copying sheet (when the color fog of the sheet was measured using a spectrophotometer, the density of the fog was 0.05 at 600 mμ). When the sheets were pressed in localized areas, colored marks were obtained.

On the other hand, when a monomer such as hexamethylene diisocyanate (e.g., not containing a free isocyanate group) was used in place of Coronate HL in the above process, the system aggregated and thus microcapsules were not obtained and further when other diisocyanate monomers such as toluene-2,4,6-triisocyanate, tolylenediisocyanate, xylylenediisocyanate, and diphenylmethane diisocyanate were used respectively in place of Coronate HL, only microcapsules which had imperfect and highly permeable walls were obtained.

That is to say, when the capsule paper prepared by applying each of these latter microcapsules and drying, was heated to 100°C for 10 hours, the color density of the marks formed on a developer sheet by applying a localized pressure to the laminate of the capsule sheet and the developer sheet was quite low.

Also, when a developer composition consisting of 300 parts of water, 100 parts of acid clay, and 20 parts of a styrene-butadiene rubber latex was applied to the layer of the microcapsules followed by drying, crystal violet lactone and benzoyl leucomethylene blue in the microcapsules exuded from the capsules to cause a reaction with the acid clay, whereby blue fogs appeared over the entire surface of the developer sheet (when the fog density was measured as in the above case, the fog density was 0.60 where xylylenediisocyanate, was used, 0.14 where diphenylmethane diisocyanate was used and 0.21 where tolylenediisocyanate was used).

On the other hand, 40 g of water containing 6 g of Epikure U was added to 55 g of water having dissolved therein 3 g of carboxymethylcellulose and 3 g of polyvinyl alcohol and while stirring the mixture, 30 g of dipropylnaphthalene containing 0.6 g of crystal violet lactone, 0.5 g of benzoyl leucomethylene blue, and 6 g of Coronate HL was added to the mixture, whereby the viscosity of the entire system increased greatly, the entire system was aggregated, and thus desirable microcapsules were not obtained.

Example 2: 10 g of a perfume oil, Emerald Jasmin was added to 20 g of an oily liquid, trichlorodiphenyl, and then 6 g of Coronate HL was added as a wall-forming material to the oily liquid. The oily liquid prepared was added to 55 g of water containing 2 g of carboxymethylcellulose and 2 g of gum arabic with vigorous stirring to form oil droplets having diameters of 20 to 30 μ.

Afterwards to the dispersion was added 90 g of water, 50 g of water containing 3 g of Epikure U and 0.5 g of hexamethylenediamine to the diluted dispersion with stirring and then the temperature of the system was increased to 70°C to finish the encapsulation, whereby perfume oil-containing microcapsules having quite strong shells were obtained.

The obtained capsule-containing composition was applied to a paper and dried. When the microcapsule paper was allowed to stand for 3 months at room temperature, no perfume oil evaporated from the microcapsules and only when the microcapsules were ruptured by pressing, did they give off a sweet smell of Emerald Jasmin. On the other hand, when capsule compositions were prepared in the same manner as described above using polyisocyanate monomers such as hexamethylene diisocyanate, diphenylmethane diisocyanate, etc., in place of the Coronate HL and were applied to papers, the perfume oil was evaporated at drying due to the imperfect capsule walls to give the smell of Emerald Jasmin in every case. When these coated papers were allowed to stand for 3 months at room temperature, almost no perfume component remained in the microcapsules and when the microcapsules were ruptured by pressing, they gave off almost no perfume smell.

Crosslinked Hydroxypropylcellulose

D.R. Shackle; U.S. Patent 4,025,455; May 24, 1977; assigned to The Mead Corporation describes a process for forming microcapsules which comprises the steps of preparing an aqueous solution containing a hydroxypropylcellulose wall-forming compound, the hydroxypropylcellulose wall-forming compound containing reactive hydroxyl groups and being characterized by having decreasing solubility with increasing temperature in aqueous solution.

An oil solution is prepared containing an oil-soluble crosslinking agent for the hydroxypropylcellulose wall-forming compound in an oil to be encapsulated, the oil-soluble crosslinking agent being a polyfunctional isocyanate containing more than one group capable on reacting with hydroxyl groups to provide crosslinkage with the hydroxypropylcellulose wall-forming compound.

The aqueous solution containing hydroxypropylcellulose is mixed with the oil solution containing a crosslinking agent in a manner such that an emulsion is formed having droplets of the oil solution dispersed in the aqueous solution. The mixture is heated to a temperature of about 45° to 52°C to cause the formation of a precipitate of the hydroxypropylcellulose wall-forming compound on the droplets of the oil solution, the precipitate resulting from the interaction of the hydroxypropylcellulose wall-forming compound and the polyfunctional isocyanate crosslinking agent to form microcapsule walls. The temperature of the heated mixture is maintained at a temperature and for a time (1 to 16 hours) sufficient to permit the microcapsule walls to become substantially oil and water impermeable.

Preferably, a second crosslinking agent for the hydroxypropylcellulose wall-forming compound is added to the first solution prior to heating the emulsion to a temperature above the precipitating temperature of the hydroxypropylcellulose wall-forming compound. The second crosslinking agent further promotes wall-formation when the appropriate precipitating temperature has been reached.

In the preferred form of this process, a minor amount, up to about 25% (preferably 10%) based on the weight of the wall-forming compound of a water-soluble crosslinking agent is added to the aqueous phase either before, during or after the emulsifying step. The water-soluble crosslinking agents may be dimethylolurea, a polyfunctional aziridine, stearato chromyl chloride complex, methoxymethylmelamine, melamine-formaldehyde resin prepolymers and urea-formaldehyde resin prepolymers.

Hydroxypropylcellulose is a film-forming cellulosic ether polymer soluble in cold water, but insoluble in hot water. The commercially available polymers have a molar substitution (MS) of about 3 to 5 hydroxypropyl units to each cellulose unit. A particular group of hydroxypropylcelluloses are the Klucels. These polymers precipitate out of a water solution at a temperature of about 45°C and preferably at about 45° to 52°C as a finely divided solid precipitate.

The polymers are available in a variety of viscosity types. The lower viscosity types, G, J, L and E are suitable for use in this process. Of these, Type L having a molecular weight of approximately 75,000 and an MS of approximately 3 has been found to be particularly useful.

The following are crosslinking agents used in the examples: Desmodur N-100 (Mobay Chemical Co.) is a liquid biuret made by reacting hexamethylene diisocyanate with water in 3 to 1 molar ratio, Mondur MRS (Mobay Chemical Co.) is a polymethylene polyphenylisocyanate, Cymel 301 (American Cyanamid Co.) is a hexamethoxymethylmelamine, Ionac PFAZ-300 (Ionac Chemical Co.) is a polyfunctional aziridine.

Example 1: An oil phase monoisopropylbiphenyl (MIPB solution) was prepared by dissolving 7 g of crystal violet lactone, 0.9 g of 3,3-bis(1'-ethyl-2'methylindol-3-yl)phthalide, 1.8 g of 3-N,N-diethylamino-7-(N,N-dibenzylamino)fluoran and 2.9 g of 3-N,N-diethylamino-6,8-dimethylfluoran, all as color precursors in 190 ml of MIPB at 85°C. This oil phase was then cooled to 15°C. An aqueous phase was prepared comprising 11 g of Klucel L dissolved in 400 ml of room temperature water. 1 g Cymel 301 crosslinking agent and 1 g of Turkey Red Oil emulsifier were added to the aqueous phase and the pH was adjusted to 4 with 16% acetic acid.

To the oil phase, which had been cooled to 15°C, 7.5 g of Desmodur N-100 oil-soluble crosslinking agent and 6 g of Mondur MRS crosslinking agent were added. This solution in turn was added to the aqueous phase and mixed in a Sunbeam blender. The mixing was continued for 3 minutes until an emulsion was formed and the mixture was then stirred at 50°C for 16 hours. The pH was then adjusted to 7 with 10% NaOH. Microcapsules so prepared were coated on paper and the paper was used as the CB (coated back) part of a carbonless copy paper system.

Example 2: An oil phase was prepared as in Example 1 using 150 ml instead of 190 ml of MIPB. An aqueous phase was prepared comprising 11 g of Klucel L dissolved in 400 ml of room temperature water. 2 g of Ionac PEAZ-300 crosslinking agent and 1 g of Turkey Red Oil emulsifier were added to the aqueous solution.

To the MIPB solution which had been cooled to 15°C, 10 g of Desmodur N-100 and 3.5 g of Mondur MRS, both crosslinking agents, were added. This solution in turn was added to the aqueous phase and mixed in a Sunbeam blender. The mixing emulsification was continued for 3 minutes resulting in the formation of an emulsion and the mixture was then stirred at 50°C for 16 hours. The pH was then adjusted to 7 with 10% NaOH. Microcapsules so prepared were coated on paper and the paper worked well as the CB part of the carbonless copy paper system.

Partially Condensed Formaldehyde Condensation Product

A process is provided by *A.E. Vassiliades; U.S. Patent 3,993,831; November 23, 1976; assigned to Champion International Corporation* for the formation of microcapsules in the absence of coacervation comprising solid walls of a hydrophobic, partially condensed, thermosetting resin and containing minute droplets of an oily material. The process may be described briefly as a simple admixing of:

(A) a partially condensed, formaldehyde condensation product in an aqueous medium, e.g., water, the condensation product being capable of being separated from the aqueous medium in solid particle form as a precipitate, upon further dilution with water; and

(B) an oil-in-water emulsion comprising a water-immiscible oily material selected from the group consisting of liquid and low melting oils, fats and waxes, as the disperse phase and an aqueous, colloidal solution of an amphiphilic emulsifying agent as the dispersion medium, the water of the emulsion being present in a quantity at least sufficient to cause the separation of the condensation product from the aqueous medium.

The admixing causes the condensation product to separate from the aqueous medium in solid particle form as a precipitate about a nucleus of oil in water upon dilution with the water of the emulsion. The dilution takes place slowly and under conditions of brisk agitation.

The thermosetting resins which can be used comprise that broad class of compositions defined as partially condensed formaldehyde condensation products. The term partially condensed as employed herein is intended to include resins not having reached the infusible or insoluble stage, e.g., B-stage resins. The preferred formaldehyde condensation products are partially-condensed melamine-formaldehyde, phenol-formaldehyde and urea-formaldehyde resins. The B-stage melamine and urea-formaldehyde resins are especially preferred.

By water immiscible oily material is meant lipophilic materials which are preferably liquid, such as oils, which will not mix with water and which are inert with regard to the components of the particular system. In making a transfer sheet record material, a low viscosity-low vapor pressure oil is preferred. Among the materials which can be used are: natural oils, such as cottonseed oil, soybean oil, petroleum lubricating oils, fish liver oils, drying oils and essential oils, synthetic oils, and halogenated biphenyls. A preferred class of water immiscible oily materials are the halogenated biphenyls, with chlorinated biphenyl being especially preferred.

For transfer sheet record material, the process may be used to encapsulate an oily printing ink, such as may be used in smudge-proof typewriter ribbons or carbon papers. In such a use, it has been found expedient to encapsulate a colorless, water-insoluble leuco dye intermediate dissolved in the oil phase of the emulsion, thus avoiding the necessity of removing the residual colored matter from the external surfaces of the capsules prior to coating as is required in the encapsulation of printing inks. Exemplary of the colorless dye intermediates for use are leuco dyes, such as crystal violet lactone, benzoyl leucomethylene blue, derivatives of bis(p-dialkylaminoaryl)methane such as disclosed in U.S.

Patents 2,981,733 and 2,981,738 and mixtures of the foregoing dyes. These dye intermediates are colorless in an alkaline medium and react to form a visible color in an acidic medium. Thus, when a capsule containing such a compound is ruptured and the compound is discharged onto an adsorbant, acidic electron-acceptor material, such as a paper web coated with an organic or an inorganic acid material, a visible color appears on the adsorbant material at the point of contact.

The emulsions to be encapsulated must be stable at least for the duration of the microcapsule formation. Since it is known that oil-water mixtures will not stabilize of their own accord, an emulsifying agent must be incorporated into the system. Selection of the appropriate emulsifier can be based on trials or, preferably, by reference to the hydrophile-lipophile balance (HLB) of the specific materials intended to be used.

The emulsifying agents to be used are said to be amphiphilic. That is, while the emulsifiers are generally preferentially soluble in one phase of the emulsion, they do possess an appreciable affinity for the other phase. It can be said, then, that an amphiphilic emulsifier gives oil a more hydrophilic nature than it had before and conversely, gives water a more lipophilic nature.

Exemplary of the amphiphilic emulsifying agents which can be used are: naturally occurring, lyophilic colloids including gums, proteins and polysaccharides such as gum arabic, gum tragacanth, agar, gelatin and starch; and synthetic materials such as methylcellulose, polyvinyl pyrrolidone, polyvinyl alcohol and copolymers of methyl vinyl ether and maleic anhydride. One preferred emulsifying agent is methylcellulose.

Brisk agitation is required in order to obtain very small droplets of the emulsion, and, ultimately, very small capsules. Thus, microcapsules having diameters ranging from about 0.1 μ to several hundred can be produced. Preferably, the microcapsules have an average particle size of between 3.5 and 7 μ, with about 4.5 μ being especially preferred. If the microcapsules are too small, they are difficult to break and the density of the resulting mark in a transfer copy system is reduced. If the microcapsules are too large, premature rupturing occurs and this results in smudging.

Example 1: (a) A water-soluble B-stage urea-formaldehyde resin is prepared by refluxing a mixture comprising 120 g of urea and 324 g of formalin (37% by weight aqueous solution of formaldehyde) neutralized to a pH of 7.0±0.1 with a sodium carbonate solution. The mixture is then refluxed for about 10 min and 0.52 g of acetic acid is added and heating under reflux is continued for about 3½ hours.

The resultant pH of the mixture is approximately equal to 4.3 and is then adjusted to 7.0 with a sodium carbonate solution. The urea-formaldehyde resin is cooled to room temperature and is in the form of a water-soluble resinous solution.

(b) Crystal violet lactone and benzoyl leucomethylene blue in an amount of 2.1 pbw and 0.9 pbw, respectively, are dissolved in 97 pbw of a hot chlorinated biphenyl, which is at a temperature of about 100°C. The hot dye solution is agitated for approximately 45 min and is then cooled to room temperature. The solution is then filtered through a 5 μ filter to remove any undissolved dye particles.

Meanwhile, methylcellulose is slowly added to cold water and the mixture is agitated until the methylcellulose completely dissolves. The agitation is stopped and the solution is permitted to stand overnight so as to eliminate any foam. 300 parts of a 10% methylcellulose (10 centipoises) solution (per 100 parts of oil) in water are transferred to a tank provided with a homomixer. Meanwhile, 100 parts of the dye solution are introduced, slowly, into the tank and are agitated with the homomixer over a period of approximately 5 to 7 min. Emulsification is continued until the particle size of the droplets is reduced to an average of about 4 to 5 μ.

Once the desired particle size is obtained, encapsulation is induced by slowly injecting 13 pbw of a 60% aqueous solution of the B-stage, urea-formaldehyde resin of Example 1(a) per 100 parts of oil into the tank slowly. 10 g of hydroxyethylcellulose (a 5% aqueous solution) are added to the microcapsular solution and the resulting dispersion is coated onto a paper web and is dried at a temperature of about 50° to 60°C.

Example 2: A mixture is prepared comprising 3 g of 1-[bis(p-dimethylaminophenyl)methyl] pyrrolidine and 97 g of cottonseed oil. The dye-oil mixture is agitated and is then passed through a filter as before.

Partially hydrolyzed polyvinyl alcohol is added to cold water and agitated to form a solution. 250 parts of the polyvinyl alcohol solution per 100 parts of oil are introduced into a tank containing an agitator. Meanwhile, 100 parts of the dye solution are introduced into the tank over a 10 min period. Emulsification is continued until the particle size of the resulting droplets is about 6 to 7 μ.

Next, 17 parts of the urea-formaldehyde resin solution employed in Example 1(b) are introduced, slowly, into the mixing vessel with brisk agitation. Microcapsules having structural integrity are immediately formed having capsule walls comprising urea-formaldehyde. A slurry is prepared comprising 10 parts of cellulosic pulp in 50 parts of 5% aqueous hydroxyethylcellulose solution. The resultant slurry is added to the microcapsular solution and the dispersion is coated onto a paper web.

Acid-Treated Gelatin plus CMC Coacervated at pH 4.8 to 6.0

H. Iwasaki, S. Shioi and J. Kouno; U.S. Patent 4,010,038; March 1, 1977; assigned to Kanzaki Paper Manufacturing Co., Ltd., Japan describe a process for producing microcapsules of complex hydrophilic colloid material enclosing fine particles of a hydrophobic substance. The process is characterized in that an acid-treated gelatin and at least one of carboxy-modified cellulose derivatives are used as the hydrophilic colloid materials, the amount of the cellulose derivative being $\frac{1}{7}$ to $\frac{1}{40}$ the amount of the gelatin by weight, the cellulose derivative having an average polymerization degree of 50 to 1,000 and a carboxyl substitution degree of 0.4 to 1.5 and that the coacervation of colloid material solution is effected at a pH of 4.8 to 6.0.

Preferable among acid-treated gelatins are those having an isoelectric point of about 7 to 9 and gel strength of about 70 to 250 g Bloom, especially of 90 to 200 g Bloom, as determined by a gel strength meter of the Bloom type according to PAGI method. The concentration of the aqueous solution of gelatin, is usually 0.25 to 10 wt %, preferably 1 to 5 wt %.

Of the carboxy-modified cellulose derivatives, carboxymethylcellulose is preferable for the formation of unclustered capsules. An aqueous solution of formaldehyde, glyoxal or glutaraldehyde may be added according to the usual process to harden the gelled coacervate.

All parts and percentages used in the examples below are by weight unless otherwise indicated. In the examples, microcapsules and pressure sensitive manifold paper prepared are evaluated by identifying the defects and determining the characteristic values as stated below.

Clustered Microcapsules in Microcapsule Dispersion: The diameter of the largest cluster of microcapsules and the number of clusters per 100 capsules produced are microscopically determined.

Tests of Microcapsules for Use in Pressure Sensitive Manifold Paper: To the microcapsule dispersion obtained in each of the examples are added 100 parts of 20% aqueous solution of oxidized starch and 15 parts of cellulose powder to prepare a color former coating composition, which is applied in an amount of 5 g/m^2 when dried, to a paper substrate weighing 40 g/m^2 to obtain transfer sheets (top sheets). A color acceptor coating composition is separately prepared from 100 parts of acidic clay, 10 parts of 20% aqueous solution of sodium hydroxide, 40 parts of 50% styrene-butadiene copolymer latex (styrene:butadiene is 60:40), 50 parts of 1% aqueous solution of sodium alginate and 200 parts of water.

The color acceptor coating composition is then applied, in an amount of 6 g/m^2 when dried, to a paper substrate weighing 40 g/m^2 to obtain copy sheets (bottom sheets). The same color former coating composition as above is applied, in an amount of 5 g/m^2 when dried, to the rear surface of each of the same copy sheets prepared in the same manner as above to obtain middle sheets. The three kinds of sheets thus prepared are tested in the following manner.

Color Forming Ability – The transfer sheet is superposed on the copy sheet with the coatings facing each other, and the set of sheets is subjected to pressure of 600 kg/cm^2 to form a color mark on the copy sheet. The density of the mark is measured by Hitachi Spectrophotometer, Model-124 at a light wavelength of 610 mμ. The result is given in terms of absorbancy (D_1).

Resolving Power – Seven middle sheets are fitted together in layers with the color former coatings facing the color acceptor coatings respectively, and the pile of sheets is pressed by electric typewriter. The sharpness of the color characters formed on the color acceptor coating on the lowermost sheet is inspected with the unaided eye and evaluated according to the following criteria: A, excellent; B, good; C, acceptable; and D, reject.

Pressure Resistance – The transfer sheet is superposed on the copy sheet with the coatings facing each other, and the set of sheets is subjected to pressure of 40 kg/cm^2 to form a color mark on the copy sheet. The density of the mark is measured by the same spectrophotometer as above at a light wavelength of 610 mμ. The result is given in terms of absorbance (D_2), which relates to smudging caused in the course of coating and winding-up operations for the production of middle sheet or when the sheet is cut or printed. The lower the value, the less is the susceptibility of manifold paper to smudging.

Frictional Smudge Resistance – The transfer sheet is superposed on the copy sheet with the coating facing each other, and the transfer sheet is moved back and forth five times over a distance of 5 cm at a speed of 450 cm/min while applying pressure of 55 g/cm^2 to the transfer paper on its uncoated surface. The color smudge formed on the copy sheet is inspected with the unaided eye and evaluated according to the following criteria: A, excellent; B, good; C, acceptable; and D, reject.

Fogging Characteristics – Expressed in terms of $D_2/D_1 \times 100$, namely the ratio of the color density produced at pressure of 40 kg/cm^2 to that produced at pressure of 600 kg/cm^2. The higher the value, the more susceptible is the manifold paper to fogging, hence less amenable to processing.

Example 1: To 225 parts of water is added 25 parts of acid treated gelatin (isoelectric point, 8; gel strength, 180 g Bloom) and after leaving the mixture at 10°C for 1 hour, 530 parts of water is added thereto. The mixture is then heated at 60°C to prepare a solution. Separately, 2 parts of crystal violet lactone and 1 part of benzoyl leucomethylene blue are dissolved in 30 parts of kerosene and 70 parts of isopropylnaphthalene, and the solution is heated to 60°C and then added to the gelatin solution.

The mixture is stirred to prepare an emulsion containing oily droplets 5 to 10 μ in mean particle size. Further separately, 5% aqueous solution of carboxymethylcellulose (average polymerization degree, 150; substitution degree, 0.6) is prepared, and 50 parts of the solution (amount of the carboxymethylcellulose: $\frac{1}{10}$ the amount of the gelatin by weight) is added to the emulsion with stirring to obtain a system having a pH of 4.3. The system is adjusted to a pH of 5.5 with a 5% aqueous solution of sodium hydroxide and then cooled to 10°C.

After adding 25 parts of 10% aqueous solution of formaldehyde to the system, the mixture is left to stand for 5 minutes. Adjustment of the mixture to a pH of 10 with dropwise addition of 10% aqueous solution of sodium hydroxide gives a dispersion of highly hardened capsules. Microscopic inspection of the dispersion reveals that it contains loose and unclustered capsules with uniform particle size distribution and entirely free from clusters. The pressure sensitive manifold paper prepared with the use of the capsule dispersion gives a color image of uniform and high density and is free of any smudging when stored for a long period of time. The table on the following page shows the characteristics of the microcapsule dispersion and the properties of the manifold paper prepared with the use of the dispersion, along with the results achieved in Examples 1 through 9.

Example 2: In 530 parts of water is dissolved 2.5 parts of carboxymethylcellulose (polymerization degree, 150; substitution degree, 0.6), and the solution is heated to 60°C. A mixture of 30 parts of kerosene and 70 parts of isopropylnaphthalene having dissolved therein 2 parts of crystal violet lactone and 1 part of benzoyl leucomethylene blue is added to the solution to prepare an emulsion, which is then adjusted to a pH of about 7 with dropwise addition of 10% aqueous solution of sodium hydroxide. To the emulsion is thereafter added 250 parts of 10% aqueous solution of acid treated gelatin (isoelectric point, 8; gel strength, 150 g Bloom) at 60°C. Adjustment of the resulting system to a pH of 5.5 with a 10% acetic acid, cooling of the system and addition of formaldehyde solution are followed by the same procedure as in Example 1 to obtain a capsule dispersion.

Example 3: To 700 parts of water are added 25 parts of acid treated gelatin (isoelectric point, 8; gel strength, 130 g Bloom) and 2.5 parts of carboxymethylcellulose (average polymerization degree, 150; substitution degree, 0.6), and the mixture is heated to 60°C to prepare a solution having a pH of 4.7. To the solution thereafter adjusted to a pH of 5.5 with a 5% aqueous solution of sodium hydroxide is added a mixture consisting of 30 parts of kerosene, 70 parts of isopropylnaphthalene, 2 parts of crystal violet lactone and 1 part of benzoyl leucomethylene blue to formulate an emulsion, which is cooled to 10°C and further treated in the same manner as in Example 1, whereby a capsule dispersion is prepared.

Examples 4 through 7: Various capsule dispersions are prepared by the process of this method following the same procedure as in Example 1 except that acid treated gelatin and carboxymethylcellulose are used in the proportions listed in the table.

Examples 8 and 9: For comparison, capsule dispersions are prepared in the same manner as in Example 1 except that acid treated gelatin and carboxymethylcellulose are used in the proportions given in the table below.

		Capsule Dispersion		..... Pressure Sensitive Manifold Paper				
Ex. No.	Carboxymethylcellulose Proportion*	Maximum Diameter of Clusters (μ)	No. of Clusters**	Color Forming Ability	Resolving Power	Pressure Resistance	Frictional Smudge Resistance	Fogging Characteristics
1	1/10	–	0	0.96	A	0.05	A	5.2
2	1/10	–	0	0.96	A	0.05	A	5.2
3	1/10	–	0	0.95	A	0.05	A	5.3
4	1/7	15	1	0.95	A	0.08	B	8.4
5	1/15	–	0	0.97	A	0.05	A	5.2
6	1/20	–	0	0.96	A	0.05	A	5.2
7	1/40	15	3	0.96	B	0.09	B	9.4
8	1/6	50	15	0.97	D	0.23	D	23.7
9	1/50	60	20	0.95	D	0.27	D	28.4

*Based on the weight of acid-treated gelatin.
**Per 100 capsules.

The table indicates that the dispersions of Examples 1 through 7 contain loose and unclustered capsules with uniform particle size distribution and almost free from clusters. The manifold papers prepared are also satisfactory in various properties. With Examples 8 and 9, the dispersions contain many clusters of capsules and it is impossible to obtain unclustered capsules with uniform particle size distribution. The manifold papers prepared with use of such dispersions are not satisfactory for use.

Gelatin plus Phytic Acid as Coacervate-Forming Agent

The method of *A. Nakazawa and M. Ono; U.S. Patent 4,066,568; January 3, 1978; assigned to Nippon Pulp Industry Company Limited, Japan* relates to producing microcapsules by use of gelatin aqueous solution, and particularly to producing microcapsules by use of phytic acid and/or its alkali metal salt or alkaline earth metal salt as coacervate forming agent. Such microcapsules can be used for noncarbon paper, pressure sensitive adhesives, and heat-sensitive recording material.

Example 1: Copy Papers – 20 g of acid treated gelatin (isoelectric point 8.8) was added to 220 g of water, and left as it was for 1 hour, and thereafter heated so as to dissolve at 60°C. On the other hand, 2.5 g of crystal violet lactone and 1.5 g of benzoyl leucomethylene blue were dissolved in 30 g of kerosene and 100 g of high boiling point aromatic hydrocarbon compound by heating at 60°C, and then this was added to the gelatin solution and also, 10g of 4% caustic soda aqueous solution was added thereto, and this was agitated so as to cause an emulsion dispersion of oil drops of an average grain size of 1 to 3 μ, and 400 g of dilution warm water was added to the emulsion as it was agitated.

Then 32 g of 10% phytic acid aqueous solution was added dropwise and it was confirmed that the pH was 3.5. In this stage, the phase separation was caused, and the thick phase thereof was deposited around the oil drops. The liquid mixture was further cooled to 10°C. Next 15 cc of 25% glutaraldehyde was added thereto and the agitation is continued for about 5 hours. The pH of the system was adjusted to 10.0 by 5% NaOH aqueous solution. The dispersion liquid of oil-including capsules thus obtained has moderate fluidity and viscosity as a coating liquid for pressure sensitive copying paper, and it could be directly used as the coating treatment.

These microcapsules include scarcely any clusters under microscopic observation. The capsule dispersion liquid thus obtained was coated and dried on a raw paper surface of 45 g/m^2 to obtain a 6 g/m^2 by dry weight of coating. This paper was overlapped to a reception paper having a principal component of acid clay and novolak type phenol resin so as to be opposed to the reception paper surface, and copying was performed on a plurality of such papers, and as a result clear color development images were obtained on the reception papers.

Moreover, this coated paper was left for 20 hours at 105°C and thereafter color development was caused, however, the concentration of the image was the same as that before the heating treatment. Also, the coated paper was overlapped onto the reception paper surface so as to be opposite to each other and subjected to a pressure of 5 kg/cm^2 in an atmosphere of 60% RH and 25°C and left for 1 hour as it was, however, any dirt due to rupturing of the capsules was scarcely observable.

Example 2: Adhesives – 200 cc of 3% acid treated gelatin (isoelectric point 8.8) aqueous solution was heated to 50°C. On the other hand, a pressure sensitive adhesive composition was prepared which was composed of 450 g of toluene, 50 g of polyisobutylene (average molecular weight, 90,000), 25 g of terpene system thermoplastic resin (melting point, 115°C) and 20 g of mineral oil. 40 g of this adhesive solution was added to the gelatin solution and emulsification is effected by means of a homogenizing mixer.

To the resultant emulsion was added 2.7 ml of phytic acid-5 sodium salt solution so as to adjust pH to 3.5 while agitating the emulsion. In this step, the phase separation was caused, and the coacervate rich in gelatin content was deposited around the adhesive oil drops. Subsequently this mixture liquid was cooled, and treated with 5 cc of 25% glutaraldehyde solution thereby effecting the hardening treatment for about 3 hours at room temperature, and microcapsules were obtained. The coated paper of these capsules was nonadhesive; however, when the capsules were broken by heat and pressure, it showed good adhesive property to the surface of paper, wood, metal, and plastic film.

Encapsulation Within Cells of Microorganisms

J.L. Shank; U.S. Patent 4,001,480; January 4, 1977; assigned to Swift & Company found that microorganisms can provide an encapsulation means that is suitable for the encapsulation or microencapsulation of any substance that is fat soluble and thus that can be absorbed into fat-containing cells of microorganisms such as yeasts or fungi. Any microorganism that synthesizes fat within itself, such as yeasts, molds, or other fungi, are suitable for producing the cells into which the substances to be encapsulated may be absorbed.

Among the numerous substances that may be absorbed into and encapsulated within the fat globules of the yeasts, molds, or other fungi, or within protozoa are various dyes. Of particular commercial importance are leuco dyes that are especially suitable for carbonless carbon paper applications.

In addition to such dyes, any substance that is fat soluble or permeable through the cell wall of protozoa can be encapsulated. Such substances may be drugs such as analgesics, antipyretics, decongestants, and the like, e.g., Malathion, phenylbutazone, caffeine, aspirin, etc. Also capable of encapsulation are various fat soluble condiments, flavors and aromas, including essential oils and flavors, citric acid, as well as fat soluble vitamins.

Example 1: Encapsulation of Leuco Dye – The yeast *Torulopsis lipofera* is placed within a nutrient medium that is low in nitrogen content, also having a high carbohydrate content. The yeast is permitted to grow until approximately 50% by weight of the cells is fat. This volume of fat is identified under a microscope as a large glistening globule occupying a substantial portion of the cytoplasm of the grown yeast. Crystal violet lactone, a leuco dye, is then put into solution with ethyl alcohol and placed into contact with this high fat content yeast for several minutes or until the cells are observed as being infused with the dye.

The dyed cells are then harvested by centrifugation. Thereafter, the cells are resuspended in an alcoholic solution as a slurry and then cast upon a paper, utilizing a small quantity of a 10% starch solution adhesive. This paper is previously treated with a suitable clay that is acidified with a mineral acid. Thus prepared is a so-called carbonless carbon paper. When pressure is applied to this product, e.g., by a pen or a typewriter character, the pressure crushes the cells which in turn releases the leuco dye so that it comes into contact with the carrier paper treated with the acid clay, thereby transforming the dye from its colorless state to its violet color. The dye's coming into contact with the acidified clay causes a pH change in the dye which effects the color change.

Example 2: Encapsulation of Sodium Sulfite – Sodium sulfite is encapsulated within a yeast in accordance with Example 1 and cast upon a web of paper treated with lead acetate. These cells are ruptured with a rod to produce a permanent black marking upon the web at the locations on which the rod was used.

Example 3: Encapsulation of Aspirin – Acetylsalicylic acid (aspirin), an acetyl derivative of methyl salicylate, is encapsulated in accordance with Example 1. The final product is an aspirin formulation in which the aspirin is not released until the yeast cell has been digested.

INTERNAL PHASE SOLVENTS FOR DYES

Phenyl-Substituted Indans

It is known to use microcapsules containing dyes for making copying papers, the microcapsules generally being ruptured by the pressure applied during a writing operation so that the liberated dye is transferred to an acid-reacting layer where, if a leuco compound has been used, the actual dye is developed. In the formation of the dye on the acid-reacting layer, a developer is required, since the dyes are generally only capable of being adsorbed on the acid-reacting layer when in solution.

The developers described for the dyes, which are at the same time solvents for the dyes and core materials for the microcapsules, are, e.g., hydrocarbons such as naphthas, xylenes, diphenyls and/or chlorinated compounds. The mixture of chlorinated hydrocarbons, particularly mixtures of chlorinated diphenyls are almost exclusively used. However, these chlorinated compounds have a number of drawbacks. On account of its high density, the microcapsule dispersion shows a relatively strong tendency to sedimentation with the formation of agglomerates, this greatly hampering the handling of the capsule dispersion in storage, metering or in the further processing thereof to form a paper coating composition.

The chlorinated diphenyls also have the drawback that in their presence, dye development takes place comparatively slowly. It is also known that chlorinated diphenyls, in particular, show a certain degree of toxicity, cannot be degraded chemically or microbiologically and tend to accumulate in certain organs of living creatures. Complete destruction of residues is only possible by incineration, which produces undesirable hydrogen chloride gas. When the papers are reused as salvage paper, there is the risk of these materials passing into foodstuffs via packaging materials. They also have an unpleasant odor. Thus there is a need for other solvents or developers for use as core materials in dye-containing micro capsules.

W. Sliwka, W.-R. Gaefke and T. Korth; U.S. Patent 3,939,095; February 17, 1976; assigned to Badische Anilin- & Soda-Fabrik AG, Germany found that microcapsules containing as core material a water-immiscible liquid and at least one dye, the water-immiscible liquid substantially consisting of one or more mono- or polyalkyl-substituted indans in which the alkyl side-chains are linear or branched and may contain from 1 to 11 carbon atoms do not suffer from the above drawbacks.

The preferred indan compounds are phenyl-substituted indans having linear or branched alkyl side-chains preferably of from 1 to 6 carbon atoms. These are, in particular, alkyl-substituted 3-phenylindans and mixtures of alkyl-substituted phenylindans or mixtures thereof with other solvents or developers. Most preferred are 1-methyl-3-phenylindan and 1-methyl-3-phenyl-5-isopropylindan.

It is surprising that in a 6% w/w mixture of a conventionally used reactive dye mixture, e.g., a mixture of crystal violet lactone and N-benzoyl leucomethylene blue in a ratio of about 3:1, the dye precursors are contained in a dissolved state to an extent of only 5.28% by weight in 1-methyl-3-phenylindan, of only 3.05% by weight in 1-methyl-3-phenyl-5-isopropylindan and of only 2.48% by weight in 1-methyl-3-(p-isopropylphenyl)-5-isopropylindan and yet produce copies having the same color intensity as given by a 6% w/w solution of said dye precursor mixture in chlorinated diphenyl. This fact shows that even undissolved dye precursor is assisted in development by the solvent in the copying operation. Previously there has been the belief that only those solvents showing very high solubility for the dye precursors and thus ensuring complete solution of the latter are capable of guaranteeing good dye development.

Another advantage of alkyl-substituted phenylindans over dichlorodiphenyl is that they have virtually no solvent or plasticizing effect on the polymeric capsule wall materials generally used, the result being that in some cases leakage through the capsule walls is less despite the lower boiling points. This means, e.g., that copying papers may be manufactured which show better storage stability. The alkyl-substituted indans used are also virtually nontoxic and, surprisingly, have only a very weak odor in comparison with chlorinated diphenyl. Thus they are less of an environmental problem than liquid developers previously used.

Another advantage of these solvents is that their density is only slightly above 1 g/cc. For example 1-methyl-3-phenylindan has a density of 1.023 g/cc. This means that aqueous capsule dispersions are virtually intrinsically stable with the result that they are simpler to store and easier to process. The solvents are also good solvents for conventional UV absorbers such as Tinuvin P, so that light stabilization of the encapsulated dye precursors is readily possible.

The phenylindans are inexpensively available from styrene as starting material. They are reaction products of styrene with itself (dimerization) or with appropriate alkyl-substituted styrene compounds. It is not necessary to use the indans as pure compounds. In the following examples, parts are by weight.

Example 1: Preparation of Copolymers for the Wall Material – In a stirred vessel equipped with a temperature bath 500 parts of a mixture of 478 parts of butanediol monoacrylate acetyl acetate, 380 parts of methyl methacrylate, 140 parts of acrylamide and 2 parts of the sodium salt of 2-sulfoethyl methacrylate, which mixture has been previously neutralized to pH 4 with 10% caustic soda solution, is mixed with 7.5 parts of azodiisobutyronitrile and 1,000 parts of isopropanol and the mixture is heated at 80°C. 15 minutes after the commencement of polymerization the remainder of the mixture is steadily added to the reaction mixture over 1 hour at from 80° to 85°C.

Polymerization is continued to completion over 3 hours at this temperature, after which the reaction mixture is cooled to room temperature and the polymer solution is diluted with 500 parts of chloroform to give a 36.8% w/w polymer solution. A 1% w/w solution in chloroform gives a K value of 44 for the polymer.

Preparation of Microcapsule Dispersion – 60 parts of the resulting solution of wall material are dissolved, together with 67 parts of 1-methyl-3-phenylindan, in 180 parts of chloroform containing 0.5 part of tributylamine, 1 part N-benzoyl leucomethylene blue, 3 parts of 3,3-bis(dimethylamino)-6-dimethylamino phthalide (crystal violet lactone) and 6 parts of isopropanol with stirring to form a homogeneous solution.

In a vessel having a capacity of 800 parts and equipped with an Ultraturrax T 45 adapted to dip into the liquid, there are placed 200 parts of water and 50 parts of a 10% solution of a polyvinylpyrrolidone having a K value of 90 and stirring is effected at a speed of 10,000 rpm. The above solution is then added over about 5 minutes. Stirring is continued until the average particle size is from 10 to 12 μ. The temperature rises to about 45°C. In this way there is obtained an emulsion which is stable for a prolonged period.

250 parts of water are placed in a stirred vessel having a capacity of 2,000 parts and equipped with a flat-paddle agitator (120 rpm) and fitted with a descending condenser, and the above emulsion is added with stirring. From the thus diluted emulsion the chloroform is distilled off over about 75 minutes. To the dispersion, which is heated at 80°C, there are added 7 parts of 40% formaldehyde solution for hardening purposes, and the mixture is maintained at 70°C for about 1 hour.

On cooling there is obtained a stable microcapsule dispersion in a yield of more than 98% based on the wall material used, the microcapsules having an average diameter of from 5 to 8 μ. The microcapsules may be readily obtained as a free-flowing powder by filtration, repeated washing with water to remove the protective colloid and drying. The simplest method of drying is to spray the microcapsules through nozzles.

Tests on the Microcapsules for Leakage — The resulting microcapsule dispersion is brushed with a fine hair-brush onto paper weighing 5.7 g/m^2 which has been stretched taut in a frame in a moist condition and then dried. The dispersion on the paper is then dried at room temperature. The coating consists of 5.6 g/m^2 of microcapsules. The papers are odorless. A portion of the papers is stored at room temperature, a portion at 80°C and a further portion at 95°C, storage being for 16 hours in all cases.

After storage, the papers thus coated are each placed with the coated side against a paper the surface of which is coated in the usual manner with an acid bentonite acting as acid-reacting layer for the dye. The sheets of paper are then placed in an electric typewriter and are typed on with the pressure lever at setting 2.

The recording properties of the coating are then assessed according to the following scale: grade 5, intensely blue, very sharply defined characters, very legible; grade 4, strongly blue, very legible; grade 3, blue, legible; grade 2, bluish, just legible and grade 1, no coloration, no copy, illegible.

The coated paper stored at room temperature immediately gives a blue copy (grade 5). The papers stored at 80° and 95°C also immediately give copies of the same intensity (grade 5). This test shows that the microcapsule wall is so well sealed that the copying properties of the paper remain unchanged despite storage under hot conditions, which means that these microcapsules may be used for making copying papers stable on storage at room temperature for prolonged periods.

Example 2: In a repetition of Example 1, 67 parts of 1-methyl-3-phenyl-5-isopropylindan are used as solvent for the dye precursor in place of methylphenylindan. This solvent is a reaction product of styrene and p-isopropylstyrene. The solution is prepared by adding 180 parts of chloroform and there is produced, at a yield of more than 98%, a stable dispersion containing microcapsules having an average diameter of 7 μ. Paper coated with the resulting microcapsules is completely odorless, even when stored in a stack for a long period. When stored at room temperature, these papers give grade 5 copies. Storing for 16 hr at 80° and 95°C did not change the grading of the copies.

Ethyldiphenylmethane

E.C. Porter, Jr.; U.S. Patent 3,996,405; December 7, 1976; assigned to NCR Corporation provides record material comprising paper sheets coated with isolated liquid droplets, comprising ethyldiphenylmethane. The isolated liquid droplets are associated on the record material with at least two color-producing reactants, at least one of which is soluble in the liquid. The liquid is associated with the reactants by either being in close proximity to both reactants or by having one of the reactants dissolved therein and being in close proximity to the other.

Of the color-producing reactants, one is a chromogenic dye-precursor and one is a coreactant material capable of developing the color of the chromogenic dye-precursor when the two reactants are brought into reaction contact by rupture of the isolating medium. Isolation of the liquid droplets is accomplished by encapsulation of the droplets with pressure-rupturable, solid, polymeric, film material. Capsule-wall materials and capsule manufacture are not critical to this process.

In making pressure-sensitive record material with liquid-containing-microcapsules, successful commercial applications have made use of crystal violet lactone (CVL) as the chromogenic dye-precursor material, an acidic coreactant material such as attapulgite clay or an oil-soluble, para-substituted phenol-aldehyde novolak resin, and a liquid solvent that is at least in part isopropylbiphenyl as disclosed in U.S. Patent 3,627,581.

Isopropylbiphenyl has a low vapor pressure and good solvent power and is readily retained by gelatin films (the most widely used capsular wall material). Isopropylbiphenyl has, therefore, served well as the solvent in pressure-sensitive record material systems of the type disclosed. Ethyldiphenylmethane has been found to provide better print intensities and better fade resistance than the previously known isopropylbiphenyl.

Nonhalogenated diluent oils may be added to the ethyldiphenylmethane without adversely affecting the performance of the record systems made therewith. High-boiling aliphatic hydrocarbons and C_{10-15}-alkylbenzenes have been used successfully as ethyldiphenylmethane diluents. Since these diluents are generally cheaper than ethyldiphenylmethane, their use is in the interest of economy.

Dye-precursor materials in addition to CVL which may be dissolved in ethyldiphenylmethane for encapsulation purposes include any colorless, chromogenic dye-precursor materials such as those disclosed in U.S. Patent 3,672,935, and dialkylamino fluoran chromogenic compounds such as disclosed in U.S. Patent 3,681,390.

Example 1: Encapsulation of CVL-Ethyldiphenylmethane Solution – A solution of CVL, 1.7%, in ethyldiphenylmethane, was chosen for use as the internal phase of the capsules. The following formulation was emulsified in a Waring Blendor at 55°C to give internal phase droplets of 4 μ diameter: 150 g of internal phase, 150 g of 10% gelatin at pH 6.5 and 62 g of deionized water. Coacervation was accomplished by addition to the above emulsion, under continued agitation at 55°C, of 100 g of 10% gum arabic solution, 10 g of 5% PVM/MA, poly(vinyl methyl ether/maleic anhydride) and 600 g of deionized water. With continued agitation and temperature maintenance, the mixture was treated with sufficient

20% sodium hydroxide solution to adjust the pH to 9.0 and then with 12.5 ml of 14% acetic acid, dropwise. The mixture was then cooled slowly, with continued agitation, to 12°C and treated with 7.5 ml of 25% glutaraldehyde. After 4 hours of stirring, 12.0 ml of basic 5% PVM/MA (pH 9.0) is added, dropwise, to the mixture which is then stirred for an additional 2.5 hours while it gradually warms, up to about room temperature. The pH of the mixture, which is now a suspension of microcapsules, was finally adjusted to 9.5 with 20% sodium hydroxide. The microcapsules may be used as is, as an aqueous suspension or they may be isolated by filtration and air-dried.

Example 2: Encapsulation of CVL-Ethyldiphenylmethane-Hydrocarbon Oil – According to the procedure of Example 1, microcapsules were made wherein a 2:1 mixture of ethyldiphenylmethane and a saturated hydrocarbon oil (distillation range 370° to 500°F) was substituted for the ethyldiphenylmethane of that example.

Example 3: Encapsulation of CVL-Ethyldiphenylmethane-Alkylbenzene – According to the procedure of Example 1, microcapsules were made wherein a 1:2 mixture of ethyldiphenylmethane and a mono-C_{11-12} alkylbenzene was substituted for the ethyldiphenylmethane of that example.

Example 4: Record Material Sheets Coated with the Capsules of Examples 1, 2 and 3 – An aqueous coating slurry of the following composition was made up by stirring the following ingredients.

Ingredient	Parts Wet	Parts Dry
Capsules	465	100
Arrowroot starch granules	24	24
Cooked cornstarch	50	10
Water	41	-

Paper sheets were coated with the above slurry with a No. 15 Mayer rod to give a dried coating weight of about 3.5 pounds per ream (500 sheets, measuring 35 x 38 inches). Coatings made with the capsules of Examples 1, 2 or 3 gave record material sheets that yielded intense blue marks when marked on against acid-sensitized receiving sheets. The test receiving sheets were standard commercial receiving sheets sensitized according to U.S. Patent 3,663,256. The so-produced marks were more intense and provided better fade resistance (when exposed to light and air) than similar marks made with coated sheets having 2:1 isopropylbiphenyl-hydrocarbon oil as the capsular internal phase solvent for the CVL.

Capsules and capsule-coated sheets were made up according to Example 2 and this example and were compared quantitatively to sheets that were identical except that isopropylbiphenyl was substituted for the ethyldiphenylmethane of this process. When marks of the same pressure were made on the two above-described capsule-coated sheets against receiving sheets (sensitized with p-phenylphenol-formaldehyde resin according to U.S. Patent 3,672,935), the concentration of colored material developed on the receiving sheet by CVL in ethyldiphenylmethane was about 30% greater than that developed on the receiving sheet by CVL in isopropylbiphenyl.

Hydrogenated Petroleum Decomposition By-Product

Polychlorinated biphenyls have been widely utilized as the solvent for use in microcapsules for pressure sensitive copying paper. These compounds, however, accumulate in the human body and can exhibit significant toxicity. The process of *A. Sato; U.S. Patent 4,039,712; August 2, 1977; assigned to Nippon Petrochemicals Company Ltd., Japan* relates to another solvent for use in microcapsules for pressure-sensitive copying paper.

The process comprises hydrogenating a hydrocarbon mixture with a boiling range of 290° to 400°C, which is obtained as a by-product in the decomposition of petroleum, etc. and which contains polycyclic aromatic hydrocarbon compounds, at a temperature within 100° to 400°C in the presence of a hydrogenating catalyst capable of catalyzing nuclear hydrogenation so as to hydrogenate the aromatic rings of the compounds which contain at least three aromatic rings and are principal components of the polycyclic hydrocarbon compounds, leaving at least two aromatic rings therein intact.

Hydrogenation is carried out in the presence of a hydrogenation catalyst having an activity capable of nuclear hydrogenation, for example, nickel-cobalt-molybdenum, nickel-molybdenum, nickel-tungsten, cobalt-molybdenum, or sulfide thereof, platinum catalysts or copper-chromium catalysts. Hydrogenation should be carried out under such a condition as to realize partial nuclear hydrogenation on polycyclic aromatic hydrocarbons since complete nuclear hydrogenation will result in the products which are unusable as the solvent in the microcapsules. Preferred ranges of temperature and pressure for such hydrogenation are 100° to 400°C and 15 to 100 kg/cm^2 gauge respectively. Also the ratio of hydrogen to the starting material is maintained within 100 to 1,000 m^3 H_2/kl, preferably 400 to 600 m^3 H_2/kl.

Figure 7.1 shows the flow sheet of the process. A high-boiling fraction with a boiling range of 200° to 460°C containing polycyclic aromatic hydrocarbons is introduced from a pipe **1** into a flush drum **2**, and the high-boiling fraction from which heavy fraction (pitch and tar) is removed through a pipe **4** is further introduced, through a pipe **3** into a predistillation tower **5** and then through a pipe **7** into a predistillation tower **8**. A light fraction and a heavy fraction are respectively removed from the top of the tower **5** through a pipe **6** and from the bottom of the tower **8** through a pipe **9'**, and a fraction with a controlled boiling range of 290° to 400°C is taken out from the top of the tower **8**.

Figure 7.1: Flow Sheet for Hydrogenation Process

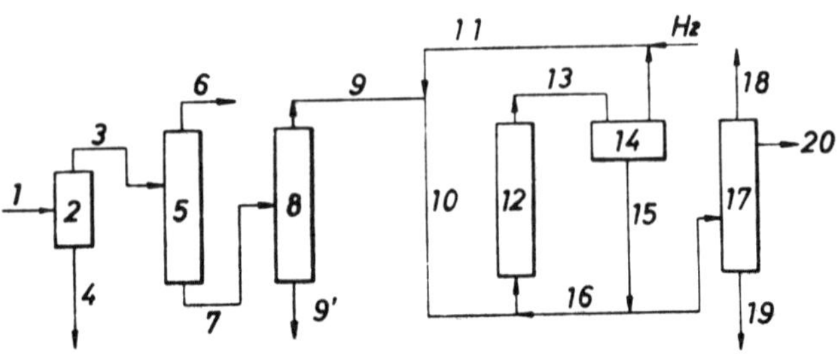

Source: U.S. Patent 4,039,712

The predistillation towers **5** and **8** are maintained at a reduced pressure in order to prevent the decomposition of the fraction. The predistillation towers **5** and **8** can be employed in the inverted order, or can be replaced by any other means or equipment capable of providing a fraction with a boiling range of 290° to 400°C by means of distillation.

The fraction obtained through the pipe **9** is mixed with hydrogen introduced through a pipe **11** and forwarded through a pipe **10** to a reactor **12** provided with a fixed catalyst bed. At this reaction it is also possible to employ a suitable diluent. The reaction mixture is taken out from the top of the reactor **12** through a pipe **13** and separated in a gas-liquid separator **14** into hydrogen and reaction product, which is forwarded through a pipe **15** into a distillation tower **17**.

A part of the flow in the pipe **15** is recycled to the reactor **12** through a pipe **16**. Light fraction and heavy fraction by-products at the hydrogenation are removed respectively from the top of the tower **17** through a pipe **18** and from the bottom of the tower **17** through a pipe **19** respectively, and the final solvent is obtained through a pipe **20**. The distillation in the tower **17** is preferably carried out under a reduced pressure. The removal of heavy fraction from the pipe **19** and of light fraction from the pipe **18** respectively improves the color and odor of the solvent. The light fraction removed from the pipe **18** is returned to and utilized again in the reactor **12**.

Example: A fraction with a boiling range of 290° to 400°C obtained by distillation from a fraction with a boiling range of 200° to 460°C, a by-product of an ethylene plant, was hydrogenated according to the flow sheet shown in Figure 7.1. The hydrogenation was carried out under the conditions of: temperature 300° to 320°C, pressure 17 kg/cm^2 gauge, SV 0.5, and a ratio of hydrogen to raw material 400 to 600 m^3 H_2/kl and in the presence of a fixed bed catalyst of nickel-cobalt-molybdenum. The solvent obtained by distillation after the hydrogenation was an excellent solvent for various dye precursors, had improved color and odor, and was free from toxic components.

The extent of hydrogenation was confirmed by mass spectrometer, and the solvent was found to be principally composed of components containing two aromatic rings represented by the general formulas C_nH_{2n-18}, C_nH_{2n-16} and C_nH_{2n-14} in which n ranges from 14 to 16.

Production of a pressure-sensitive copying paper utilizing coacervation process microcapsules utilizing the abovementioned solvent was performed as follows. Crystal violet lactone was used as the color forming agent, and the solvent, therefor was solely composed of the solvent obtained as described above. The color-forming solution was prepared by dissolving CVL in a 3% concentration in the solvent. A 1 wt % aqueous solution of polyvinyl methyl ether-maleic anhydride copolymer, water and an 11% aqueous solution of gelatin were placed in a blender, and the color-forming solution was added under agitation and mixed until the dispersed particle size of the solution reached 5 μ or less.

The emulsion thus obtained was added with a solution of gum arabic, and the mixture was regulated to a pH value of 9 and then diluted with water under agitation. Coacervate was precipitated around the dispersed particles by gradually lowering the pH value to 4.6 by means of the addition of 10% acetic acid.

After the encapsulating step, the capsule shells were hardened by a known process adding glutaraldehyde. A first sheet material, A, of pressure-sensitive copying paper was prepared by coating thus obtained microcapsules on a paper sheet. The microcapsules thus prepared were identical in performance with those prepared with prior process employing polychlorinated biphenyl. Two sheet materials, B and C, of pressure-sensitive copying paper respectively coated with clay and phenol-aldehyde copolymer were respectively superposed with the first sheet material A so that the capsule coating on the sheet material A and the coating on the second sheet materials B or C face each other.

Upon application of handwriting pressure on the noncoated surface of the first sheet material A, a blue image was obtained immediately on the second sheet material B and C. The obtained copy was sharp and clear, and the color developing speed was recognized to be sufficiently fast.

STILT MATERIALS

Alkali-Swollen Crosslinked Starch Granules

Carbonless copy paper employs chromogenic ink capsules coated on the copy paper which rupture under typewriter or similar impact pressure to release the marking material to make a copy without the necessity of carbon paper. Such coatings usually employ stilt materials, or protective materials in the coating which prevent premature rupture of the microcapsules during normal handling prior to use of the copy paper in making a data record copy.

The stilt material should be slightly larger than the microcapsules, and should be as inexpensive as possible. Most inexpensive starch granules which have the desirable uniformity of shape are too small in average size to effectively eliminate smudging of typical microencapsulated ink coatings on carbonless copy paper. One material which has the desired uniformity of shape, and a large enough average particle size is arrowroot starch. However, arrowroot starch is both scarce and expensive, so substitute stilt materials have been developed.

The process of *S. Rogols and J.W. Salter; U.S. Patent 4,139,505; February 13, 1979; assigned to General Mills Chemicals, Inc.* relates to an enlarged granular starch material obtained from smaller size starch granules which are first caused to enlarge without a complete loss of birefringence, and are then treated to retain the enlarged intact discrete granular structure through subsequent coating and processing operations. Enlargement of average granule size may be as much as 25 to 35% without loss of birefringence. The initial controlled swelling of the granules is obtained by treating an aqueous slurry of the undersized granules with an alkali such as sodium hydroxide at a level of alkalinity and for a time sufficient to swell the granules without loss of birefringence.

When a bimodal starch such as wheat is being treated, it can be obtained from wheat flour second clears without drying, or a previously dried wheat starch can be used. The bimodal wheat starch can be subjected to a single-pass through a hydrocyclone of the type described in U.S. Patent 3,901,725 to separate out only the smallest granule portion so that the average subsieve particle size of the starch granules to be alkali treated is at least 12.5 μ. After the single-pass hydrocyclone separation, the underflow stream contains the slightly larger granule portion and comprises about half of the original weight of the starch. This underflow stream is treated with sodium hypochlorite to oxidize the granules slightly and enhance the alkali-swelling. The usual alkali treatment period is about two hours. Care must be taken throughout the treatment of the starch granules to preserve granule birefringence and retain cold water insolubility of the granules.

The swollen granules are then strengthened against dissolution or fragmentation by crosslinking them with a polyfunctional crosslinking agent such as phosphorus oxychloride, epichlorohydrin, sodium hexametaphosphate or urea-formaldehyde. The crosslinked granules are resistant to heat, and can be slurried in water during the copy paper coating process without dissolving. The enlarged granules are sufficiently large to provide effective protection to ink microcapsules during handling of coated carbon copy paper.

Undersized starch granules can be enlarged and made into effective stilt materials by the process, thereby substantially increasing the proportion of usable granules in a starch having bimodal granule size distribution. The smallest granules of wheat starch are difficult to swell sufficiently without loss of birefringence to attain a particle size which is useful as a typical stilt material, in which the average subsieve particle size should be more than 14 μ, and preferably, at least 14.5 μ. As presently practiced, by combining the single-step hydrocyclone separation, the alkali-swelling and crosslinking, approximately 50% by weight of the starch in a prime grade wheat starch can be utilized as stilt materials by using this process.

Example 1: A slurry of wheat starch was cooled to 70° to 74°F (21.1° to 23.3°C), and the pH was adjusted to 4. The slurry was then treated by adding dilute sodium hydroxide (4.5° Bé) until the titer was 13.3 ml. An alkaline titer procedure was used in all examples which employed 0.1 N HCl added dropwise to a 10 ml starch slurry sample containing phenolphthalein until the sample reaches the phenolphthalein end point (solution changes from red to clear), as described in U.S. Patent 3,876,629.

The temperature increased during this addition to about 80°F (26.7°C). The above addition of sodium hydroxide caused the starch granules to swell without losing their birefringence. After one hour of the above treatment, 0.36% by weight phosphorus oxychloride based on the weight of the starch was added to crosslink the enlarged granules. The addition of phosphorus oxychloride caused the titer to drop to about 9.8 to 10.0 ml.

A sample of the swollen granules showed an average subsieve particle size above 13 μ, compared to an initial subsieve value of about 11 μ for the original prime grade starch. The Kofler hot stage pasting temperature for this product was 122° to 125.6°F (50° to 52°C). When observed microscopically, the granules appeared to have retained their shape and integrity, but were large and rounder, and exhibited birefringence under polarized light. The product was used as a stilt material for carbonless copy paper, and provided acceptable smudge (friction staining) values above 80 and typewriter intensity values below 55.

Example 2: In a typical production process, a quantity of first-pass underflow wheat starch slurry is collected from a hydrocyclone system. The hydrocyclones are type P Doxie Impurity Eliminators and have the following dimensions.

Diameter, cylindrical section	1.02"
Height, cylindrical section	19/32"
Diameter, feed aperture	3/16"
Diameter, vortex finder	21/64"
Length, vortex finder (inside)	7/8"
Diameter, discharge aperture	350"
Apex angle	16°

Typical Baumé of the feed slurry is 7.5° Bé. The feed slurry may be made from either previously dried wheat starch, or from native colloid wheat starch slurry which is substantially free of fiber and gluten and has never been dried. It is important that the slurry of starch granules be substantially free of broken or damaged granules and fragments of granules, and that the granules be effectively nonagglomerated after the pretreatment and before commencing the alkali-swelling.

The slurry is placed in a reactor tub at 70° to 72°F (21.1° to 22.2°C) and about 0.44% by weight based on the starch dry weight of chlorine (added as sodium hypochlorite) is added and reacted for 1.5 to 2 hours. This oxidation treatment is believed to open the granules slightly to make the granules more susceptible to the alkali-swelling. The slurry temperature is then kept below 80°F (26.7°C) while being agitated and 4° to 5° Bé sodium hydroxide is added until 10 ml of slurry requires 13 to 14 ml of 0.1N HCl to titrate to a phenolphthalein end point (that is, when the titer solution just turns clear from red).

Approximately 1.8% by weight NaOH (dry solids) is required, based on the dry weight of the starch. The alkali treated slurry is stirred for about a two hour reaction time, and a sample is removed and observed under a polarized light microscope. Birefringence of the granules should be present. The sample is also observed for subsieve value. The alkali-swelling should be continued until the subsieve value is 15.8 μ or more, but the granules should retain their birefringence. The usual time is about two hours.

Then the slurry is adjusted to a titer of 9 ml by adding phosphorus oxychloride. About 0.36% $POCl_3$ based on the weight of the dry starch is required. After the titer is adjusted to 9 ml, the slurry is allowed to react for 0.5 to 1 hour. The slurry is then adjusted to 5 to 7 pH with concentrated sulfuric acid, about 2.3% by weight H_2SO_4 based on the starch dry weight is required. The slurry is then screened, filtered, washed and dried. The dried swollen starch is then ground in a Jeffrey mill, taking care to preserve the intact granules.

The resulting product has an average subsieve particle size of at least 14.0 μ, and the birefringence of the granules is retained. The crosslinking insures that the granules will remain intact during normal carbonless copy paper coating applications. The slightly crosslinked granules have a Kofler hot stage pasting temperature of 12° to 18°F (5° to 8.3°C) higher than the prime grade wheat starch from which they were made.

Starch Derivatives from Legume Sources

D.L. Johnson; U.S. Patent 3,996,060; December 7, 1976; assigned to A.E. Staley Manufacturing Company describes several new starches which are useful stilt materials having the required properties of particle size, TI and FS values and which can replace scarce arrowroot starch granules.

These new stilt materials are starches derived from certain species of legumes now being cultivated in the Great Plains provinces of Canada, where the cool climate is particularly suited for the growing of faba bean (*Vicia faba L.*) and yellow field pea (*Pisum sativum* var.).

The particle size of the starches derived from these legumes falls in the highly desirable range of 20 to 75 μ. It is further expected that these starch particles will have an ideal balance of TI (typewriter intensity) value of 55 or less when tested according to the test procedure set forth in Dutch Patent 7,005,045 and an FS (friction stain) value of 85 or more.

The pasting temperatures of these large granule starches can be increased as necessary to meet the higher temperatures used in at least one of the coating processes. The pasting temperatures may be increased by at least 20°F by means of a highly alkaline, two step $POCl_3$ crosslinking process which retains the granular discrete particle structure of the starch. Other crosslinking agents which may be used for increasing the pasting temperature of these starches include epichlorohydrin, urea-formaldehyde, mixed anhydrides (from adipic acid and acetic anhydride), and other polyfunctional crosslinkers including polyphosphate salts.

The highly alkaline $POCl_3$ crosslinking process is preferred because it has a rapid reaction, and gives a substantial increase in pasting temperature. When yellow field pea starch was $POCl_3$ crosslinked according to the highly alkaline method, the pasting temperature was increased 20°F in one test (Kofler hot stage pasting temperature). The faba bean starch, crosslinked by the alkaline $POCl_3$ reaction, had an increase in pasting temperature of about 20°F. It is believed that this substantial increase in temperature stability obtained with both of these starches makes them ideally suited for coating processes in which the drying temperature in the coating reaches as high as 158°F, with complete retention of the protective function of the stilt starch particles. The types of starches which are believed useful as stilt materials and for other applications, such as antioffset lithograph powders, include the following.

Type of Plant Source	. . . Starch Granule Size, μ . . . Average	Largest
Varieties of pea:		
Yellow field pea	20-40	60
Shell pea	20-40	60
Chickling pea	15-30	45
Wrinkled pea	5-25	25*
Varieties of bean:		
Faba bean	25-50	50
Common bean	20-50	60
Kidney bean	20-40	60
Runner bean	20-40	60
Lima bean	8-50	75
Adzuki bean	30-65	90
Jack bean	20-40	55*
Cultivated vetch	20-35	55
Moon bean	20-50	75
Lentil	20-40	55*

*Estimated.

The above average granule sizes are taken, in part from the literature, and in part from actual measurements. It must be appreciated that particular samples and other varieties of legumes may have some different average granule sizes, with less or more large granules, and the actual size of the large granules observed in a particular sample can differ from sample to sample.

Example 1: Samples of starch derived from yellow field pea, *Pisum sativum* var. Trapper 1973 and Century 1972 were tested for Kofler hot stage pasting temperature, and DSC pasting temperature, following the procedure described in U.S. Patent 3,876,629. Similar tests were run for starches derived from faba bean, *Vicia faba L.* (Leguminosae). The test results are set forth below in tabular form.

Type of Starch	DSC Pasting Temperature, °C Start	Peak	End	Kofler Hot Stage, °C
Yellow field pea	62	67	74	60
Faba bean	62	67	73	60

When the above starches were $POCl_3$ crosslinked using the highly alkaline process, the Kofler hot stage pasting temperatures increased to 71°C for crosslinked yellow field pea starch and 70°C for crosslinked faba bean starch. This represents an increase in pasting temperature by means of the $POCl_3$ crosslinking of better than 20°F. These crosslinked products can be used in coating equipment which dries the coating at surface coating temperatures up to 158°F. The alkali fluidity values for those crosslinked starches, again following the test procedure set forth in U.S. Patent 3,876,629, and using 15 g dry substance starch product, 25 ml distilled water, and 80 ml 2 N NaOH, were as follows.

Type of Starch	Alkali Fluidity
Yellow field pea	80
Faba bean	55

It does appear that the starches derived from faba bean will require some color improvements, as by bleaching, depending on the particular color requirements in use. The Coulter counts performed on the subject starches showed the following.

Type of Starch	Percent Larger than 10 μ	Percent Larger than 20 μ	Percent Larger than 30 μ
Yellow field pea	96	60	10
Faba bean	100	55	5

D.L. Johnson; U.S. Patent 3,996,061; December 7, 1976; assigned to A.E. Staley Manufacturing Company also found that although the starches disclosed above have the desirable starch particle size, they have relatively large amounts of protein and fiber, which can interfere with the use of these starches as stilt materials for pressure sensitive microencapsulated coatings. It has been found important to remove the protein and fiber from these large granule legume starches to obtain the required functionality, particularly when yellow field pea starch is used. For this purpose, the starches of Example 1 were subjected to additional processing as set forth below.

Example 2: The yellow field pea starch of Example 1 was slurried in water to make a 30% solids suspension. A small amount of a dispersing aid, such as a nonionic surfactant (Pluronic L-61) was added. The slurry was then screened through a 140 mesh screen to remove fiber, and the screen was washed with water. The screened material was then filtered with no added washing. The filter cake, containing about 46% by weight water was then reslurried with sufficient added water to make a 30% solids suspension. The pH was about 6.8, or nearly neutral.

The slurry was then treated with an amount of NaOCl which was sufficient to provide 2% by weight chlorine based on the starch dry substance to remove substantially all traces of protein from the screened and filtered starch slurry. During the chlorine treatment, the pH of the slurry dropped from 10.5 to 8.8.

To stop the action of the chlorine, sodium metabisulfite was added to the slurry. The pH dropped further, down to about 5.3, and was then adjusted to nearly neutral with soda ash (Na_2CO_3). The slurry was then filtered and washed, and the filter cake was dried to about 9.8% moisture. The resulting large granule pea starch was substantially free of fiber and protein. The Gardner Color Index for this product was 7.6, and the Coulter Count Test revealed that at least 50% by weight of the granules were 27.5 μ in size, or larger.

The resulting product was tested in a carbonless copy paper coating, and provided superior protection for the microencapsulated ink granules, as evidenced by handling tests (smudge value and friction staining). The improved protein and fiber free yellow field pea starch so obtained comprised about 87% by weight of the total weight of the unimproved starch from which it was prepared. The preferred Gardner Color Index should be below about 9, and the maximum acceptable percentage nitrogen (indication of protein) is about 0.1% by weight (Kjehldahl analysis) and the preferred maximum nitrogen is about 0.05% by weight.

Example 3: Another sample of yellow field pea starch as described in Example 1 was subjected to the following additional processing to remove fiber and protein. These additional steps are preferably completed prior to any crosslinking or other derivatization.

The yellow field pea starch was slurried at 30% solids and screened to remove all fiber as before, through a 140 mesh screen. The screened slurry was then filtered, reslurried at 30% solids, and refiltered. The filter cake was reslurried at 30% solids and the pH was adjusted to 4.0 with dilute HCl. About 0.03% by weight $KMnO_4$ in dilute solution was added to the slurry and reacted for about 1 hour with stirring. Then 0.18% by weight dry sodium metabisulfite was added to stop the oxidation. The slurry was neutralized with soda ash, filtered, washed and dried. The resulting product had a Gardner Color Value of 7.5 or less, and a N_2 analysis (Kjehldahl) of 0.12% by weight.

Other oxidation agents could be used, provided that the desirable granular structure, and the desirable Gardner Color Values are obtained. For example, hydrogen peroxide, sodium hypochlorite, chlorinated lime, and 1% sodium hydroxide with 0.5% NaOCl are all considered useful in varying degrees as oxidation agents to effectively remove the excess protein, and improve the color of the starch granules to a level acceptable for these stilt material containing coatings.

Large Granule Wheat Starch

The need for improving the yield of usable protective material derived from wheat starch becomes evident when the selling price of the by-product small granule portion is compared to the much greater value of the large granule protective material which is used in carbonless copy paper coatings.

R.W. Best; U.S. Patent 4,141,747; February 27, 1979; assigned to General Mills Chemicals, Inc. describe a method of obtaining a large granule starch material having a weight average particle size of 20 μ or larger. The bulk of the large granule starch material is obtained from a prime grade wheat starch which normally has a typical granule size distribution with 20 to 22% by weight of the granules ranging in size from 20 to 32 μ and 50 to 55% by weight of the granules ranging in size from 16 to 32 μ, and 45 to 50% are 2 to 16 μ.

The process employs a wet separation system in which the slurried starch is passed through a plurality of hydrocyclones which are connected to recirculate certain by-product streams back into the system as a part of the feed stream to increase the yield of large granule starch product by 15 to 25%. For every 100 parts by weight of feed starch, the yield of useful product which can be obtained is 40 parts or better.

An important feature of the process is the careful balancing of the recirculation feed streams so that the proportion of large granules and small granules substantially matches the proportion of such granules found in the feed stream. The system is most effective when the feed stream is kept in careful balance by careful control of the recirculation feed streams.

There is thus obtained the best possible yield of a particular average granule size from a starch feed stream having a plurality of possible particle size fractions. A primary hydrocyclone supplies a second and third hydrocyclone. One stream is recirculated from each of the second and third hydrocyclones and they are added to the feed starch slurry which is supplied to the first hydrocyclone. The particle size distribution of the recirculated streams should substantially match, or nearly match, the input starch feed stream particle size distribution.

If the recirculated streams fall below the particle size distribution of the feed stream, the product particle size distribution gradually drops below specification. If the recirculated streams are higher than the feed stream in particle size distribution, the system requires adjustment to remove more large granules on the first and second pass underflows. Otherwise, the particle size distribution of the product will vary considerably, with some collected product exceeding product specification, which represents an economic loss, since less product is produced for a given amount of feed stream starch. The process can improve the yield of product fraction by as much as 15 to 25%.

The resulting product may be further improved by adding and blending a predetermined amount of another starch with it, which starch has a different particle size distribution, to change the particle size distribution of the final product in the direction of the particle size distribution of the added starch. For example, when the average particle size of a large granule wheat starch fraction is slightly lower than desired, it may be increased by blending a predetermined amount of refined, large granule pea starch, arrowroot starch, or specially fractionated potato starch having a higher particle size distribution than the fractionated wheat starch to obtain the desired increase in overall particle size of the blended, large granule product. The product can be dewatered and dried and used as a protective material in carbonless copy paper. Details for obtaining the large granule starch are presented. No specific proportions are given for its use in carbonless copy paper.

Incorporation of Epoxy or Polystyrene Resin in Fill Material

In accordance with the process of *G.E. Maalouf; U.S. Patent 4,000,087; December 28, 1976; assigned to Moore Business Forms, Inc.* unintended CF (coated front) discoloration is substantially avoided in colorless copying systems utilizing CB (coated back) coatings comprising microencapsulated dye precursor solutions through the use of an additive which is included in the encapsulated liquid fill material.

The microcapsules comprise minute discrete droplets of liquid fill material including an initially colorless chemically reactive color forming dye precursor and a carrier therefor encapsulated within individual, rupturable, generally continuous polyamide shells. These microcapsules are produced by incorporating in the fill material, an amount of an epoxy or polystyrene resin effective to render the microcapsules resistant to inadvertent release and transfer of the fill material. The polyamide shells are formed by interfacial polycondensation from a polyterephthalamide and the resin which is added to the fill is an epichlorohydrin/bisphenol A epoxy resin.

The process has been found to be particularly useful in conjunction with microcapsules which contain a dye precursor such as Michler's hydrol, p-toluene sulfinate of Michler's hydrol, methyl ether of Michler's hydrol, benzyl ether of Michler's hydrol and the morpholine derivative of Michler's hydrol.

The preferred polystyrene resin is Styron 666U, a general purpose polystyrene having a Vicat softening point of 212°F (ASTM method D1525) and an Izod impact strength of 0.2 ft-lb/in of notch at 73°F (ASTM method D256). This material also has a specific gravity of 1.04 (ASTM method D792) and a melt viscosity of 1,800 poises (ASTM method Rate B D1703). The preferred epoxy resin is Epon 1002, an epichlorohydrin/bisphenol A-type solid epoxy resin. Epon 1002 has a viscosity of 1.7 to 3.0 poises when measured at 25°C by the Bubble-Test method (ASTM D154), and an epoxide equivalent of 600 to 700 (ASTM D1652-59T).

Example 1: Control – Microcapsules having a fill material which does not contain a polystyrene or epoxy resin were produced for comparison purposes. 1.00 gram of p-toluene sulfinate of Michler's hydrol (PTSMH) were admixed with 20.0 g of dibutyl phthalate (DBP) solvent and this admixture was warmed slightly on a hot plate until a clear solution (A) was obtained.

Thereafter solution A was allowed to cool to room temperature. Then, 3.26 g of terephthaloyl chloride were added to 10.0 g of DBP solvent and this mixture was also warmed slightly on a hot plate until a clear solution (B) was obtained. Solution B was then also allowed to cool to room temperature. After solutions A and B were prepared, 100 ml of an aqueous solution containing 2.0 wt %

Elvanol 50-42 (a polyvinyl alcohol having a hydrolysis of 87 to 89% and a viscosity of 35 to 45 cp in a 4% aqueous solution at 20°C as determined by the Hoeppler falling ball method) were placed in a semimicro Waring blender and then solutions A and B were mixed together at room temperature and the resultant solution was added to the Elvanol solution in the blender. The blender was activated and high shear agitation was continued for about 2 minutes until an emulsion having a dispersed phase particle size of 5 to 6 μ was obtained.

In this emulsion, the continuous phase was the aqueous solution containing the Elvanol polyvinyl alcohol and the dispersed phase was the DBP solution of PTSMH and terephthaloyl chloride. The emulsion was then transferred to a suitable container, such as a beaker, and was stirred with a variable speed mechanical stirrer at 300 to 500 rpm while an aqueous solution containing 1.86 g of diethylene triamine, 0.96 g of sodium carbonate and 20 ml of water was added. Stirring was continued at room temperature for about 24 hours until a stable pH was observed.

By this time, the dispersed phase particles had become individually encapsulated in a polyamide shell. The slurry containing the microcapsules and having the Elvanol polyvinyl alcohol binder in the continuous phase was then drawn down on a 13 lb neutral base continuous bond paper sheet at a coating weight of 2.34 to 3.04 g/m^2 and the coated sheet was oven dried at a temperature of 110°C for 30 to 45 seconds.

Example 2: The procedure was identical with that in Example 1 except that, in this instance 1.0 g of Epon 1002 was incorporated in solution A and the preparation of solution A was varied slightly in that the Epon 1002 and the dibutyl phthalate were first mixed and the admixture was warmed slightly on a hot plate until a clear solution was obtained. This solution was allowed to cool to room temperature before the PTSMH was added.

The PTSMH was then added at room temperature and the admixture was again warmed slightly on a hot plate until a clear solution was obtained. Solution A containing Epon 1002, PTSMH and DBP was then allowed to cool to room temperature. The capsules thus produced, which include a fill material containing Epon 1002, were coated onto a paper substrate in accordance with the procedure outlined in Example 1.

Example 3: The exact procedure outlined in Example 2 was repeated except that the quantity of Epon 1002 included in solution A is 2.0 g. The microcapsules thus produced were coated onto a paper substrate outlined in Example 1.

Example 4: The procedure outlined in Example 2 was repeated identically except that 1.0 g of Styron 666U was utilized in solution A rather than the Epon 1002. The resultant microcapsules were coated onto a paper substrate as outlined in Example 1.

Example 5: Coated paper was produced by a procedure identical with that in Example 4 except that solution A contained 2.0 g of Styron 666U.

The CB papers produced in accordance with Examples 2 through 5 above were compared with the CB paper in Example 1. The papers were evaluated and compared with regard to the intensity of the image produced in an eight-part manifolded set when the latter is subjected to normal usage, with regard to ghosting and with regard to blush. In each instance where CF sheets are utilized or referred to in the following evaluation and comparison procedures it should be understood that the acidic coatings thereon consist of acid-leached bentonite-type clay layers.

Ghosting is defined as a secondary image transfer from a CB sheet to a CF sheet. The primary image is the original image produced on a CF sheet as a result of an imaging process such as typing, printing, etc. Secondary image transfer occurs subsequently to the original image producing operation. To measure the secondary image transfer (or ghosting), a fresh CF sheet is mated with the CB sheet in place of the original imaged CF sheet and the secondary image thus produced is examined visually at different periods. Ghosting could occur during ordinary handling of carbonless paper and is objectionable in carbonless copying systems.

Blush is an unintentional coloration of a CF coating caused by contact with free precursor from a CB coating. Blush can result from the presence of a small amount of dye precursor which initially escaped encapsulation, from leaky capsules or from capsules which are ruptured during processing or handling of the carbonless paper.

It was determined that the papers produced in accordance with Examples 2, 3 and 4 were capable of generating an image having an intensity comparable with the intensity of the image generated by the paper produced in Example 1 while the image generated by the paper produced in Example 5 had slightly less intensity than the intensity of the image from the paper of Example 1 although the intensity of the image from the paper of Example 5 was acceptable.

With regard to blush, the samples were evaluated 5 days, 9 days and 19 days after production. The papers produced in accordance with Examples 2 through 5 clearly exhibited less blush than the papers produced in accordance with Example 1 at all stages of the blush evaluation and comparison tests.

With regard to ghosting, the papers were tested for ghosting after 5 days and after 20 days. At the end of 5 days, none of the papers produced in accordance with Examples 1 through 5 exhibited a significant tendency to ghost. After 20 days, however, each of the papers tested showed some ghosting, although in no instance was the ghosting experienced with the papers produced in accordance with Examples 2 through 5 greater than the ghosting which was experienced with the paper produced in accordance with Example 1 and in fact the paper produced in accordance with Example 2 (low concentration Epon) showed less ghosting than the paper of Example 1.

Since blush was substantially reduced and image intensity was not significantly diminished, it was concluded that the paper produced in accordance with Examples 2 through 5 was superior to the paper produced in accordance with Example 1.

COATING COMPOSITIONS

Hot Melt Suspending Medium with Microencapsulated Chromogen

The process of *G.T. Davis, G. Schwab and D.R. Shackle; U.S. Patents 4,137,343; January 30, 1979 and 4,143,890; March 13, 1979; both assigned to The Mead Corporation* relates to a pressure-sensitive carbonless transfer sheet comprising a paper substrate having a front and back surface and a coating composition adhered to at least one of the front and back surfaces of the paper substrate. The coating composition is set to a flexible, tack-free coat. The coating composition includes a solvent free nonaqueous hot melt suspending medium which is characterized by being substantially water insoluble, being characterized by the presence of one or more functional groups selected from the group consisting of carboxyl, carbonyl, hydroxyl, ester, amide, amine, heterocyclic groups and combinations thereof to impart polarity thereto and having a melting point of 60° to 140°C and a melting point range of less than 15°C.

In addition, the coating composition includes an encapsulated, chromogenic material which is substantially dispersed therein, the hot melt suspending medium being compatible with the color forming characteristics of the capsular chromogenic material. This process further includes a liquid chromogenic coating composition which comprises a hot melt suspending medium in combination with a microencapsulated chromogenic material. The chromogenic material is a color precursor of the electron donating type which is mixed with a carrier oil to form an oil solution of the chromogenic color precursor material which is then combined with one or more wall forming compounds.

A process for producing a pressure-sensitive carbonless transfer sheet comprises the steps of preparing a hot melt suspending medium, the hot melt suspending medium being water insoluble and having a melting point of 60° to 140°C and a melting point range of 0° to 15°C. A microencapsulated chromogenic material is prepared and dispersed in the hot melt suspending medium, the chromogenic material being a color precursor of the electron donating type.

A coating dispersion is prepared by combining the hot melt suspending medium with the microencapsulated chromogenic color precursor material, the hot melt suspending medium being compatible with the color forming or developing characteristics of the chromogenic material. The coating dispersion is then applied to a substrate, the coating dispersion being applied at a coat weight of 1.0 to 8.0 lb/3,300 ft^2 of substrate at a coat thickness of 1 to 50 μ. The coated substrate is set by cooling the coating dispersion.

The preferred group of electron donating color precursors includes the lactone phthalides, such as crystal violet lactone and 3,3-bis(1-ethyl-2-methylindol-3-yl)-phthalide, the lactone fluorans, such as 2-dibenzylamino-6-diethylaminofluoran and 6-diethylamino-1,3-dimethylfluoran, the lactone xanthenes, the leucoauramines, the 2-(omega substituted vinylene)-3,3-disubstituted-3-H-indoles and 1,3,3-trialkylindolinospirans. Microencapsulated oil solutions of color precursors are used. The color precursors are preferably present in such oil solutions in an amount of from 2 to 7%. The hot melt suspending media include waxes and resins. The preferred group of compounds useful as hot melt suspending media include deresinated, oxidized mineral waxes such as the montan waxes, amide waxes such as bisstearamide wax, stearamide wax, behenamide wax, fatty acid waxes, hydroxylated fatty acid waxes, hydroxy stearate waxes, oxazoline waxes, amine waxes and mixtures thereof. The hot melt suspending medium is characterized by having a penetration hardness of less than or equal to 0.1 to 20.0, a melting point of 60° to 140°C, a narrow melting range of less than 15°C, a low viscosity when molten, a certain amount of polarity and a light color.

Included in the preferred group of hot melt suspending media are the following waxes: 2-n-heptadecyl-4,4-bis-hydroxymethyl-2-oxazoline, N,N'-ethylenebisstearamide, N-(2-hydroxyethyl)-12-hydroxystearamide, glyceryl monohydroxystearate and ethylene glycol monohydroxystearate and mixtures thereof.

Another type of preferred hot melt suspending media is a nonpolar hydrocarbon wax, such as Be Square 170/175 which includes a small amount of dispersing agent. The dispersing agent may, for instance, be sulfated castor oil, more commonly known as Turkey red oil. The preferred waxes have a penetration hardness of from 0.1 to 20, preferably 0.1 to 3, measured by the needle penetration test given an ASTM designation of D1321-61T.

Example: The apparatus used in the example is a four-necked round bottom flask fitted with stirrer, vacuum take-off, addition funnel and manometer. For Run A, the abovementioned four-necked flask containing 60 g oxazoline wax (Oxawax TS-254AA) was immersed into an oil bath at a bath temperature of 210° to 220°F. The wax melted and an aspirator was connected to produce reduced pressure (26 mm Hg). An aqueous HPC (hydroxypropylcellulose) capsule slurry (60.5 g, 24.2 g dry weight) was added over a period of several hours during which time the water was removed.

The final hot melt dispersion was of low viscosity, about 400 cp at 85°C and easy to apply to paper with a heated Mayer bar. The coated sheet appeared smooth and white with a slightly waxy feel. It marked very well when typed against a novolak coated record sheet.

For Run B, into the same apparatus a mixture of 56 g Oxawax TS-254AA and 14 g Oxawax TS-254A was melted. 30 g HPC capsules (dry weight) were slowly added to the melt under reduced pressure and agitation. To the final hot melt 20 g of dry arrowroot starch was added. The mixture had a viscosity of 600 cp at 85°C. It was coated on paper to form a white slightly waxy surface. This CB surface formed clear and intense images when typed against a novolak coated record sheet.

The oxazoline waxes used above contain the heterocyclic oxazoline group and some hydroxy groups. Oxazoline waxes are available under designations including Oxawaxes TS-254, TS-254A, TS-254AA and TS-970.

This illustrates a preferred species of hot melt suspending media wherein polarity is imparted to the waxes by the presence of one or more functional groups such as carboxyl, carbonyl, hydroxyl, ester, amide, amine, heterocyclic groups and combinations thereof. In addition to the oxazoline wax, others used successfully include those of the modified mineral type (synthetic waxes) or of vegetable origin. Specific synthetic waxes are Hoechst waxes S, LP and L, which are acid waxes based on montan wax, further modified by oxidation to obtain carboxylic acid groups in the final grades (some original ester groups are kept intact);

Duroxon waxes J–324 AM, H 111 and E 421 R, which are oxygenated and esterfied Fishcher-Tropsch waxes; Paricin waxes which are glyceryl monohydroxy stearate, ethylene glycol monohydroxystearate, stearyl 12-hydroxystearate and N-(2-hydroxyethyl)-12-hydroxystearamide. Further polar waxes include Ceramid (hydroxyethylstearamide) from Glyco Chemicals, Inc.; Advawax (bisamide waxes) from Cincinnati Milacron; and Ceramer (a maleic anhydride-ethylene glycol-modified oxidized hydrocarbon wax) from the Bareco Division of the Petrolite Corporation.

All of these waxes can be used singly or in combination. Another bonus of most of the above mentioned polar waxes is their high melting point and their great hardness which eliminates wax transfer to the developing sheet, thus improving image clarity, increases blocking temperature and diminishes picking problems.

It should also be noted that the method of preparation of the dispersion in this example is one in which the hot melt phase is melted and stirred in molten form at reduced pressure while an aqueous slurry of microcapsules is added slowly and continuously. This technique results in an almost instantaneous removal of water. The upholding of nearly anhydrous conditions is important in this particular process because the microcapsules used have been found to degrade considerably in hot (about 70°C) aqueous mixtures, but to be thermally stable at about 95°C for about 18 hours under nearly anhydrous conditions.

Alternatively, the dispersion can be made by a process wherein the HPC microcapsules in an aqueous slurry are spray dried to form a free flowing powder. This free flowing powder is stirred into a molten phase of a single wax or of a mixture of waxes to form a smooth dispersion of microcapsules in the continuous molten phase. The hot melt can be coated or printed onto the paper substrate. It sets immediately after application to the substrate and forms excellent marking sheets. Total coat weights of 3 to 4 lb/3,300 ft^2 are used in the best examples of this method.

While this example establishes the use of HPC capsules in various polar hot melt suspending media as one preferred type CB coating, other microcapsules may be used and a nonpolar hot melt suspension medium may also be used as long as a dispersing agent is also present.

Dispersion of Microcapsules in Radiation Curable Binder

A process is provided by *Y.-S. Lee and D.R. Shackle; U.S. Patent 4,110,511; August 29, 1978; assigned to The Mead Corporation* for the production of a coating composition containing microcapsules having a hydrophilic core for use in the manufacture of pressure-sensitive carbonless transfer papers comprising the following steps. A hydrophilic emulsion component is prepared by dispersing at least one chromogenic material in a hydrophilic liquid, the chromogenic material being soluble in the hydrophilic liquid.

A hydrophobic emulsion component is prepared by dispersing an emulsifier in a radiation curable hydrophobic liquid. A first wall-forming material and a second wall-forming material are added to the hydrophobic emulsion component, with mixing. The first and second wall-forming materials are soluble in the hydrophobic emulsion component, and the first wall-forming material is reactive with the second wall-forming material to form a polymeric capsule wall. The resultant polymeric capsule wall is substantially insoluble in the hydrophilic and the hydrophobic emulsion components. The hydrophobic emulsion component is mixed together with the hydrophilic emulsion component to form an emulsion containing droplets of the hydrophilic emulsion component dispersed in the hydrophobic emulsion component.

Mixing is maintained for a period of time sufficient to allow the first and second wall-forming materials to react to form a dispersion of microcapsules in the hydrophobic emulsion component. The formed microcapsules have capsule walls substantially impermeable to the hydrophobic and the hydrophilic emulsion components.

The pressure-sensitive carbonless transfer paper may be produced by applying the dispersion of the microcapsules prepared as above to a substrate, and curing the dispersion by subjecting the dispersion on the substrate to radiation for a period of time sufficient to cure the radiation curable hydrophobic liquid, thereby producing a tack-free, resinous film on the substrate.

The dispersion of microcapsules is prepared in situ in the radiation curable hydrophobic liquid by reaction of a first wall-forming material and a second wall-forming material both present in the radiation curable hydrophobic liquid. The term chromogenic refers to materials such as color precursors, color developers, and color formers. The coating composition can also contain photoinitiators.

To prepare pressure-sensitive transfer sheets, the most preferred hydrophilic liquid is a mixture of water and glycerin. The hydrophilic liquid also contains at least one chromogenic material dissolved therein. Besides being soluble in the hydrophilic liquid, the chromogenic materials should be essentially insoluble in the hydrophobic liquid and should not be substantially reactive to any appreciable degree with the other ingredients of the coating composition, such as the hydrophilic liquid, the radiation curable substance and the wall-forming materials.

The chromogenic material can be selected from any color-forming pair in which one chromogenic material reacts with another chromogenic material in the presence of the hydrophilic liquid to form a color. Following are pairs in which the first mentioned chromogenic material is particularly useful. A most preferred chromogenic material is sodium orthovanadate.

Color Former Pairs	Color
Ammonium ferric sulfate-potassium ferrocyanide	Blue
Ammonium ferric sulfate-potassium thiocyanate	Red-brown
Ammonium ferric sulfate-salicylaldoxime	Brown
Ammonium ferric sulfate-gallic acid	Black
Ammonium ferric sulfate-tannic acid	Black
Ammonium ferric sulfate-catechol	Black
Ammonium ferric sulfate-8-hydroxyquinoline	Black
Ferric oleate-catechol	Violet-black
Ferric oleate-sodium diethyldithiocarbonate	Black
Sodium orthovanadate-2-ethylhexyl gallate	Black
Sodium orthovanadate-gallic acid	Black
Ammonium metavanadate-gallic acid	Black

(continued)

Color Former Pairs	Color
Ammonium metavanadate-tannic acid	Black
Ferric sulfate-2,4-dinitro-1-napththol	Black
Cupric sulfate-dithioxamide	Black
Cupric oleate-dithioxamide	Black

The chromogenic materials are present in the hydrophilic liquid in an amount from 0.2 to 10%, preferably 0.5 to 4.0% based on the weight of the hydrophilic liquid. The radiation curable liquids comprise the free radical polymerizable ethylenically unsaturated organic compounds. These compounds contain at least one terminal ethylenically unsaturated group per molecule.

These compounds are hydrophobic liquids and function as a continuous hydrophobic phase during the in situ preparation of the microcapsules and as a dispersing medium for the microcapsules and other ingredients of the coating composition prior to the coating operation. They are nonreactive with the wall-forming materials and they are curable to a solid resin when exposed to ionizing or ultraviolet radiation. Thus the cured resin acts as a binder for the microcapsules to a substrate such as paper.

A group of useful radiation curable compounds are the polyfunctional ethylenically unsaturated organic compounds which have two or more terminal ethylenic groups per molecule. Due to the polyfunctional nature of these compounds, they cure rapidly under the influence of radiation by polymerization, including crosslinking, to form a hard, dry, tack-free film.

Included in this group of radiation curable compounds are the polyesters of ethylenically unsaturated acids such as acrylic acid and methacrylic acids, and a polyhydric alcohol. The radiation curable hydrophobic liquid can be present in the microcapsular coating composition in an amount of 25 to 75%, preferably 40 to 55% by weight of the composition.

The first wall-forming material can be selected from the group consisting of polyols, epoxy compounds, polythiols, polyamines, acid anhydrides, and polycarboxylic acids, and mixtures thereof. The preferred first wall-forming materials are the polyols. The second wall-forming material is a polyisocyanate and may include diisocyanates, triisocyanates, tetraisocyanates, and isocyanate prepolymers.

The radiation curable hydrophobic liquid may also contain a catalyst to promote the reaction of the first and second wall-forming materials. Such catalysts include amines, organo-metallic compounds and various organic acid salts of metals. A photoinitiator is added to the coating composition if the composition is to be cured by ultraviolet radiation. The preferred photoinitiators are the benzoin alkyl ethers, such as Vicure 30 (a mixture of alkylbenzoin ethers), benzoin butyl ether (Vicure 10), benzoin methyl ether, and α,α-diethoxyacetophenone.

Photoinitiation synergists can be added to enhance the initiation efficiency of the photoinitiators. The preferred synergists are the chain transfer agents, such as the tertiary alcoholamines and substituted morpholines, triethanolamine, N-methyldiethanolamine, N,N-dimethylethanolamine and N-methylmorpholine. The amount of photoinitiation synergist added can be 0.2 to 10%, preferably 3 to 8% by weight of the coating composition. The Brookfield viscosity of the hydrophobic emulsion component can be from 0.5 to 1,000 cp, preferably from 1 to 50 cp.

A catalyst to promote the reaction of the first and second wall-forming materials, such as dibutyltin laurate, may be added if desired to the hydrophobic emulsion component prior to emulsification. Preferably, the radiation curable hydrophobic liquid is divided into two portions and the first portion is present in the hydrophobic emulsion component prior to the emulsification step. A second portion of the radiation curable hydrophobic liquid containing, in particular, faster curing polyfunctional oligomers and prepolymers may be added after the microcapsules are formed.

At this point, other materials such as the photoinitiation synergists may be added to give a coatable composition. Stilt material may be added, if desired, to prevent premature rupture of the microcapsules. The microcapsular coating composition can be applied to a substrate, such as paper or a plastic film by any of the common paper coating processes such as roll, air knife, or blade coating, or by any of the common printing processes, such as offset, gravure, or flexographic printing.

The rheological properties, particularly the viscosity, of the coating composition, can be adjusted for each type of application by proper selection of the type, molecular weight and relative amounts of the liquid radiation curable compounds. These coating compositions can be cured by any free radical initiated chain propagated addition polymerization reaction of the terminal ethylenic groups of the radiation curable compounds.

The preferred curing process is by exposure of the coating composition to ultraviolet radiation having a wavelength of 2000 to 4000 A. For curing to occur the composition must contain suitable ultraviolet absorbing photoinitiators which will produce polymerization initiating free radicals upon exposure to the radiation source.

A typical ultraviolet source is a Hanovia 200 watt medium pressure mercury lamp. Curing efficiencies of the coating composition are dependent on such parameters as the nature of the radiation curable substance, atmosphere in contact with the coating, quantum efficiency of the radiation absorbed, thickness of coating and inhibitory effects of the various materials in the composition.

Example 1: In 30 parts of distilled water was dissolved 2.1 parts of vanadium pentoxide, 3.9 parts of sodium hydroxide, 60 parts of glycerin and 40 parts of sodium bromide (Liquid A). The vanadium pentoxide and sodium hydroxide combine to form the chromogenic material, sodium orthovanadate. The glycerin and sodium bromide are added to prevent loss of the aqueous phase.

To 150 parts of 2-ethylhexyl acrylate (radiation curable compound) was added 1.5 parts of a mixture of glycerol stearate and polyoxyethylene stearate (an emulsifying agent – Arlacel 165) and stirred at room temperature. A cloudy mixture (Liquid B) was obtained. The Brookfield viscosity of Liquid B at 25°C was 12 cp.

A solution of 22.5 parts of Mondur CB-60 (a 61% solution in a mixture of xylene and 2-ethoxyethyl acetate of a toluene diisocyanate-based adduct) and 2.4 parts of dipropylene glycol (polyol) were dissolved in 75 parts of 2-ethylhexyl acrylate at room temperature to give a clear solution (Liquid C).

Liquid B was placed in a Waring Blender. Liquid A was slowly added to Liquid B in the Waring blender while running at high speed. The emulsification was continued for 2 minutes. Liquid C was then added slowly at high speed and mixed for 3 more minutes. The resultant emulsion was then transferred to a 3-neck glass reactor which was equipped with a condenser and a mechanical stirrer. The emulsion was stirred overnight (about 16 hours) at 40°C to yield a dispersion of microcapsules.

To 60 parts of this microcapsular dispersion was added 8 parts of Ucar Actomer X-80 (a polyfunctional acrylate oligomer), 10 parts of Keestar 339 (an anti-smudge agent), and 2.4 parts of Vicure 30 and the mixture (coating composition) was applied on a sheet of polyvinyl alcohol base-coated paper with a #19 Mayer bar. The sheet was exposed to ultraviolet light, light which was generated by the ultraviolet QC 1202 AN Processor.

Another coating composition was made as mentioned above except that the Vicure 30 was omitted. This coating composition was then coated with a #22 Mayer bar to a polyvinyl alcohol base-coated paper and cured by a linear cathode electron beam processor which was operated at 5 Mrad, 230 kV, and a speed of 50 ft/min using a nitrogen blanket. The ultraviolet light cured and electron beam cured transfer sheets each performed satisfactorily as transfer sheets of a carbonless paper system using a 2-ethylhexyl gallate coated record sheet.

Example 2: In 30 parts of distilled water, 2.1 parts of vanadium pentoxide, 3.9 parts of sodium hydroxide, 60 parts of glycerin and 40 parts of sodium bromide were dissolved (Liquid A). To 175 parts of 2-ethylhexyl acrylate was added 2 parts of Arlacel 165, 2.4 parts of dipropylene glycol (polyol) and 22.5 parts of Mondur CB-60 (polyisocyanate) and the mixture was stirred at room temperature. A cloudy mixture (Liquid B) was obtained.

Liquid A was then emulsified into Liquid B for 4 minutes in a Waring blender at high speed. The emulsion was then transferred into a glass reactor to cure overnight (about 16 hours) at 40° to 44°C. To 60 parts of this microcapsular dispersion was added 8 parts of Ucar Actomer X-80, 10 parts of Keestar 339 and 2.4 parts of Vicure 30 and the mixture was applied on a sheet of polyvinyl alcohol base-coated paper with a #19 Mayer bar. The sheet was exposed to the ultraviolet QC 1202 AN Processor.

Another coating composition was made as mentioned above except no Vicure 30 in the mixture. This coating composition was then coated with a #22 Mayer bar to a polyvinyl alcohol base-coated paper and cured by a linear cathode electron beam processor, which was operated at 5 Mrad, 230 kV and a speed of 50 ft/min using a nitrogen blanket. The ultraviolet light cured and electron beam cured transfer sheets each performed satisfactorily as a part of a carbonless paper system using a 2-ethylhexyl gallate coated record sheet.

Load Bearing Agent with Polymeric Core Partially Grafted to Shell

Certain polymeric products including thermoplastics such as polystyrene, are normally nonadherent with respect to cellulosic materials such as paper substrates. However, for many applications it would be highly desirable to provide a cellulosic substrate with such a plastic coating. Such coatings possess certain desirable physical and chemical properties not possessed by cellulosic substrates, such as paper.

A.E. Vassiliades, D.N. Vincent and S. Shroff; U.S. Patent 4,115,474; Sept. 19, 1978; assigned to Champion International Corporation found that cellulosic substrates may be successfully coated and/or permeated with polymeric materials that are normally nonadherent to cellulosic substrates in their particulate form by treating such substrates with discrete, substantially spherical microcapsules, which have a solid, polymeric shell and a solid, nontacky, polymeric core that is at least partially grafted to the shell.

The polymeric shell of the microcapsules is composed of material or materials that are compatible with cellulosic materials, while the core is a nontacky polymer and is at least partially grafted thereto. These microcapsules may be fused, if desired, and thus form a polymeric film that is compatible with a cellulosic substrate. Thus, such microcapsules may be coated onto a cellulosic substrate or permeated into the cellulosic substrate, and the substrate may be heated to bond the capsules to the cellulosic fibers.

The microcapsules are provided by forming precursor microcapsules having a monomeric core that is capable of being polymerized in situ to form a solid, nontacky polymer. During polymerization, the polymeric core becomes at least partially grafted to the solid, polymeric shell which surrounds the core. Any monomeric material which is capable of being encapsulated in a microcapsule and polymerized therein to form a solid, nontacky polymer may be employed. Suitable monomeric materials include ethylenically unsaturated monomers, for example, acrylic esters, vinyl esters, vinyl monomers, olefins, alone or mixtures thereof to provide the desired properties.

The quantity of polymer-containing microcapsules to be employed will depend upon the qualities desired in the ultimate product. Thus, for example, between 1 and 15% or 20% by weight of the resulting substrate may be comprised of the polymer-containing microcapsules and the product will still retain its paper-like qualities. On the other hand, if a more rigid, plastic-like product is desired, the percentage of microcapsules may be increased. The grafted, polymeric microcapsules may be employed as load-bearing agents in record systems wherein image-forming microcapsules, e.g., microcapsules containing colorless dye precursors are employed.

Preferably, the polymeric shell of the microcapsular load-bearing agents of the process is formed of the same polymer as is the shell of the pressure-rupturable, image-forming microcapsules. In this manner, the microcapsular load-bearing agents are made compatible with the same binder materials, such as methyl cellulose, starch, etc., that are selected for the image-forming microcapsules.

Preferably, the polymeric wall is formed of a hydroxylated polymer, such as methyl cellulose, a substituted starch, polyvinyl alcohol, or crosslinked by a formaldehyde condensation product, such as melamine or urea-formaldehyde. Preferred polymeric core materials are the thermoplastic and crosslinked thermoplastic polymers, such as polystyrene, polyvinyl chloride, or polyvinyl acetate.

Polymerization of the precursor microcapsules may be initiated thermally, e.g., by the application of heat alone, or with the aid of a polymerization catalyst, such catalyst being either an oil-soluble material, e.g., benzoyl peroxide, incorporated in the dispersed monomer phase, or a water-soluble material, e.g., potassium persulfate, incorporated in the continuous aqueous phase. Thus, the microcapsules may be provided with a core containing the monomer, styrene, and an effective amount of a polymerization catalyst for the styrene, such as benzoyl peroxide. Alternatively, the monomer may be encapsulated and the polymerization catalyst then dissolved in the continuous phase, whereupon polymerization occurs when such an initiator radical diffuses into the capsule. A vital feature of this process is the ability to graft at least a portion of the polymer formed inside the capsule to the capsule wall.

The portion of the solid polymer core that is grafted to the capsule wall may be varied over a wide range. For example, it may be between 20 and 80% of its weight depending upon the particular application. Thus, when the microcapsules are to be employed as spot welds a higher degree of grafting is preferred, e.g., between 50 and 80%.

For fused coatings a moderate degree of grafting, e.g., between 40 and 60%, is preferred. Depending upon the ratio of the wall material to core initially used to prepare the microcapsules and on the extent of grafting occurring during polymerization, the product, i.e., the solid-walled microcapsules having an essentially solid polymeric core, may contain from less than 10 to over 60% of the total capsule weight as free (ungrafted) polymer in the core.

An especially preferred method of providing the monomer system-containing microcapsules comprises admixing the following:

(a) a water-immiscible, polymerizable monomeric material containing an oil-soluble, cross-linking agent; and
(b) an aqueous solution of a hydroxyl group-containing polymeric, emulsifying agent.

The admixing is conducted under conditions to form an oil-in-water emulsion, wherein the monomeric material is dispersed in the form of microscopic droplets in an aqueous continuous phase. The crosslinking agent is reacted with the polymeric emulsifying agent thereby surrounding each of the droplets with a solid, crosslinked capsule wall of the crosslinked emulsifying agent.

The reaction of the crosslinking agent with the polymeric emulsifying agent, i.e., the curing step, may be conducted at any suitable temperature, for example, between ambient temperature and 100°C for periods of between 1 and 24 hours. The upper temperature at which the curing step may be conducted is only limited by the temperature at which the emulsion will break, i.e., the stability limit of the emulsion. Preferably, the crosslinking reaction is conducted at a temperature of 40° to 80°C, for about 1 to 3 hours.

The ratio of polymeric emulsifying agent to crosslinking agent that is provided in the emulsion is at least one part by weight of emulsifying agent per part of crosslinking agent. Thus, suitable ratios of emulsifier to crosslinking agent include between 1 and 100 parts by weight of emulsifying agent per part of crosslinking agent, preferably between 4 and 20 parts by weight of emulsifying agent per part of crosslinking agent.

In this system, the capsule walls are formed solely by the reaction of the crosslinking agent with the polymeric emulsifying agent. Thus, the emulsifying agent is the sole coreactant for the crosslinking agent.

Example 1: 50 g of undistilled styrene monomer containing 1.0 g of benzoyl peroxide are emulsified in 183 g of an 8.2% aqueous solution of methyl cellulose in a Waring blender. Agitation is continued until the desired particle size is attained, whereupon 30 g of a partially condensed (B-stage) urea-formaldehyde resin (65% solids) are added with brisk agitation. The microcapsules thus formed have an average particle diameter of about 0.7 μ.

The microcapsular suspension is then heated at 60°C for 3 hours thereby forming microcapsules containing a polystyrene core. The average particle diameter of these polymer-containing microcapsules is about 0.7 μ, or essentially the same as the microcapsules prior to polymerization.

The capsular suspension is then dried, the recovered solids pressed under 10,000 lb at 150°C to rupture the capsules. The resultant film is ground and extracted with refluxing benzene. About 10% of the dry capsule weight is recovered as soluble polystyrene having a viscosity average molecular weight of 685,000.

Example 2: 50 g of distilled styrene monomer without an added polymerization catalyst are encapsulated as described in Example 1, thereby yielding microcapsules with an average diameter of 2.5 μ. ½ g of a water-soluble initiator, potassium persulfate, is added to the aqueous phase and the suspension is heated at 60°C for 24 hours to effect polymerization. The capsules are isolated by drying the suspension and then hot pressed, ground, and extracted with refluxing benzene. About 36% of the dry capsule weight is recovered as soluble polystyrene having a molecular weight of 951,000. A weight balance indicates that more than 80% of the styrene monomer is converted to polymer.

Example 3: For comparative purposes, a polystyrene latex is prepared by standard emulsion polymerization techniques. Thus, 200 g of distilled styrene monomer are emulsified in 360 g of water containing 5 g of potassium oleate. 1 g of potassium persulfate is added to the aqueous phase, the emulsion is purged with nitrogen and heated at 60°C for 5 hours. The particle size is estimated at about 0.1 μ and the polymer has a molecular weight of 957,000.

A film of this latex is deposited on a paper substrate using a 0.0005 inch Bird applicator. In a similar manner, films of the microcapsular suspensions prepared in Examples 1 and 2 respectively are also deposited on paper substrates. These coatings are first air-dried and then further dried in an 80°C force draft oven for 10 minutes.

The latex coating is very chalky and easily rubs off on the fingers, whereas the two microcapsular coatings exhibit good adhesion to the substrate. The coated papers are hot pressed at 160°C under 2,000 psi between chrome plated steel sheets. The microcapsule coated papers yield a glossy smooth surface whereas the latex coated paper exhibits a splotchy surface.

Example 4: A solution consisting of 80 parts by weight of styrene monomer, 20 parts of a 50% solids solution of an oil-soluble melamine-formaldehyde condensation product, and 1 part benzoyl peroxide are emulsified in 400 parts by weight of a 7.5% aqueous solution of a benzylated starch (commercially available as Emulsicote 87). Agitation is continued in a Waring blender to yield particles having a 15 to 20 μ average diameter. The resulting dispersion is then heated while under conditions of mild agitation for a period of 2 hours at a temperature of 60° to 65°C in order to cure the capsule wall. Next, the dispersion is heated for an additional 2 hours at a temperature of 85° to 90°C to polymerize the styrene monomer core. The resulting capsules are then admixed with microcapsules containing a dye intermediate and the resulting admixture is coated onto a paper substrate to provide a transfer copy sheet.

Example 5: 80 parts of styrene monomer, 20 parts of a 50% solids solution of an oil-soluble melamine-formaldehyde condensation product, and 1.6 parts of benzoyl peroxide are admixed to provide a clear solution. The resulting solution is then emulsified in 533 parts of a 7.5% by weight aqueous solution of polyvinyl alcohol (commercially available as Elvanol 50-42) until particles having an average diameter of 15 to 20 μ is provided.

Next, 1.6 parts by weight of a water-soluble melamine-formaldehyde condensate (60% solids) is added to the aqueous phase and the resulting dispersion is heated at a temperature of 75° to 80°C under mild agitation for a period of 6 hours to polymerize the styrene monomer and provide microcapsular load-bearing agents. The resulting capsules are then composited with dye intermediate-containing capsules having an average particle diameter of about 5 μ and the resulting dispersion is coated onto a paper substrate to provide the transfer copy sheet.

OTHER

Dye Comprising Ureidofluoran Chromogenic Compounds

D.N. Vincent and C.-H. Chang; U.S. Patent 4,104,437; August 1, 1978; assigned to Champion International Corporation describe a chromogenic compound, which can be encapsulated and used in pressure sensitive copy systems. The chromogenic compound has the structural formula

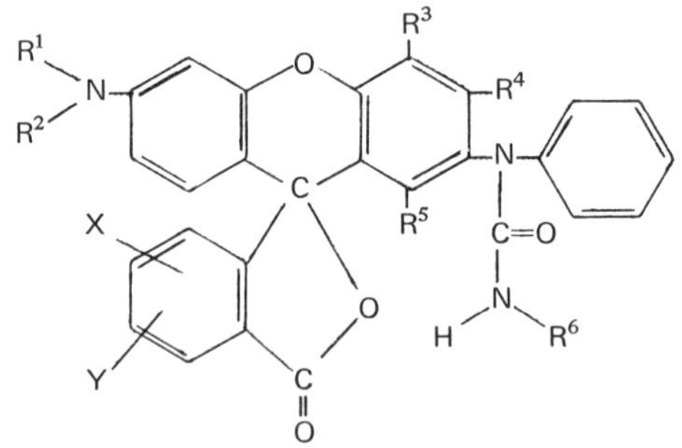

wherein R^1 and R^2 each represent an alkyl group; R^3 and R^4 each represent a hydrogen atom, a halogen atom, an alkyl group, a nitro group, an amino group, an acyl group, or a carboalkoxy group; R^5 represents a hydrogen atom or an alkyl group, with the proviso that R^5 represents an alkyl group only when R^4 represents a hydrogen atom; R^6 represents an alkyl group, an aryl group or an aralkyl group; and X and Y each represent a hydrogen atom, a halogen atom, a nitro group, a lower alkyl group, an aryl group, an alkoxy group or a carboalkoxy group.

Where R^1 and R^2 represent an ethyl group, R^3, R^4, R^5, X and Y represent hydrogen and R^6 represents a phenyl group, the compound is 2-(N'-phenyl-N-phenylureido)-6-diethylaminofluoran. The microcapsules can in addition contain the dialkylaminofluoran precursors.

The fluoran chromogenic compounds are employed in pressure-rupturable copy systems wherein the fluoran compounds are enclosed in microcapsules that are formed by a reaction involving a polyfunctional isocyanate. The preferred system for forming microcapsules involving the fluoran compounds is described in U.S. Patent 3,875,074. According to the system described therein, pressure-rupturable oil-containing microcapsules are provided by admixing the following.

(a) A water-immiscible, oily material containing the fluoran compound and an oil-soluble, nonpolymeric crosslinking agent in the form of a polyfunctional isocyanate; and

(b) Thereafter an aqueous solution of an organic, polymeric emulsifying agent containing a plurality of hydroxyl groups.

The water-immiscible oily material and the aqueous solution of the emulsifying agent are admixed under conditions to form an oil-in-water emulsion, wherein the oily material is dispersed in the form of microscopic emulsion droplets in an aqueous, continuous phase.

The emulsifying agent aids in the formation of the emulsion and additionally, possesses crosslinkable hydroxyl groups that are capable of reacting with the crosslinking agent to form a crosslinked capsule wall at the oil/water interface. The crosslinking agent is reacted with the hydroxyl groups of the polymeric emulsifying agent and in such manner surrounds each of the droplets with a solid, crosslinked capsule wall.

The dialkylaminofluorans provide a red color upon contact with an electron-accepting Lewis acid material—any of the well-known acidic materials including bentonite, kaolin, acidic clays, talc, aluminum silicate, calcium citrate, metal oxides, metal chlorides or the like.

Various concentrations of fluorans may be utilized in the formation of ureidofluoran-containing microcapsules for use in copy systems. The fluorans can be used in amounts of between 1 and 6 parts by weight per 100 parts by weight of the oily core material of the microcapsules. Preferably, between 2 and 4 parts by weight per 100 parts by weight of oil may be used.

The ureidofluorans may also be used in combination with other colorless chromogenic compounds. For example, the precursor fluoran compound, crystal violet lactone (CVL), and benzoyl leuco methylene blue (BLMB) may be added to provide an excellent black imaging system.

The total quantity of the dyes per 100 parts by weight of the oily core material of the microcapsules can be in amounts of between 2 and 8 parts by weight, while the molar ratio of ureidofluoran:precursor fluoran:CVL:BLMB can be, 2.0:3.0:0.1:0.2. Preferably, between 4 and 6 parts by weight per 100 parts by weight of oil may be used.

Example 1: Production of 2-Anilino-6-Diethylaminofluoran – Into 500 g of 97% sulfuric acid are dissolved 31.3 g of 2'-carboxy-4-diethylamino-2-hydroxy-benzophenone at room temperature. The solution is cooled to 10°C and 18.5 g of 4-anilinophenol are slowly added. The solution is then stirred at 20°C for 65 hours to provide a reaction mixture containing a sulfate of 2-anilino-6-diethylaminofluoran.

Example 2: 2-(N'-Phenyl-N-Phenylureido)-6-Diethylaminofluoran-Precursor Mixture – The reaction mixture of Example 1 is poured into 2,000 g of ice-water, basified to pH 9 with 20% sodium hydroxide solution, and extracted with xylene. The xylene solution is washed with 5% sodium hydroxide until the aqueous layer is nearly clear and finally with water 3 times. After concentrating to 300 ml, 11.9 g of phenyl isocyanate are added.

The solution is heated at 60°C for 2 hours, and subsequently, 100 ml of water are added while the stirring is continued for 1 hour. The organic phase is separated, dried over anhydrous sodium sulfate, and poured into 900 ml of heptane to precipitate 43.6 g of the product, 2-(N'-phenyl-N-phenylureido)-6-diethylaminofluoran and its 2-anilino-6-diethylaminofluoran precursor.

Example 3: 2-(N'-Phenyl-N-Phenylureido)-6-Diethylaminofluoran – The reaction mixture of Example 1 is poured into 2,000 g of ice-water, basified to pH 9 with 20% sodium hydroxide solution, and extracted with xylene. The xylene solution is washed with 5% sodium hydroxide until the aqueous layer is nearly clear and finally with water 3 times. After concentrating to 300 ml, 11.9 g of phenyl isocyanate are added.

The solution is refluxed at 145°C for 4 hours and subsequently, 100 ml of water is added while the stirring is continued for 1 hour. The organic phase is separated, dried over anhydrous sodium sulfate, and poured into 900 ml of heptane to precipitate 51.6 g of the product, 2-(N'-phenyl-N-phenyl-ureido)-6-diethylaminofluoran, having a melting point of 129° to 131°C.

Example 4: Encapsulation and Use – To a dye solution of 2 parts of 2-(N-phenyl-N-phenylureido)-6-diethylaminofluoran in 100 parts of mono-isopropylnaphthalene are added 6 parts of a toluene diisocyanate adduct of hexanetriol (3:1 molar, 75% solids, Mondur CB-75). The solution is then emulsified in 214 parts of a 7% polyvinyl alcohol (87 to 89% hydrolyzed) aqueous solution. The emulsion is cured at 60°C for 2 hours to complete the encapsulation.

The resulting microcapsules are coated onto a sheet of paper to form 1 part (CB sheet) of a pressure-rupturable transfer system. The second part of the system is a receiving sheet (CF sheet) coated with acidic clay. Rupture of the microcapsules by a stylus pressure releases the dye intermediate solution which is absorbed onto the receiving sheet, producing an intense red image.

Example 5: Encapsulation and Use – To a dye solution of 2.0 parts of 2-(N'-phenyl-N-phenylureido)-6-diethylaminofluoran, 3 parts of 2-anilino-6-diethylaminofluoran, 0.1 part of a crystal violet lactone and 0.2 part of benzoyl leuco methylene blue in 100 parts of mono-isopropylnaphthalene are added 6 parts of a toluene diisocyanate adduct of hexanetriol (3:1 molar, 75% solids, Mondur CB-75). The procedure of Example 4 is followed to encapsulate the dye solution and prepare a pressure-sensitive copying system. Rupture of the microcapsules produces an intense black image on the receiving sheet.

Reducing Smudge by Application of Microcapsules to Rough Surface of Machine Glazed Paper

One known clean-to-handle pressure-sensitive copying system comprises an upper sheet, known as a CB sheet, which is coated on its lower surface with pressure-rupturable microcapsules containing a solution of a color former material, and a lower sheet, known as a CF sheet, which is coated on its upper surface with a color reactant material, such as an acidic clay or a phenolic resin.

For most applications, a number of intermediate sheets, known as CFB sheets, are also provided each of which is coated on its lower surface with microcapsules and on its upper surface with color reactant material. The pressure exerted on the sheets by writing or typing ruptures the microcapsules, thereby releasing the color former solution onto the reactant material on the next lower sheet and giving rise to a chemical reaction which develops the color of the color former. The microcapsules are usually applied in aqueous suspension. The above described pressure-sensitive copying system will herein be called "a pressure-sensitive copying system of the kind referred to".

It has become a normal practice to coat the microcapsules onto the surface together with a so-called stilt material, such as cellulose fibers or starch granules, the dimensions of which are such that the stilt material protrudes further from the base paper than the microcapsules. The stilt material, therefore, serves to protect the microcapsules against accidental rupture while still allowing rupture under typing or writing pressure. The presence of stilt material adds to the expense of CB and CFB sheets, and may also lead to problems in coating the base paper with microcapsule suspension.

L. Westcott; U.S. Patent 4,081,188; March 28, 1978; assigned to Wiggins Teape Limited, England has found that the use of machine glazed (MG) paper as the base paper obviates the need for stilt materials, or at least renders their presence necessary in smaller amounts, and affords a number of other advantages.

The process provides a coated paper for use in pressure-sensitive copying systems of the kind referred to, of which the base paper has been machine glazed, the color reactant, when present, being on the glazed surface of the base paper, and the microcapsule coating, when present, being on the rough surface of the base paper.

The coated paper may be a CF sheet, in which case color reactant will be present and microcapsules will be absent, or a CB sheet, in which case color reactant will be absent and microcapsules will be present, or a CFB sheet in which case color reactant and microcapsules will both be present.

A process for manufacturing coated paper for use in a pressure-sensitive copying system of the kind referred to comprises the steps of drying a paper web which has been formed on a papermaking machine wire by means of a machine glazing cylinder, and applying a coating of a color reactant material to the glazed surface of the web, and/or applying a coating of microcapsules to the rough surface of the web. The process is described with reference to Figure 7.2.

Figure 7.2: Reducing Smudge by Application of Microcapsules to Rough Surface of Machine Glazed Paper

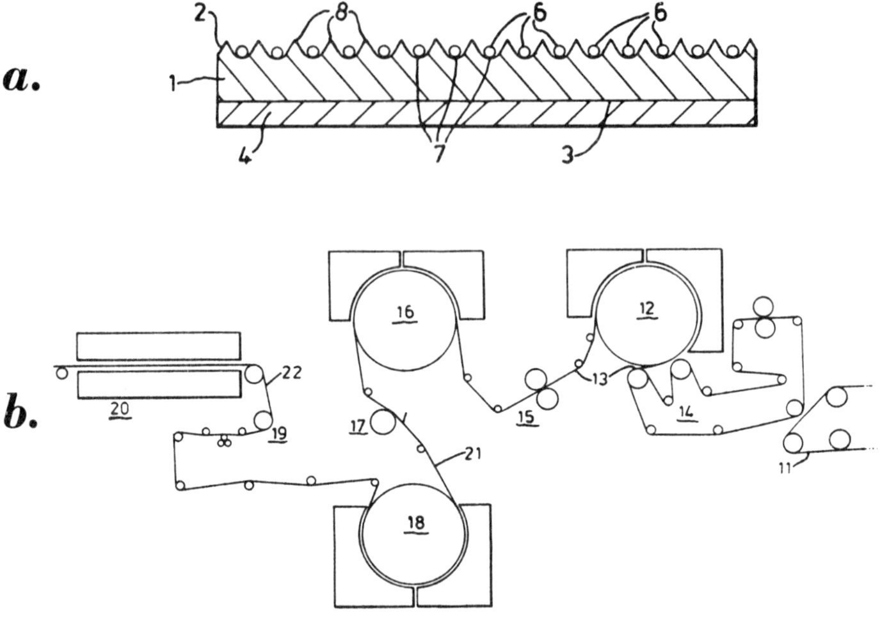

(a) CFB sheet having MG paper base.
(b) Apparatus for manufacturing CFB sheet of Figure 7.2a.

Source: U.S. Patent 4,081,188

In Figure 7.2a there is shown a CFB sheet which has been manufactured from an MG paper **1** by coating a color reactant material coating **4** on its glazed surface **3**, and a coating of microcapsules **6** on its unglazed surface **2**. Although the rough surface is shown as being uppermost, in use, the smooth surface will be uppermost to provide the writing surface, and the rough surface will be face down.

As seen in Figure 7.2b, a paper web **13** produced on a papermaking machine wire **11** is passed to a first MG cylinder **12** (a highly polished, heated drying cylinder) by means of a felt and roller arrangement **14**. After drying on the cylinder **12** the paper web **13** passes through a conventional size press apparatus **15** where it is sized and dyed as desired. After being sized and dyed the paper web **13** is passed around a second unfelted MG cylinder **16** to dry the sized and dyed web.

From the cylinder **16** the paper web is passed to a conventional coating apparatus, e.g., a Bill-blade **17** or a trailing blade, where a color reactant material coating is applied to the glazed surface of the paper web to produce a coated paper web **21**. From the coating apparatus **17** the coated paper web

21 is passed around a third MG cylinder **18** which dries the applied color reactant material coating. The web **21** is then passed to an air-knife coating apparatus **19** by means of which a microcapsule coating is applied to the unglazed uncoated surface of the paper web **21** to produce a web **22** which is coated on both surfaces. From the coating apparatus **19** the web **22** is passed through a drying apparatus **20**, for example an air-suspension drying apparatus, and is then reeled up at a reel-up station, in the form of CFB paper as shown in Figure 7.2a. Instead of the third MG cylinder **18**, an air-suspension drying apparatus may be used if desired.

By omitting the coating apparatus **19** and the drying apparatus **20** the machinery described above can be used to manufacture CF paper containing only color reactant material **4** and by omitting the coating apparatus **17** and the cylinder **18** the machinery can be used to manufacture CB paper containing only microcapsules **6** on unglazed surfaces. The size press apparatus **15** and the cylinder **16** may if desired be omitted in which case the paper web **13** may be sized and dyed as necessary by suitable additions to the stock from which the paper web **13** is manufactured.

ADDITIONAL USES FOR ENCAPSULATED PRODUCTS

AGRICULTURAL CHEMICALS

Microporous Capsule Walls for Controlled Release

D.A. Hofacker; U.S. Patents 4,002,458; January 11, 1977; 3,977,992; August 31, 1976 and 3,985,840; October 12, 1976; all assigned to Minnesota Mining and Manufacturing Company provide capsules which have permeable or semipermeable walls, i.e., walls having microscopic passages or interconnecting pores providing a release route which permits an osmosis-like effect to occur at a controllable or predetermined rate. The observed effect resembles osmosis in that the amount of liquid contained within the capsule walls does not appear to diminish significantly, but any solute dissolved in the encapsulated liquid passes out of the capsules when a moist environment (e.g., soil) containing a lower concentration of solute exists outside the capsules.

The capsules also can be used to release liquids volatile at the temperature of use, provided that, a partial pressure driving force is present as in the case when water-containing capsules are placed in a low humidity environment. The capsules are durable, crush resistant, uniformly small, substantially spherical, and nontacky, and they are particularly suited for providing controlled release of dissolved chemicals from encapsulated aqueous solutions. Among the suitable dissolved chemicals are fertilizers, pesticides, herbicides, and other agents with agricultural utility, but the process is generally useful for encapsulating liquids or solutions of any desired type. The release rate can be controlled so as to prevent groundwater pollution in agricultural applications. The filled capsules are dry and can be readily handled and shipped.

It has been found that a microporous capsule wall can be obtained when certain critical phase relationships are observed during the manufacture of the capsules. The capsule shell- or wall-forming material should comprise at least a first material which melts at elevated or moderately elevated temperatures and is capable of forming a single phase when admixed with a second material (which also melts at elevated or moderately elevated temperatures). A small amount of a high-boiling solvent or plasticizing material can be used, if desired, to facilitate this single phase formation step. After the first and second materials have been blended, heated, and formed into a homogeneous molten phase, the wall-forming composition is brought into contact with a fill material (preferably an aqueous liquid) by means of the biliquid column technique disclosed in U.S. Patents 3,423,489 and 3,389,194.

Contact with the liquid fill rapidly cools the homogeneous wall-forming phase, and as this molten phase approaches a solidified state and becomes an incipient capsule wall or shell, one of the materials present in this incipient wall begins to separate out as a discontinuous, solid phase dispersed throughout a substantially continuous wall matrix. The resulting dispersed particles are normally considerably smaller than the thickness of the capsule wall which ultimately results. The dispersed particles preferably contract, upon further cooling, at a rate which is faster than the contraction rate of the continuous matrix, but any disparity between the matrix and dispersed phase with regard to their respective rates or degrees of contraction can assist in the formation of cracks or pores in the capsule walls.

Since the dispersed phase is present in a significant quantity, e.g., at least 5 parts by weight of the total composition, the resulting capsule is characterized by microporous walls having a porosity (determined by mercury porosimetry) of at least about 3 vol %. The "microporosity" (this term being used herein to include submicroscopic porosity) imparts permeability or semipermeability to the capsule walls and effects similar to osmosis are observed when a concentration gradient across the capsule wall is present.

The capsules are on the order of about 100 to 10,000 microns, preferably about 1,000 to 3,000 microns, in diameter. Capsules of this size are readily packaged, stored, and shipped, while larger capsules are weak, fragile, and subject to breakage during packaging, handling, or shipping. Capsules smaller than 100 microns in diameter have a large shell or wall volume in comparison to liquid fill volume and are excessively expensive for most uses.

The preferred capsules comprise an aqueous fill and a microporous (including submicroscopic porosity) capsule wall wherein the capsule wall comprises three or more phases, i.e., a solid, crystalline olefinic polymer phase, an amorphous phase (e.g., a hydrocarbon resin), and a second crystalline or semicrystalline phase, e.g., a natural, paraffinic or microcrystalline petroleum wax. The wax ordinarily separates out first upon cooling, thus forming a crystalline or semicrystalline phase dispersed throughout a continuous matrix of the other phases. Microporosity results upon further cooling, due apparently to one or more phenomena, including differences in the rate of degree of contraction between two or more phases and shear forces created by the disparity in structure between the different crystal types or between the polyolefin/amorphous resin and wax phases.

The ability of the capsules to release the contained solute over a period of time is readily demonstrated by extraction techniques. 20 g of filled capsules are placed in a sealed bottle together with 100 ml of distilled water and allowed to stand for 24 hours at 25°C. A 10 ml aliquot is thereafter withdrawn, evaporated to dryness, the amount of solid residue determined, and the percent of active ingredient released during the 24-hour period calculated. The remaining solution is decanted and 100 ml of fresh distilled water added, the bottle resealed and allowed to stand for a second 24-hour interval, another aliquot removed, and the percent of active ingredient released is calculated. The procedure is then repeated at various intervals.

Example 1: An apparatus as illustrated in Figure 1 of U.S. Patent 3,423,489 was used to form capsules filled with an aqueous fertilizer solution. The apparatus contained a submerged, generally upwardly pointed nozzle for discharging fill liquid to be encapsulated. The nozzle was supplied by a conduit means provided with a needle valve to control the flow, and was immersed beneath the surface of a bath of hardenable liquid encapsulating material. The level of the liquid encapsulating material was maintained at an even distance above the nozzle orifice by means of a constant level overflow reservoir provided with a recirculating pump. Air pressure was applied to the reservoir of fill liquid and the nozzle was provided with tip windings of an electrical resistor to minimize congealing of encapsulating material around the nozzle.

The capsule shell comprised 85 parts polyolefin and 15 parts compatible hydrocarbon resin. The nozzle was inclined at an angle of 30° from the vertical, was provided with an orifice of 0.74 mm in diameter, and was immersed in the bath to a depth of 2 mm. The fill liquid had the following composition:

	Parts by Weight
Water	34.0
Urea	27.6
11-37-0 analysis fertilizer (TVA liquid base solution)	12.0
10% solution of an interpolymer of methyl vinyl ether and maleic anhydride (Gantrez AN-169)	25.3
25% solution of the sodium salt of alkyl aryl polyether sulfonate (Triton X-200)	1.1

The shell composition contained 85.0 parts by weight polyolefin, 1,500 MW, 102°C softening point, 0.91 specific gravity, 145 cp viscosity at 140°C (Polyethylene AC617A, Allied Chemical Co.); and 15.0 parts by weight hydrocarbon resin, 95°C softening point, 0.93 specific gravity (Wing-Tack 95).

Four liters of filtered fill solution were placed in the reservoir to which 0.34 atm gauge pressure was applied. The temperature of the fill liquid was 22°C. The shell composition temperature was 250°C and the tip winding was heated to about 700°C. The needle valve was opened and the fill solution was discharged at a rate of 133 cm/min. The polyolefin-hydrocarbon shell composition solidified at a distance approximately 100 cm from the orifice, this time being sufficient to permit the biliquid column to form a string of capsules and then to separate into individual discrete capsules. Capsules were produced at the rate of about 40,000/min. The total trajectory length was about 10 ft after which the capsules were allowed to fall into a water-filled collecting trough.

The capsules collected were 2,125 microns in average diameter and had a shell wall thickness of about 120 microns. The fill liquid comprised about 79% of the total capsule weight and the shell material about 21%. The release properties of these capsules were demonstrated by extraction as previously described, the results being shown in the following table.

Example 2: This example illustrates the encapsulation of liquid fertilizer in a capsule shell comprising 60 parts of the polyolefin of Example 1, 37.5 parts of the hydrocarbon resin of Example 1, and 2.5 parts of hydrocarbon wax having a melting point of 84°C, and a specific gravity of 0.94 at 15°C (Shellwax 700).

Four liters of filtered fill solution were placed in the reservoir to which 0.34 atm gauge pressure was applied. The temperature of the fill liquid was 20°C. The temperature of the shell composition was 241°C and the temperature of the tip winding was about 700°C. The needle valve was opened and the fill solution was discharged at a rate of 149.5 cm/min. Capsules were produced at the rate of about 40,000/min. The capsules collected were about 2,360 microns in average diameter and had a shell thickness of about 140 microns. The fill liquid comprised about 75.6% of the total capsule weight and the shell material about 24.4%. These capsules were extracted as previously described, the results being shown in the table below.

Example 3: This example illustrates encapsulation of a liquid herbicide and illustrates incorporation of a mineral oil plasticizer in the capsule shell. The nozzle was inclined at an angle of about 30° from the vertical, was provided with an orifice 0.74 mm in diameter, and was immersed in the bath to a depth of about 2 mm. The fill liquid was 61.5 parts of a 65% aqueous solution of Diquat, 20.6 parts water, and 25.3 parts of a 10% aqueous solution of Gantrez AN-169. The shell composition was 59.8 parts of the polyolefin used in Example 2, 21.4 parts of the hydrocarbon resin used in Example 2, 14.5 parts of the hydrocarbon wax used in Example 2, and 4.3 parts mineral oil (Nujol).

Four liters of filtered fill solution were placed in the reservoir to which 0.27 atm gauge pressure was applied. The temperature of the fill liquid was 22°C. The shell composition temperature was 284°C and the temperature of the tip winding was about 700°C. The needle valve was opened and the fill solution was discharged at a rate of 106 cc/min. The capsule solidified at a distance of approximately 120 cm from the orifice which was one second travel time of the capsule in the trajectory path. This time was sufficient to permit the billquld column to first form a string of capsules and then separate into individual discrete capsules. Capsules were produced at the rate of about 35,000/min.

The total trajectory length was about 8 ft after which the capsules were allowed to fall into a water-filled collecting trough. The capsules collected were 2,360 microns in average diameter and had a shell thickness of about 82 microns. The fill liquid comprised about 81.3% of the total capsule weight and the shell material about 18.7%. The results indicated in the table below show that the capsules of this example released less than 5% of their contents during the first 24 hours and released less than 10% of the contents in five days. This was considered to be a release rate sufficient to provide an adequate initial dosage of herbicide to the plants and also allow steady release of more herbicide for a definite period of time.

Cumulative Total Percent of Fill Solution Extracted at Various Intervals

Ex.	Days									
No.	1	2	3	4	5	6	7	8	9	10
1	9.36	11.74	12.36	13.08	–	–	14.53	15.01	15.53	15.90
2	1.37	1.68	1.79	1.90	–	–	–	–	–	–
3	1.69	2.75	4.04	–	–	10.27	13.79	17.73	21.78	26.18

Posttreatment of Polyurea Microcapsules with Ammonia to Reduce Isocyanate Levels

H.B. Scher; U.S. Patent 4,046,741; September 6, 1977; assigned to Stauffer Chemical Company describes posttreatment of polyurea microcapsules with ammonia or amines to reduce the residual isocyanate level. Reduction of the residual isocyanate level, which results from the process in which the microcapsules are formed, permits flowable formulations of the microcapsules to be stored at pH values below 8 without the generation of carbon dioxide gas. Microcapsules are prepared by the process, in which polyurea capsule enclosures are formed around water-immiscible material by the interfacial polymerization of an organic isocyanate intermediate with water in the aqueous phase. The generation of carbon dioxide gas occurs when residual or unreacted isocyanate groups present after processing react with water in storage. The posttreatment of polyurea microcapsules with ammonia is also used to modify the permeability of the microcapsule wall.

The posttreatment is particularly useful for polyurea microcapsules of methyl parathion and the organic phosphate insecticide-acaricide having as its active ingredient the compound N-(mercaptomethyl)phthalimide S-(O,O-dimethylphosphorodithioate).

Example 1: The use of posttreatment of the process for polyurea microcapsules with ammonia or amines to reduce residual isocyanate levels, was carried out with polyurea microcapsules of Sutan (S-ethyl diisobutyl thiocarbamate). The purpose was to prepare polyurea microcapsules including a core material and to treat these microcapsules with ammonia or an amine and to eliminate or substantially decrease the generation of gaseous carbon dioxide at pH values lower than about 7. This was to determine the storage capabilities of flowable formulations of polyurea microcapsules stored at pH values of less than about 7.

Microcapsules were typically prepared as follows: Water (2,104 g) containing 2.0% of neutralized poly-(methyl vinyl ether/maleic anhydride) protective colloid and 0.2% linear alcohol ethoxylate emulsifier was placed into an open reactor vessel. In a separate container, 1,398 g S-ethyl diisobutyl thiocarbamate (a herbicide), 165.4 g of polymethylene polyphenylisocyanate (PAPI) and 82.7 g toluene diisocyanate (TDI, 80% 2,4 and 20% 2,6) were mixed together. This mixture was then added to the reactor vessel and emulsified with a high shear stirrer.

The resulting particle range was about 5 to 30 microns. Only mild agitation was required for the balance of the reaction. The temperature of the reaction was raised 50°C, over a 20-minute period. The temperature was maintained at 50°C for about 3 hours.

The polyurea microcapsule dispersion was then divided into portions. A quantity of ammonia or an amine equivalent to 10 times the unreacted isocyanate in the microcapsules was added to each portion. The pH was then adjusted. Each portion was then heated to 50°C for 6 hours. Then each portion was adjusted to pH 4.5 and placed in 500 cc stainless steel cylinders equipped with pressure gauges. These cylinders were stored at 110°F (43.5°C). Pressure readings were taken periodically for one month. The results of the pressure readings after 2 and 4 weeks are given in the table shown on the following page.

Storage Stability—Sutan*

Posttreatment	Pressure in Cylinders ....psig........... 2 Weeks	4 Weeks
Untreated	12.8	15.0
50°C, 6 hr, pH 9.5	9.5	14.0
3.2% dibutylamine, 50°C, 6 hr, pH 9.9	1.5	1.5
0.5% NH_3, 50°C, 6 hr, pH 9.6	0	1.7
1.8% diethylamine, 50°C, 6 hr, pH 11.1	2.0	3.0
2.4% dipropylamine, 50°C, 6 hr, pH 11.2	1.6	2.2

*15% wall; PAPI/TDI = 2.0.

The posttreatment of the polyurea microcapsules with ammonia or amines was effective in reducing the residual isocyanate levels as evidenced by the reduced carbon dioxide pressure in the cylinders.

Example 2: Posttreatment of the polyurea microcapsules with ammonia is especially effective in reducing the residual isocyanate levels in polyurea capsules containing methyl parathion. Since methyl parathion is susceptible to hydrolytic decomposition at pH values greater than about 7, storage of these microcapsules at lower pH values is required. Therefore, treatment with ammonia after the formation of the polyurea microcapsules is extremely valuable.

When methyl parathion microcapsules are stored at pH 11.0 for six weeks at 110°F (43.5°C), 13% methyl parathion decomposition resulted. Storage at low pH was considered in order to overcome the decomposition problem. However, when the microcapsules were stored at low pH (4.5), 23 psig carbon dioxide pressure was produced from residual isocyanate reaction with water. However, if the capsules are posttreated with ammonia and then stored at pH 4.5., there is no decomposition of the methyl parathion and only about 3.5 psig developed from the hydrolysis of any residual isocyanate.

Pyrethroid Insecticide in Polyurea Shell Containing Benzophenone Shell Stabilizer

In accordance with the process of *L.L. Barber, Jr., A.J. Lucas and R.Y. Wen; U.S. Patent 4,056,610; November 1, 1977; assigned to Minnesota Mining and Manufacturing Company*, there is provided a microcapsule insecticide composition comprising microcapsules each having a polyurea shell including as an integral part of the shell a photostable ultraviolet light absorbent compound having a log molar extinction coefficient of from 2 to 5 with respect to radiation having wavelengths in the range of from 270 to 350 nanometers and a liquid fill capable of slowly permeating the shell and comprising a pyrethroid and a biological synergist therefor.

Preferably the entire microcapsule composition consists essentially of 60 to 90% of liquid fill and 40 to 10% of shell wall, the liquid fill comprising 5 to 40% of pyrethroid, 25 to 50% of biological synergist and 20 to 40% of a water-immiscible organic solvent and the shell including as an integral part thereof 0.5 to 20% of photostable ultraviolet light absorbent compound (all percentages being based on the weight of the entire microcapsule composition).

The pyrethroid remains inside the microcapsules while the composition is packaged and in storage, i.e., in a closed container due to the partial pressure of the pyrethroid surrounding the microcapsules. When the product is applied as an insecticide, the pyrethroid releases slowly (the actual speed of release depending upon the thickness and porosity of the capsule walls). The pyrethroid is chemically stable during storage and after application until it permeates the capsule walls. At that time it becomes available as an insecticide until degraded to an inactive product. Since the fill permeates the shell wall slowly, the microcapsule product has a long effective insecticidal life and may be stored for extended periods (e.g., for 6 months and more).

Insect pest activity can be controlled by contacting insects with an effective level of the compositions directly, by atomization of the composition into the air in the form of a spray so that it contacts the insect directly or indirectly by applying the composition to surfaces upon which the insects alight or crawl. Alternatively, compositions may be provided in various other forms, for example, in sheet materials carrying the microcapsules (e.g., tapes coated or impregnated with the microcapsules) that may be placed in areas where the insects may alight or crawl. Moreover, animals infested with insects, for example, dogs and cats infested with fleas and poultry infested with lice, can be treated by contacting the fur or feathers of the animal with the compositions.

The microcapsules obtained comprise a distribution of spherical capsules generally ranging from 1 to 100 microns, preferably from 1 to 30 microns in diameter. Suitable pyrethroids for use in the liquid fill include both the naturally occurring pyrethrum esters derived from the dried flower heads of *Chrysanthemum cinnerariaefolium* and *Chrysanthemum coccineum* and the synthetically prepared esters of chrysanthemic acid. Biological synergists for inclusion in the liquid fill generally have little or no insecticidal activity by themselves, but significantly increase the insecticidal activity of the pyrethroids when combined therewith. A preferred class of shell stabilizers comprises substituted benzophenone sulfonic acids, particularly 2-hydroxy-4-methoxybenzophenone-5-sulfonic acid.

Example: 36.7 parts of a 20% by weight solution of naturally occurring pyrethroids in deodorized kerosene (Premium Pyrocide 175, McGlaughlin Gormley King Co.), 36.7 parts of biological synergist (piperonyl butoxide), 0.73 part of fill stabilizer (4-dodecyloxy-2-hydroxybenzophenone), 0.73 part of antioxidant (2,6-dioctadecyl-p-cresol) and 14.6 parts of polyisocyanate (Mondur MRS, Mobay Chemical Co.) are mixed to form a liquid fill composition.

A water solution is prepared by adding 54 parts of 17% aqueous polyacrylic acid to 1,500 parts of water. The resulting solution is adjusted to a pH of 7 to 9 with 60 parts of 1 N sodium hydroxide.

The liquid fill (including the polyisocyanate) is then dispersed in the water solution in a mixer (a Dispersator, Premier Mill Corporation) operated at 3,000 rpm. After 5 minutes of mixing, 1.5 parts of polyfunctional amine (tetraethylene pentamine) are added over approximately 2.5 minutes. The resulting mixture is allowed to react for 5 minutes at room temperature (approximately 25°C) at 3,000 rpm while the microcapsule shell walls form. A shell stabilizer (9.04 parts of 2-hydroxy-4-methoxy-benzophenone-5-sulfonic acid) is added to the dispersion of microcapsules over a 2-minute period and reacted with the available amine groups of the shell wall. The reaction takes 3 to 5 minutes and goes to completion. The pH of the composition is maintained at 7 to 9 by the addition of sodium hydroxide.

The resulting composition comprises microcapsules (10 to 30 microns in diameter) each having a polyurea shell containing a photostable ultraviolet light absorbent compound (a shell stabilizer) as an integral part thereof and a liquid fill comprising a natural pyrethroid, an organic solvent, a biological synergist, an antioxidant, and a photostable ultraviolet light absorbent compound (a fill stabilizer). The composition is then coated onto polyester, at three different coating weights. The first coating has a pyrethroid concentration of 0.105 mg/cm^2 and a shell stabilizer concentration of 0.0775 mg/cm^2 on the polyester. The second coating has a pyrethroid concentration of 0.102 mg/cm^2 and a shell stabilizer concentration of 0.170 mg/cm^2, and the third a pyrethroid concentration of 0.093 mg/cm^2 and a shell stabilizer concentration of 0.294 mg/cm^2 on the polyester.

The samples are then tested for biological activity both initially and after exposure to 88 hours of simulated outdoor conditions. In all instances, each sample knocks down 100% of the houseflies within 15 minutes.

The unencapsulated liquid fill used in this example is coated onto polyester to a pyrethroid concentration of 0.22 mg/cm^2. The sample is tested for biological activity both initially and after 30 hours of exposure to simulated outdoor conditions. It knocks down 100% of the houseflies within 15 minutes initially, but after 30 hours of exposure to simulated outdoor conditions, it knocks down 0% of the houseflies within 60 minutes.

A microcapsule insecticide composition similar to the abovedescribed microcapsule composition but containing no shell stabilizer is coated onto polyester to a pyrethroid concentration of 0.11 mg/cm^2. The sample is tested for biological activity both initially and after exposure to 39 hours of simulated outdoor conditions. It initially has 100% knockdown of the houseflies within 15 minutes. After exposure to 39 hours of simulated outdoor conditions, it knocks down 0% of the houseflies within 60 minutes.

Parathion Encapsulated with a Crosslinked Polyamide-Polyurea Wall

C.B. DeSavigny; U.S. Patent 3,959,464; May 25, 1976; assigned to Pennwalt Corporation found that microcapsules of methyl parathion or ethyl parathion contained within a wall of crosslinked polyamide-polyurea are improved insecticidal compositions having more effective and extended toxicity to insects and decreased toxicity to mammals. The compositions are stable in aqueous carriers.

The average particle size of the microcapsules will generally range from 30 to 130 microns with a preferred average particle size of 80 to 100 microns. Such relatively fine particles are advantageous to prevent plugging of orifices in the spraying equipment used for field application of the pesticide compositions. The wall thickness of the crosslinked polyamide-polyurea capsule will range from 0.5 to 4 microns, with from 1 to 3 micron thickness preferred. The thickness of the capsule wall, as well as the degree of crosslinking of the polymer constituting same, will affect the rate of diffusion of the parathion insecticide therethrough, and thereby influence the performance of the insecticide in the field relative to extended life and insect kill rate.

The weight ratio of the pesticide to the polymer in the encapsulated composition will generally range from about 2:1 to 10:1 with a ratio of 5:1 being preferred. A convenient water dispersion, suspension or slurry for shipping and storage will consist of from 10 to 30% by weight, preferably about 25%, of the pesticide-containing microcapsules, which will be diluted to about 1% for spraying.

An exemplary recipe for preparing the crosslinked polyamide-polyurea encapsulating polymer wall for the methyl and ethyl parathion is as follows: Polyfunctional isocyanate (such as polymethylene polyphenylisocyanate known as PAPI), x mols, where x equals 0.1 to 0.5; diacid chloride (such as sebacoyl dichloride), 1 minus x mols, difunctional amine (such as ethylene diamine), n minus y mols, where n equals 1 to 3; diethylene triamine (a difunctional polyamine), y mols, where y equals 0 to 1.5; in addition, 1 minus x mols of sodium carbonate may be included in the recipe to neutralize the hydrochloric acid generated during the polycondensation reaction. Excess amine may be present in the recipe.

The diacid chloride and isocyanate are added to the insecticide which acts as a water-insoluble organic solvent. The organic material is dispersed in water and amine is charged to the reaction as an aqueous solution. The procedure of U.S. Patent 3,577,515 is employed to produce the encapsulated parathion product.

Example: The following solutions are prepared: (A) Stock solution of polyvinyl alcohol, a 4% aqueous solution of which has a viscosity of 35 to 45 cp at 20°C determined by Hoeppler falling ball method (Elvanol 50-42 G, E.I. DuPont de Nemours & Company) in warm water with high speed stirring.

(B) Amine solution of 14.6 g ethylene diamine, 16.6 g diethylenetriamine, 25.6 grams sodium carbonate, anhydrous and 200 ml water.

(C) Organic phase, prepared just prior to use. 200 g technical methyl parathion, 29.0 g sebacyl chloride and 10.8 g PAPI which has the following properties.

Isocyanate equivalent (dibutylamine)	135 maximum
Viscosity (cp at 25°C)	400 maximum
Acid value (ppm of H^+)	200 maximum
Volatile content (100°C/20 mm)	0.3% maximum
Specific gravity (20/20°C)	1.2
Average molecular weight	380 to 400
Flash point (Cleveland Open Cup)	425°F
NCO content by weight	31% minimum

600 ml of 0.5% polyvinyl alcohol solution (A) is placed in a 2-liter baffled flask and stirred vigorously with a Dispersator unit (Premier Mill Corp.) equipped with a 1-inch duplex head. The organic phase, solution (C), is added, followed immediately by amine solution (B). A paddle stirrer is substituted for the dispersion stirrer and the mixture is agitated slowly to maintain suspension for 2 hours. The microcapsules are recovered by vacuum filtration, washed with water to a neutral pH, and redispersed in water to produce a slurried product containing the equivalent of 17% active methyl parathion.

A commercial methyl parathion concentrate is diluted and emulsified with water to provide a composition containing 10% active methyl parathion as control. Both materials are applied to cotton plants in the greenhouse at the same concentrations of 1 lb/acre active ingredient, using conventional spray equipment. At selected time intervals, 25 bollworms are placed on the treated leaves and the percentage kill noted. Encapsulated methyl parathion gives effective, long-lasting control (100% kill after 7 days and 75% kill after 10 days) while the control shows rapid decrease in activity (giving only about 5% kill after 7 days, and no kill after 10 days).

Toxicity tests on mammals show that the encapsulated methyl parathion product has about 0.1 of the toxicity to mammals of the unencapsulated, emulsifiable concentrate control, and that the ethyl parathion capsule has about 0.01 the toxicity of the unencapsulated control.

Stable Water Dispersions of Encapsulated Malathion

H.C. Nemeth; U.S. Patent 4,107,292; August 15, 1978; assigned to Akzona Incorporated is concerned with aqueous dispersions of polymer-encapsulated insecticides (e.g., phosphorothioates and phosphorodithioates) wherein xanthan gum is used as a dispersing agent. It has been found that by use of the xanthan gum, the aqueous dispersions are highly stable, even for periods as long as two years or more.

The insecticidal compositions consist essentially of an aqueous dispersion of:

(a) from 1 to 40% by weight of composition of capsules of a member of the group consisting of a phosphoromonothioate and a phosphorodithioate insecticide encapsulated in a skin selected from the group consisting of a polyamide, a polyurea, and a mixed polyamide-polyurea crosslinked with a crosslinking agent selected from the group consisting of a polyalkylene polyamine and a polyfunctional isocyanate;

(b) from 0.1 to 0.5% by weight of composition of a xanthan gum dispersant for the capsules; and

(c) balance water.

The preparation of capsules of polymer-encapsulated insecticides is well known. See, for example, U.S. Patent 3,577,515 (Pennwalt Corporation) which describes suitable methods involving interfacial polymerization. The actual methods used to form capsules wherein the skins are crosslinked polyamide, polyurea, or mixed polyamide-polyurea are set forth in Examples 11, 12, 14, and 17 from the above patent.

Preparation of Insecticide Capsules: The reactions were carried out in a 1-liter resin flask fitted with a Kraft Nonaerating Stirrer and 2 dropping funnels. All reactions were carried out at ambient temperature and pressure. To facilitate the formation and increase the stability of the initial oil-in-water suspension during the encapsulation process, a dispersing aid, such as Gelvatol 20/90 (Monsanto) a polyvinyl alcohol resin was used in the aqueous phase at a level of 0.5%. To reduce foaming, a defoaming agent, e.g., Antifoam B (Dow Corning) was also employed.

Example: In this example, an organic liquid pesticide, malathion was encapsulated in a polyamide-polyurea skin crosslinked by employing a polyfunctional isocyanate for the polyurea reaction. The flask contained 450 ml aqueous 0.5% Gelvatol 20/90 solution and 9 drops Antifoam B. The first funnel contained 44.7 g malathion (technical grade), 19.5 g azeloyl chloride and 3.0 g PAPI. The second funnel contained 30 g diethylenetriamine, 15 g sodium carbonate monohydrate and 150 ml distilled water.

The flask, charged as indicated above, was agitated at 6,000 to 7,000 rpm and contents of the first and second funnels were added rapidly and consecutively thereto. Following addition, the agitation speed was reduced and continued for approximately one hour. During the addition and agitation stages, small droplets were clearly visible in the reaction mixture and the reaction proceeded rapidly to produce the insecticide capsules. After standing, the capsules settled to the bottom of the reaction vessel and were additionally concentrated by centrifugation and the supernatant was removed. The capsules were washed twice with deionized water with removal of the liquid phase following centrifugation.

Subsequently, the capsules were air dried at room temperature on a filter paper. When suspended in a water slurry, microscopic examination revealed that the capsules ranged in diameter from about 5 to 40 microns with the majority being in the 20 to 30 micron range. For use in pesticide preparations, these pesticide-containing capsules can release their contents by gradual diffusion, or by leaching action.

In preparing aqueous dispersions of the process, it has been found that small amounts of xanthan gum within the narrow range of from 0.1 to 0.5% are sufficient to stabilize aqueous dispersions containing from 1 to 40% solids. The term percent is based upon the total weight of the formulation. Percent solids or solids loading is the weight percent of capsules present and is determined by separating the insecticide capsules from the water and other ingredients present in the liquid phase and determining the weight of the dry capsules which is equal to the weight of the polymeric skin plus the encapsulated insecticide.

A stable aqueous dispersion is one where nonseparation is discernable immediately after formulation and up to 24 hours thereafter, and where after 2½ years, at least 95% of the capsules remain dispersed based on visual observation. A dispersion which is readily redispersable, such as in the process, is one wherein even after prolonged standing (e.g., at least 2 years), any material which has separated and formed a third phase on the bottom of the dispersion container, is redispersable by gentle agitation. For samples contained in 4 to 8 oz sample bottles, redispersion can be accomplished in 5 seconds or less just by manual shaking of the bottle.

With the above definitions in mind, it has been found that 0.1% xanthan gum is sufficient to stabilize 40% solids or more with the advantages set forth above. At 30% solids and 0.1% Xanthan gum, a small amount of separation (e.g., 15%) is observed after 24 hours. At solids levels below 30% (e.g., 15%), the dispersions are less stable where the amount of gum employed is very small, i.e., use of small amounts of gum is of use primarily in stabilizing high solids loadings. Similarly, at 0.2% gum concentration, medium levels of solids loading (e.g., 15%), were found to be stable. At gum concentrations of 0.3 to 0.5%, solids loadings as low as 1% are stable. To form stable dispersions by using low concentrations of gum (e.g., 0.3%) as compared to common practice, it is necessary simply to increase the solids loading until stability is achieved, it being understood from the above example that the stability at high solids loading can be achieved with low gum levels.

The stable aqueous dispersions are prepared by admixing insecticide capsules with water until the desired loading is obtained, e.g., from 1 to 40% by weight based on the total composition weight and preferably from 10 to 40% by weight. Where the material is to be diluted prior to application and also to avoid shipment of large volumes of water, it is desirable to have a solids loading of from 20 to 40%, and preferably about 30%. Soon after forming the capsule/water admixture, and before the capsules have had time to cake together, the xanthan gum dispersing agent is added with sufficient stirring to form a homogenous dispersion.

As discussed above, the amount of gum employed is from 0.1 to 0.5 wt %. For relatively high solids loadings, e.g., 30 to 40%, the amount of gum employed can be as little as 0.1% which certainly constitutes a commercial advantage. However, for lower solids levels, e.g., less than 15%, the dispersions may be unstable. This can be corrected by raising the gum level to 0.3% or more, or by increasing the solids content.

Another method of forming the dispersions involves addition of the xanthan gum directly to commercially available formulations such as Penncap M (Pennwalt Corporation) aqueous dispersions of polyamide-polyurea encapsulated methyl parathion. In this case, the material as received may be caked and may require strenuous mixing to initially redisperse the capsules. However, once dispersed, the xanthan gum is added as described above to form a stable aqueous dispersion. Xanthan gum as employed in the process includes the available commercial forms of gum such as Keltrol (Kelco), Kelzan (Kelco), and Biopolymer (General Mills).

Fertilizer Particles Encapsulated in Water-Insoluble Metallic Carbonate Salts

F.T. Kawar; U.S. Patent 4,013,442; March 22, 1977; assigned to Exxon Research and Engineering Company found that a hard, crystalline-like, continuous, metal carbonate capsule of low porosity is obtained if the particle, rather than being dusted with the finely divided metal carbonate salt, is coated initially with the corresponding hydroxide or oxide of the specific metal carbonate salt intended as the encapsulating material and then carbonated by subjecting the coating to treatment by a source of CO_2, thereby resulting in an in situ conversion of the hydroxide or oxide to the corresponding carbonate on the surface of the particle. The encapsulated particles resist caking.

The particulate matter for encapsulation includes various fertilizer compositions containing urea, substituted ureas, ammonium phosphates, ammonium nitrate, superphosphates, etc.; various inorganic salts such as sodium chloride, potassium chloride, sodium nitrate, potassium nitrate, sodium iodide, potassium iodide, ammonium chloride, etc.; and in general, various solid substances, organic and inorganic in nature, which are subject to caking.

The most preferred carbonate salts are those derived from calcium and magnesium. Additionally, there can be used a mixture of the abovementioned group of carbonates, or a combination with a fine ground inert material such as limestone or phosphate rock. Also, calcium oxide, magnesium oxide and mixtures thereof as found naturally occurring such as calcitic quicklime, dolomitic quicklime, dolomitic single hydrated lime, dolomitic double hydrated lime, calcitic hydrated lime, etc., are useful since they will undergo carbonation to produce the desired product.

However, when an oxide is used as the initial coating material, it is necessary to add water in an amount of at least 0.1% preferably between 0.1 to 20% of the total weight of oxide and particles used in order to initiate conversion of the oxide to the hydroxide form. Addition of a greater amount of water will result in dissolution of particles. Gaseous CO_2 is utilized to effect carbonation of the coated particle. While pure carbon dioxide gas is the most preferred, CO_2-containing combustion gases, or diluted CO_2 from any conventional CO_2 source can also be utilized.

The encapsulating process comprises:

(a) adding to a conventional coating drum the particles to be encapsulated along with the metallic oxide or hydroxide which is to coat the particles and to be carbonated to form the encapsulating material,

(b) rotating the drum so as to achieve adherence of the coating material to the particles,

(c) introducing carbon dioxide into the coating drum by means of a sparger, an apparatus emitting carbon dioxide directly into the rotating bed of particles, and

(d) removing the encapsulated particles from the coating drum.

Examples 1 through 5: In each of the following examples, 60 lb of prilled urea were added to a conventional coating drum along with varying amounts of finely divided calcium hydroxide and 30 g of water to achieve maximum adherence of the powder to the prilled urea particles. The drum was rotated until uniform coating of the urea prills by the calcium hydroxide powder was achieved. The temperature of the drum was maintained at 110°F. An amount of carbon dioxide, as specified in the accompanying table, added at the rate therein specified, was injected into the rotating bed of coated urea prills. After completion of the carbon dioxide addition, the encapsulated particles were removed. The data and results from these examples are shown below.

Ex. No.	$Ca(OH)_2$ (lb)	CO_2 (lb)	Addition Rate CO_2 (lb/min)	Urea Prills (lb)	Encapsulated Products (lb)	Coating (%)	Empty Capsules (wt %)
1	3*	1.84	0.084	60	62.8	4.5	4.5
2	3**	1.84	0.084	60	63.3	5.3	5.3
3	3**	1.84	0.084	60	63.6	5.6	5.6
4	1.25	0.8	0.084	60	61.7	2.7	2.7
5	1.25	0.8	0.084	60	61.8	2.9	2.9

*In three 1 lb additions.
**In two 1½ lb additions.

To determine the weight of the capsule, 100 g of the product of each example was introduced into 500 g of water, whereupon the entrained urea dissolved, leaving the empty calcium carbonate capsules as individual entities within the urea-water solution. The empty capsules of the individual examples were separated from the water, washed, dried and weighed.

Rapid Encapsulation in Polyurea Using Phase Transfer Catalyst

H.B. Scher; U.S. Patent 4,140,516; February 20, 1979; assigned to Stauffer Chemical Company describes a method for the production of discrete polyurea microcapsules containing various core materials by the addition of a phase transfer catalyst to the organic phase.

It has been found that effective encapsulation by interfacial polymerization of an organic isocyanate intermediate can be effectively enhanced by the addition of a phase transfer catalyst in the process which utilizes two substantially heterogeneous immiscible liquids, one termed an aqueous phase and the other termed an organic phase, and which comprises establishing a physical dispersion of the organic phase in the aqueous phase, the organic phase containing the organic isocyanate intermediate for the polyurea capsule skin or enclosure. The interfacial polymerization of the process to form the capsular wall involves hydrolysis of an isocyanate monomer in the presence of a catalytic amount of phase transfer catalyst to form an amine which in turn reacts with another isocyanate monomer to form the polyurea enclosure.

The addition of no other reactant is required once the dispersion establishing droplets of the organic phase within a continuous liquid phase, i.e., aqueous phase, has been accomplished. Thereafter, and preferably with moderate agitation of the dispersion, the formation of the polyurea capsule skin or enclosure around the dispersed organic droplets is enhanced by the catalytic action of an agent known as a phase transfer catalyst capable of increasing the rate of isocyanate hydrolysis, thereby effecting the desired condensation reaction at the interface between the organic droplets and the continuous phase without external heating of the dispersion.

The product from the process is particularly suitable for direct agricultural pesticidal applications, additional agents can be added such as thickeners, biocides, surfactants and dispersants to improve storage stability and ease of application.

The procedure involves first, producing, as by simple agitation, a solution of water, a suitable surfactant and protective colloid. These three ingredients comprise the aqueous phase or continuous phase of the process. The aqueous or continuous phase is essentially free of any components that will react with the material therein or any of such groups of materials. The surfactant and protective colloid in the aqueous phase do not enter into the polycondensation reaction by which the capsule wall is formed.

A second phase known as the organic phase, comprises the material to be encapsulated, a polyisocyanate and phase transfer catalyst. The preferred amount of organic phase is about 25 to 50% by volume. The nature of the organic polyisocyanate determines the release properties of the capsule formed by this process. The polyisocyanates also determine the structural physical strength of the capsular wall. The organic polyisocyanates employed include those members of the aromatic polyisocyanate class which includes the aromatic diisocyanates, the aliphatic diisocyanates and the isocyanate prepolymers.

It is desirable to use combinations of organic polyisocyanates. Such combinations as, for example, polymethylene polyphenylisocyanate and tolylene diisocyanate, containing 80%, 2,4- and 20% 2,6-isomers, produce excellent capsular enclosures with exceptional controlled release properties.

The use of a phase transfer catalyst allows the use of aliphatic isocyanates, such as hexamethylene diisocyanate for capsule wall formation at 25°C or ambient temperatures. Without a phase transfer catalyst the aliphatic diisocyanates react too slowly even at elevated temperatures. This permits favorable blending of aliphatic and aromatic isocyanates to thereby modify the permeability of the microcapsule wall.

The amount of organic polyisocyanate used in the process will determine the wall content of the capsules formed therein. The preferred range is from about 5.0 to 50.0% wall content. Certain organic quaternary salts of Group V-A of the Periodic Table of the Elements have been found effective as "phase transfer catalyst" useful in the rapid formation of microcapsules according to the process.

Examples of such catalysts are quaternary salts having the formula $(R_3R_4R_5R_6M)^+X^-$ wherein R_3, R_4, R_5 and R_6 are hydrocarbon radicals having a total sum of 18 to 70 carbon atoms selected independently from the group consisting of alkyl, alkenyl, aryl, alkaryl, aralkyl and cycloalkyl radicals; M is a pentavalent ion selected from the group consisting of nitrogen, phosphorus, arsenic, antimony, and bismuth, preferably nitrogen or phosphorus; and X is an anion which will dissociate from the cation in an aqueous environment, preferably a halide ion or a hydroxyl ion, most preferably chloride or bromide. The number of carbon atoms in the hydrocarbon substituents may vary considerably so as to contain from 1 to 25 or more carbon atoms in each instance.

The preferred phase transfer catalysts are tetra-n-butyl phosphonium chloride, tri-n-butyl phosphonium chloride, tri-n-butyl n-cetyl phosphonium bromide, hexadecyl tributyl phosphonium bromide, benzyl triethyl ammonium chloride, benzyl triethyl ammonium bromide, trioctyl ethyl ammonium bromide, tetraheptyl ammonium iodide, triphenyl decyl phosphonium iodide, tribenzyl decyl arsonium chloride, tetranonyl ammonium hydroxide, tricaprylyl methyl ammonium chloride, and dimethyl dicoco ammonium chloride. The latter two catalysts are manufactured by General Mills Co., Chemical Division and are alternatively designated by the names Aliquat 336 and Aliquat 221, respectively.

The term catalytic amount is used herein to represent any amount of phase transfer catalyst (quaternary salt) which will enhance the progress of the reaction. The amount of catalyst normally used will range from preferably 0.2 to 2.0 wt % based on the organic phase.

While stirring the aqueous phase, the organic phase is added, preferably in a premixed state. Upon addition of the organic phase to the aqueous phase, a suitable dispersing means to disperse one liquid into the other is employed. Any high shear device can be used conveniently to obtain the desired droplet size within the range of 0.5 to 4,000 microns.

The process is capable of satisfactory performance and production of encapsulated material with easy adjustment of pH to facilitate the reaction. At a low pH value (about 2 to 5), the rate of wall formation is slow even with a phase transfer catalyst present. This is advantageous to allow time for dispersion of the organic phase. However, satisfactory dispersion can take place in the pH range of from 2 to 8. When properly dispersed to the desired particle size, the pH is raised to about pH 8 to pH 12, preferably pH 10, at which value the wall-forming reaction for the microcapsules takes place rapidly.

In an alternative procedure, the encapsulation process can be achieved by initially adjusting the pH of the aqueous phase to 5 to 10, without further pH adjustment after dispersion. In most instances, the reaction is about two-thirds complete in the initial 5 minutes after raising the pH value to about 10 at ambient temperature or about 25°C. Without a phase transfer catalyst present only about one-half completion is achieved in 60 minutes at 25°C depending upon the type of diisocyanate and material to be encapsulated. The encapsulation process will proceed most satisfactorily at a pH value of preferably between 8 and 12.

Example 1: Water (279 g), containing 2.0% of neutralized poly(methyl vinyl ether/maleic anhydride) protective colloid (Gantrez AN 119), 0.22% polyvinyl alcohol protective colloid (Vinol 205) and 0.3% linear alcohol ethoxylate emulsifier (Tergitol 15-5-7) is placed into an open reactor vessel. The pH is adjusted to about 4.3 with sodium hydroxide solution. In a separate container, 340 g of S-ethyl diisobutylthiocarbamate (a herbicide), 14.2 g of N,N-diallyl dichloroacetamide (a herbicide antidote), 15.8 g polymethylene polyphenylisocyanate (PAPI), 12.9 g tolylene diisocyanate (TDI) and 2.3 g tricaprylyl methyl ammonium chloride (a phase transfer catalyst, also known as Aliquat 336) are mixed together.

This mixture is then added to the reactor vessel and emulsified with a high shear stirrer. The resulting particle size is in the range of from 5 to 40 microns. Only mild agitation is required for the remainder of the reaction. No heating is required. The pH of the resulting mixture is adjusted to 10.0 with a 20% sodium hydroxide solution. At pH 10.0 the microcapsule wall formation is about 93.2% complete in about 2 minutes. Well formed, discrete microcapsules are observed under a microscope. In contrast, conventional polyurea microcapsule formation as described, without the phase transfer catalyst, requires about 3 hours at 50°C.

Example 2: In a similar procedure as described in Example 1, to 509 g of water containing 2.0% polyvinyl alcohol protective colloid (Vinol 205) and 0.3% linear alcohol ethoxylate emulsifier (Tergitol 15-5-7) is added 165 g S-ethyl diisobutyl thiocarbamate (a herbicide), 7.3 g polymethylene polyphenylisocyanate, 6.0 g tolylene diisocyanate and 1.0 g tri-n-butyl n-cetyl phosphonium bromide (a phase transfer catalyst). There is no initial pH adjustment. Emulsification is carried out as previous described. The particle size is established at about 5 to 40 microns. At this point the pH is adjusted to about 10.0 with sodium hydroxide solution. In about 6 minutes the formation of microcapsules is about 56.5% complete. Stirring is continued until the desired degree of completion is achieved as determined by sodium hydroxide consumption. Discrete well-formed microcapsules are observed with a microscope.

The process for encapsulation employing a phase transfer catalyst provides capsules capable of controlling release of encapsulated organic material. Representative and especially of importance are the process and capsules comprising as a constituent in the organic phase herbicides of the class thiocarbamate such as S-ethyl diisobutylthiocarbamate; S-propyl dipropylthiocarbamate, etc.; organo phosphorus insecticides of the class organo phosphoro and phosphorothioates and dithioates such as O-ethyl S-phenyl ethylphosphorodithioate, S-[p-chlorophenylthio)methyl] O,O-dimethyl phosphorodithioate, O,O-dimethyl O-p-nitrophenyl phosphorothioate, etc; and insect hormones and mimics such as: Cecropia-Juvenile Hormone-I,1-(4'-ethyl)phenoxy-3,7-dimethyl-7,7-epoxy-trans-2-octene, ethyl 3,7,11-trimethyldodeca-2,4-dienoate, etc.

Capsules of compounds useful for plant disease control provide a route to long term control of disease using compounds generally regarded to have only short term effectiveness. Similarly, herbicides, complementary herbicide antidotes, nematocides, insecticides, rodenticides and soil nutrients can be encapsulated with useful results.

Microgranules with Protective Colloid

The process of *H. Frensch, K. Albrecht and K. Hook; U.S. Patent 4,144,050; March 13, 1979; assigned to Hoechst AG, Germany* provides microgranules for pesticides which comprise a homogeneous content of a solid pesticidal active ingredient within a particle size range of from 0.075 to 0.4 mm, in addition to inert substances, wetting agents, dispersing agents and adhesion-promoting agents as well as, optionally, a protective colloid.

The process comprises grinding pesticides in the wet state together with inert substances, wetting and dispersing agents, adhesion-promoting agents and, optionally, protective colloids in ball mills to yield a particle size of a maximum of 0.01 mm, preferably of about 0.005 mm, and spray-drying the suspensions or pastes thus obtained by means of rotating disks at a circumferential speed of from 80 to 100 m/sec, preferably using single feed nozzles under a spraying pressure of from 5 to 8 atm gauge, or double feed nozzles under a spraying pressure of from 0.5 to 4 atm gauge, preferably from 0.5 to 1.5 atm gauge, at a drying gas inlet temperature of from 300° to 140°C, preferably from 270° to 180°C, and at a drying gas outlet temperature of from 50° to 120°C, preferably from 60° to 80°C.

The process allows granulation of all solid pesticidal active ingredients, for example, herbicidal, insecticidal and fungicidal compositions, together with the inert material to be advantageously used for maintaining their chemical stability and their biological activity, for example, diatomaceous earth, silicic acids, kaolinite-containing quartz, alumina, chalk, bentonites, atta-clay, inorganic salts, milk powder or starch.

An addition of dispersing and wetting agents, for example, sodium or ammonium salt of lignine-sulfonic acid, sodium salt of butylnaphthalene-sulfonic acid, oleylmethyl tauride sodium, sodium salt of an alkylphenyl-sulfonic acid, or condensation products of fatty acids and albumin permits a uniform distribution, wetting and release of the active ingredient particles. Depending on the type and dosage of adhesion-promoting agents, advantageously sodium salt of lignine-sulfonic acid, polyvinyl acetate, polyvinyl acetate copolymers and partially hydrolyzed polyvinyl alcohols or carboxymethyl cellulose having various polymerization degrees, vegetable rubber or glues, the release of the active ingredient can be accelerated or delayed.

Example 1: Microgranules of Pentachloronitrobenzene Having an Active Ingredient Content of 80% – (a) A mixture of 40 parts of pentachloronitrobenzene, 9 parts of sodium salt of lignine-sulfonic acid, 1 part of partially hydrolyzed polyvinyl acetate and 50 parts of water was ground in the wet state in a friction ball mill to yield a grain size of from 1 to 5 microns; the paste or suspension thus obtained was then spray-dried in a drying tower by means of a single feed nozzle at a pressure of from 7 to 8 atm gauge at an air inlet temperature of 240°C and an air outlet temperature of 75°C, 82 to 85% of the finest particles obtained had a size of from 0.075 to 0.350 mm. The content of active ingredient was 80%.

(b) Microgranules obtained according to the above method were mixed with 0.4 part of a polyvinyl acetate copolymer to slow down the release of the active ingredient.

Example 2: Microgranules of Linuron Having an Active Ingredient Content of 10% — In a manner analogous to Example 1, a paste or suspension containing 40% of linuron was prepared. This was stirred with further 35 parts of sodium salt of lignine-sulfonic acid, 3.5. parts of partially hydrolyzed polyvinyl acetate, 311.5 parts of kaolinite-containing quartz powder (or a mixture of 187 parts of kieselguhr and 124.5 parts of sodium hyperphosphate) and 215 parts of water in a colloid mill. The suspension thus obtained having a solids content of 60% was spray-dried. The yield of microgranules having a particle size of from 0.075 to 0.35 was 85%. The active ingredient content was 10%. By adding from 0.1 to 1.5 parts of polyvinyl acetate in dispersed form the granules obtained had a slower release of active ingredient.

PIGMENTS

Polymeric Metal Phosphate Complex

C.M. Sherman; U.S. Patent 3,946,134; March 23, 1976; assigned to The Harshaw Chemical Company found that one or more characteristics, such as the chemical, thermal or light stability, of a particle such as an inorganic chrome pigment or an organic azo pigment is improved by encapsulating each of the particles with a continuous layer or skin of a polymeric metal phosphate complex, optionally containing up to 30 wt % of fluoride ions or ions of BF_4^-. The coating, which normally constitutes between 5 and 30% by weight of the particle, has a thickness of between 25 and 300 A. The coating is typically applied by controlled polymerization from a liquid medium in which the particles are generally insoluble.

The organic or inorganic particles, in finely divided form, are made into a slurry to which is normally added aluminum acetate or other soluble basis aluminum salt, such as the dibasic formate, which is capable of forming a complex with the phosphate, and which has no tendency to dissolve the particle or otherwise adversely affect the same. The phosphate ions are then added to the slurry as an orthophosphate or a precursor thereof, after which the aluminum and the phosphate slowly begin to form a low molecular weight colloidal polymeric complex which condenses on the surface of the particles as a continuous, dense adherent coating or skin. The temperature is preferably maintained below 40°C to promote the controlled precipitation and to prevent flocculation and the formation of large particles of the complex. The pH of the slurry during the addition of the phosphate ions, the formation of the metal phosphate complex and the condensation of the coating on the particle is maintained in a range between 1 and 6 to prevent premature precipitation of the metallic salt. After the reaction is complete, the pH of the slurry is adjusted, if necessary, to a final value of between about 6 and 7.5.

The fluoride or fluoborate ions are preferably added to the slurry in soluble form. Ammonium bifluoride, hydrofluoric acid and sodium fluoride have been found to be suitable for this purpose. The fluoride ions may be added to the slurry along with or following the addition of the metal salt complexing agent. If BF_4^- ions are used in place of the fluoride ions, these are preferably added as the ammonium salt. The phosphate ions should preferably be added to the slurry in the form of ortho- or metaphosphoric acid or a precursor thereof, such as an ester of phosphoric acid.

The ratio of aluminum to phosphorus in the coating is generally between 0.8 and 1.8 with a preferred range being between 0.8 and 1.2. The ratio of aluminum to phosphorus in solution may vary from as low as 0.2 to 2.0. The higher amounts of metal in the complex appear to enhance the H_2S resistance of the coating.

The formation of the colloidal sol is also dependent upon the concentration of the aluminum salt and the orthophosphate or its precursor in solution. The formation of the sol can occur in 5 seconds or less at high concentrations of 20 mg/ml, whereas a formation time of 20 minutes is not uncommon for very dilute solutions, as low as 0.5 mg/ml. Also, undesirable floc formation is precluded at low concentrations. The particles in the sol are between 50 and 600 A in size with high Al/P ratios favoring the formation of smaller particles, typically under 200 A, considerably smaller than the size of particles produced by flocculation.

At the completion of the encapsulation, the coated particles are recovered by filtration or other suitable means and are then dried by heating to a temperature below that likely to cause the substrate to degrade. A temperature of 150°C has been found to be acceptable for lead chromate and other inorganic pigments, whereas a temperature of 50° to 150°C for organic pigments is satisfactory.

Example 1: 50 g of finely divided lead chromate is blended into water to give a 500 ml slurry. To this is added a solution of 8.37 g of aluminum acetate (Niaproof Aluminum Acetate, basic, stabilized with boric acid, Union Carbide Corporation), and a solution of 3.2 g of ammonium bifluoride, each dissolved in 50 ml deionized water. The slurry is then stirred at room temperature after which 4.73 g of H_3PO_4 (85%) diluted to 50 ml is added. A colloidal sol of aluminum phosphate slowly forms and deposits on the pigment particles in the slurry. Throughout this procedure, the pH of the slurry is controlled between 3 and 6 to prevent attack and degradation of the lead chromate by acid or alkali, and to preclude the pigment from solubilizing. Furthermore, maintaining the pH above 3 precludes the undesirable reduction of the hexavalent chromium to the trivalent form. After 15 minutes, the pH is adjusted to 7.4 with about 85 ml of 30% $(NH_4)_2HPO_3$. The slurry is pressure filtered to recover the pigment and the pigment is dried at 50°C for 16 hours.

A portion of the coated pigment is mixed into an alkyd resin vehicle in an amount of 15 wt % of pigment, and a drawdown of the same is exposed along with a drawdown of an uncoated pigment in the same vehicle, to a Fadometer test for 100 hours. One-half of each panel is shielded from light. The color retention of the coated pigment is noticeably better than that of the uncoated panel.

Another portion of the coated pigment is blended in an amount of 1% by weight with styrene granules which are heated and extruded into a first test panel which is subjected to a heat test along with a second panel containing 1% of the uncoated pigment and a third panel containing 1% of a pigment coated with a layer consisting of 20% silica, 4% alumina and TiO_2. Each panel is heated to the breaking temperature which is the temperature at which visual darkening occurs. The first and third panels are heated up to 575°F at which temperature a comparison reveals that the panel coated according to the process does not darken as much as the panel coated with $SiO_2/Al_2O_3/TiO_2$. In the second panel containing the unencapsulated pigment, darkening occurs at about 425°F.

The chemical stability of the coated pigment is compared with that of the uncoated pigment in the presence of H_2S, NaOH and HCl. In all instances, the degradation of the uncoated pigment is much more rapid than that of the coated pigment.

Example 2: A monoazo pigment, BON Maroon 1081 is encapsulated using the method of Example 1. Care is exercised during encapsulation to insure that the pH is maintained below about 6 to prevent degradation of the pigment. The encapsulated pigment is dried at 150°C for 24 hours while retaining its texture and most of its color characteristics. An untreated pigment is totally degraded to a brown sintered mass at this temperature in 1.5 hours.

Metal Phosphate Complex Microcapsules Not Requiring Dehydration

C.C. Hayman; U.S. Patent 4,110,492; August 29, 1978; assigned to The Harshaw Chemical Company provides an improved method of particle encapsulation so as to produce more dense, impervious and adherent microcapsules. The particle encapsulation is accomplished without the necessity of the dehydration step disclosed in U.S. Patent 3,946,134.

This is achieved by continuously adding to an aqueous dispersion of the substrate, at 70° to 100°C, separate aqueous solutions of: (a) aluminum and/or magnesium ions, particularly mono or dibasic aluminum ions, which are added in the form of lower alkyl carboxylates or halo substituted lower alkyl carboxylates, and (b) orthophosphoric and/or mono and/or difluorophosphoric acid which may be present as a hydroxy aluminum phosphate-boric acid complex. The resulting encapsulated particulate substrate is generally separated from the resulting dispersion. Optionally, components (a) and (b) are added in the presence of: (c) a coordinating species which may be either boric acid, H_3BO_3, or fluoride ion F^-, or a complex fluoro anion which may be fluoborate, BF_4^- or hexafluorophosphate, PF_6^-, or combinations thereof.

Component (c) can be added in a separate solution (as in the case of fluoborate or hexafluorophosphate ions) or it can be codissolved with component (b). In addition, component (c) can be present in chemical combination with either component (a) as in the case of a dibasic aluminum carboxylate-boric acid complex, or component (b) as in the case of the hydroxy aluminum phosphate-boric acid complex.

The pH of the dispersion during the encapsulation is controlled and maintained in the range 2.5 to 5.5 by maintaining the molar proportions of the magnesium and/or aluminum, the phosphorus and the other species of (c) in the coreactants (a), (b) and (c) within the range 0.8:1.0:0.0 to 1.4:1.0:10.0. Sufficient quantities of the coreactants are simultaneously added over the course of 0.5 to 5.0 hours to encapsulate the substrate in at least 5 and up to 50% of the complex metal phosphate or fluorophosphate, based on the total combined weight of substrate and capsule. The resulting encapsulated product is isolated, as by filtration, preferably washed, and may be dried at any convenient temperature below the decomposition temperature of the substrate or it may be used in the wet state.

Example: Two light yellow finely divided 65 wt % lead chromate, 35 wt % lead sulfate pigments (C.I. 77603) were prepared by standard techniques by precipitation out of aqueous solution, pH adjustment with sodium carbonate solution to 5.6 to 6.0, recovery by filtration, washing with water and drying. The first pigment A was prepared without light stabilizers, sulfuric acid being used to precipitate the excess lead in solution as lead sulfate prior to the pH adjustment.

The second pigment B was treated prior to pH adjustment by the addition to the aqueous solution at 5-minute intervals of separate aqueous solutions of aluminum sulfate, titanium sulfate and cerium nitrate such that the pigment B was calculated to have primarily as a pigment coating 2 wt % alumina, 1 wt % titania and 3 wt % ceria, the weights calculated as the hydrous oxides based on the total weight of the dried pigment.

A 23-g sample of each of pigments A and B was treated as follows in accordance with the method. For these treatments three solutions were prepared.

Solution X was 5.29 g of the aluminum acetate employed in the examples of U.S. Patent 3,946,134 (Union Carbide Corporation, Niaproof Aluminum Acetate, basic, stabilized with boric acid) dissolved in 62 ml of water.

Solution Y was boric acid stabilized aluminum phosphate prepared by adding to 80 ml of water 61.0 ml of phosphoric acid (85.5%), 5.5 g of boric acid and 25.0 g of commercial high surface area alumina, heating the resulting slurry with stirring to and at 85° to 90°C until a colloidal dispersion is formed, cooling the dispersion to 25° to 30°C and adding water to adjust the total volume to 250 ml.

Solution Z was a solution of 0.92 g of ammonium bifluoride, 0.50 g of ammonium fluoborate, 1.84 g of phosphoric acid (85.5%) and 4.6 ml of Solution Y in 62 ml of water.

Each pigment sample was added to 170 ml of water, and each resulting slurry was blended for 10 minutes in a Waring Blender to break up pigment aggregates. Each resulting slurry was then transferred to a vessel to which was begun a simultaneous addition of Solutions X and Z, each at a rate of about 0.8 ml/min. After about 10% (or 6 to 7 ml) of each solution had been added, each pigment slurry was heated rapidly to 80°C and maintained at that temperature while continuing the same additions of Solutions X and Z until completed.

Each resulting pigment slurry was neutralized to a pH of 5.0 with a 1:1 water:ammonium hydroxide solution. Each pigment while still in slurry was then coated with an aluminum rosinate by adding quickly 2.38 g of additional aluminum acetate dissolved in 15 ml of water and then adding dropwise over 5 minutes 1.65 g of a commercial rosin (basically hydrogenated abietic acid) dissolved in 60 ml of water at 85° to 95°C solubilized with a small amount of sodium hydroxide. Each pigment was then filtered out of its slurry, washed thoroughly with water and dried at 80°C.

A portion of each encapsulated pigment was mixed into an alkyd resin vehicle in an amount of 15 wt % pigment, and a drawdown of such pigmented alkyd resin was exposed to a Fadometer test for 100 hours. A portion of each encapsulated pigment was also mixed with polypropylene molding material in an amount of 1 wt % pigment, and the pigmented polypropylene was injection molded at 575°F (302°C).

Similar pigments A and B treated in accordance with the method of U.S. Patent 3,946,134 as controls were also tested in like manner for purposes of comparison. The thermal stability of the respective molded polypropylene containing pigments A and B treated in accordance with this process was better than the thermal stability of the corresponding molded polypropylene containing the corresponding control pigments. The light stability of the alkyd resin containing pigment B treated in accordance with this process was better than the corresponding alkyd resin containing control pigment B. The alkyd resins containing pigment A without light stabilizers had poor light stability after either pigment treatment.

Similar thermal stability results are achieved when the aluminum rosinate coating is omitted and the pigments are mixed and extruded with polystyrene. Similar results are achieved when magnesium acetate is substituted mol per mol for the aluminum acetate in Solution X.

Pigment Presscake Encapsulated with Ammoniacal Acrylic Resin

J. Rothmayer; U.S. Patent 4,036,652; July 19, 1977; assigned to Sun Chemical Corporation found that a superior encapsulated pigment presscake product can be produced by a process that comprises the following steps:

(1) preparing a high solids pigment presscake by any known method from a conventional presscake containing about 15 to 30% of pigment, for example, by evaporating or vacuuming off water or by displacing water with a nonmiscible solvent. The resulting presscake contains about 50 to 60% of pigment and about 40 to 50% of water;

(2) mixing the resulting high solids pigment mass with an ammoniacal resin solution, whereby the presscake is peptized by the resin into a thin, watery fluid product;

(3) removing water from the watery product by evaporation, vacuuming, decantation, or the like, while continually mixing the materials, resulting in a thick, plastic, kneadable mass; and

(4) dispersing the kneadable mass under conditions of high shear to encapsulate the pigment presscake.

The products are encapsulated pigment presscakes containing about 50 to 80 parts of pigment, about 10 to 40 parts of ammoniated resin, and about 10 to 40 parts of water. Generally, the ratio of resin to pigment is about 10 to 40 parts of resin:100 parts of pigment, and preferably the ratio is about 20 to 30:100.

The pigments require no posttreatment before use. They are easily dispersible in water- or solvent-based ink systems; they contain no surfactants, and they exhibit minimal levels of foam in ink manufacture. The process is equally applicable to organic and inorganic pigments and to dyestuffs. The resin employed in step (2) is an ammonia-soluble resin, particularly an acrylic resin, such as a homopolymer, copolymer, or interpolymer of an acrylate or methacrylate.

The amount of acrylic resin added to the high solids pigment presscake mass is about 10 to 40, preferably about 20 to 30, parts per 100 parts of pigment mass. The acrylic resin is added in the presence of ammonia, the amount of ammonia being about 5 to 50, and preferably about 15 to 25, parts per 100 parts of the pigment.

In order to obtain the encapsulated pigment presscakes, the dispersion in step (4) must take place under conditions of high shear agitation, such as, for example, by agitation in a heavy duty dispersion or sigma blade mixer, a Banbury mill, a Manton-Goulin homogenizer, or other such similar intensive dispersion equipment.

Example 1: A presscake containing 25% of phthalocyanine blue pigment and 75% of water was charged into a jacketed heavy duty sigma blade dispersion mixer. Water was evaporated (using steam in the jacket), optionally under vacuum, until the presscake contained 50% of pigment and 50% of water.

1,000 parts of the resulting high solids presscake was mixed with 40 parts of ammonia (26°Bé) and 500 parts of Acrysol 1-94 (Rohm and Haas' acrylic resin emulsion containing 30% solids), resulting in a thin, watery mixture. Mixing and removal of water by evaporation were continued until a plastic, kneadable mass was obtained.

This kneadable mass was then dispersed under high shear conditions to encapsulate the pigment presscake and yield 840 parts of a finely divided product containing 55% of phthalocyanine pigment, 17.5% of ammoniated acrylic resin, and 27.5% of water. The product was easily discharged into a closed container and was nondusting.

Example 2: A flexographic ink was prepared in a conventional manner in a ball mill for 24 hours from the ingredients shown in the table on the following page.

	Parts by Weight
Encapsulated pigment of Example 1	27.3
Water	36.2
Aqueous ammonia (26°Bé)	7.0
Acrylic resin (Joncryl 67)	18.5
Diethylene glycol monoethyl ether	5.0
Antifoam agent	1.0
Isopropanol	5.0

The pigment was easily dispersed into the system, the ink was exceptionally glossy and transparent as compared to an ink prepared as above except that the pigment was not encapsulated.

Dense Silica-Encapsulated Aluminum Flake Pigment Treated with Carboxylic Chromic Chloride

Aluminum flake pigment is widely known for its ability to impart metallic luster to coating compositions in which it is used. Although aluminum flake is used in many different decorative applications, the metallic luster characteristic of this pigment is particularly desirable in automotive finishes. While the aluminum flake pigments have proven readily useful in coating compositions based on organic solvent systems, difficulties have been encountered in attempting to use the same pigments in aqueous solvent systems, e.g., solvent systems containing about 80% water.

In aqueous medium, aluminum flake pigment can undergo reaction with water with accompanying evolution of hydrogen gas. This phenomenon, known as "gassing," can be especially troublesome when the pigment is stored in aqueous medium in sealed containers. Gassing can be lessened, to some extent, by encapsulating the aluminum flakes with dense amorphous silica.

K. Batzar; U.S. Patent 3,954,496; May 4, 1976; assigned to E.I. DuPont de Nemours and Company found that dense silica-encapsulated aluminum flake pigments can be treated with a carboxylic chromic chloride so that during preparation or when incorporated into coating compositions, the resulting pigment will have high resistance to gassing in contact with water.

Dense silica-encapsulated aluminum flake pigment is prepared by precipitating dense silica from an aqueous suspension of finely divided aluminum flake pigment which contains active silica. The improvement comprises treating this silica-encapsulated pigment with a carboxylic chromic chloride selected from the group consisting of methacrylato chromic chloride, stearato chromic chloride and myristato chromic chloride. For applications where coating compositions containing the treated aluminum flake pigment are exposed to high humidity, methacrylato chromic chloride is preferred because it imparts humidity resistance to the pigment.

The treated silica-encapsulated aluminum flake pigment permits the use of far less silica coating than is necessary on untreated pigment, while achieving much higher resistance to gassing. For example, it has been found that untreated silica-encapsulated aluminum flake pigment containing as high as 10% by weight of SiO_2 produces about ten times as much gas in aqueous medium as the same amount of treated pigment containing about only 4% by weight of SiO_2. Since silica coatings tend to decrease the luster of aluminum flake pigment, the use of lesser amounts of silica, while achieving high resistance to gassing, is commercially desirable.

The amount of carboxylic chromic chloride used should be from about 2 to 20% by weight (preferably 4 to 8% by weight), based on the weight of the pigment, to effectively inhibit gassing. The carboxylic chromic chloride is advantageously applied while the pigment is dispersed in an aqueous medium. Thus, the chromic chloride, being water-soluble, can be added to the suspension for purposes of its absorption onto the pigment particles. In any case, it is preferable that the temperature of the aqueous dispersion does not exceed 60°C or otherwise excessive hydrolysis of the chromic chloride can occur. Excessively high pH values, i.e., of 11 or greater, should be avoided.

The amount of dense silica utilized in the process should be from 2 to 30% (preferably 4 to 10%), based on the pigment weight, depending upon the degree of metallic luster or reflectivity desired in the final encapsulated pigment.

Example: 50 g of a commercially available aluminum flake pigment, having a particle size of about 2 to 50 μ, is washed free of mineral spirits with butyl Cellosolve. The pigment is washed into a conventional high-shear blending device using 500 ml of an aqueous solution containing 12.0 g sodium silicate and 0.01 gram of nonylphenoxy poly(ethyleneoxy)ethanol, a commercially available surfactant sold under the name Tergitol NP-14, to aid in dispersing the mixture. The resulting mixture is blended at low speed for 5 minutes, then transferred to a 4-neck round-bottom flask equipped with a stirrer, gas inlet tube, condenser and thermometer. The above dispersion procedure is repeated to provide an additional 50 g of suspended aluminum flake pigment which is placed in the flask to give a total of 100 g of suspended pigment.

The suspension is stirred at about 200 rpm for 45 minutes while being gradually heated to 95°C. The temperature is maintained at 95°C for 75 minutes as CO_2 is passed over the surface of the suspension at a rate of about 18 cc/min. Ice is then added to the suspension to lower the temperature to 45°C. The pH of the cooled suspension is 8.0 to 8.3. The treating agent is a 29% solution in isopropanol of methacrylato chromic chloride. 24 g of the treating solution is slurried in 25 ml of water and added with stirring to the suspension at a uniform rate to thus give 8% methacrylato chromic chloride based on the aluminum flake pigment. The solution is stirred for 2 minutes.

The pH of the suspension is adjusted to 8.0 by the use of aqueous 5% NaOH. The suspension is stirred for 15 minutes followed by readjustment of the pH to 8.0 with 5% NaOH. The suspension is filtered and washed with tap water until the resistivity is 5,000 ohm-cm. The suspension is further washed four times with 300 ml butyl Cellosolve each time. The product is dried prior to analysis and found by analysis to contain 4.0% SiO_2, dry basis.

To test the product for gassing in a typical aqueous-based dispersion, 4.6 g of the silica-encapsulated aluminum flake, dry basis, and 5.4 g of an aqueous solution containing about 50% of a low-molecular-weight (ca 8,000) carboxylic acrylic interpolymer formed by copolymerization of a mixture of 50 parts of methyl methacrylate, 30 parts of butyl acrylate and 20 parts acrylic acid, which has thereafter been neutralized with N,N-diethyl-2-aminoethanol, are added to 10 ml of water and thoroughly mixed. This dispersion is placed in a sealed container, equipped with a device for measuring the amount of gas which evolves from the composition, and held at 60°C for 24 hours. During that time, 3 ml of hydrogen gas evolves from the dispersion.

Control: 50 g of aluminum flake pigment described above is cleaned with butyl Cellosolve and then washed into a blending device using 500 ml of an aqueous solution containing 48.5 g sodium silicate. The resulting mixture is blended at low speed for 5 minutes, then transferred to the round-bottom flask described above. This procedure is repeated to give an additional 50 g of suspended flake, which is placed in the flask.

The suspension is stirred at about 200 rpm for 45 minutes while being gradually heated to 95°C. The temperature is maintained at 95°C for 5 hours as CO_2 is passed over the surface of the suspension at a rate of about 36 cc/min. The suspension is filtered and washed as above. The product is found by analysis to contain 10.2% SiO_2, dry basis.

The untreated product is tested for gassing according to the same procedure as used to test the treated product (described above) and is found to produce more than 30 ml of hydrogen gas during the testing period.

CATALYST AND CATALYST CARRIERS

Dual-Walled Hard Microcapsule Suitable for Catalysts

In accordance with the process of *W.T. Short; U.S. Patent 4,076,774; Feb. 28, 1978; assigned to General Motors Corporation,* an active agent, such as a catalyst or a cocatalyst, is encapsulated in a dual-walled microcapsule. Both walls of the microcapsule are polymerization reaction products and both are formed in one basic process. The active agent is initially dissolved in a slowly polymerizing liquid monomer mixture such as a solution of toluene diisocyanate and a polyoxyalkylene polyol. The "monomer solvent" and the active agent combination is selected so that the active agent is nonreactive but soluble in the liquid monomer and insoluble in the polymer formed therefrom. However, before the active agent precipitates, the solution is dispersed in a nonreactive medium and the outer polymeric wall is formed by vigorously stirring the dispersion and then adding a reactive polyfunctional monomer.

This polyfunctional monomer, which preferably has two primary aliphatic amine functionalities in terminal or near terminal positions, such as ethylene diamine, quickly reacts with the isocyanate of the initial monomer solution, via an interfacial polymerization reaction, to form the outer polyurea wall around each bead in the dispersion. Then the active hydrogen functionalities of the urea groups on the inner surface of the outer wall react with a portion of the nonreacted isocyanate functionality to form a biuret linkage between the outer wall and either or both the polymerizing monomer solution and the inner polymer wall which is formed therefrom. This reaction effectively bonds the outer wall to the inner wall as it forms.

As the polyurethane polymerization reaction continues, the active agent precipitates and migrates toward the center of the microcapsule, and is thereby isolated and protected by the dual-walled structure which has been formed in one basic operation.

Example: A dual-walled microcapsule was formed around an aniline-type compound which is useful as a cocatalyst in vinyl polymerization reactions. This dual-wall microcapsule structure did not require separate and distinct processes to form each individual wall. All steps were carried out at or near room temperature and atmospheric pressure.

The first step in this operation was to dissolve 24 g of a polyoxypropylene triol having a number average molecular weight ($\overline{M}n$) of about 1,500 in about 10 g of toluene diisocyanate. The triol used is TP1540 (part of the Pluracol series). The toluene diisocyanate used is Hylene T. About 0.1% dibutyltin dilaurate was added to catalyze the polyurethane forming reaction; however, seven hours was still required to form the inner wall.

The next step was to dissolve in the solution formed above about 5 g of the aniline active agent; this aniline is 4,4'-methylenebis(N,N-dimethylaniline). This is a tertiary amine which also reacts with the isocyanate, but very slowly; therefore, there was little concern about this side reaction.

The next step was to disperse or emulsify the aniline solution formed above in about 500 ml of distilled water, which for these particular solutes is substantially an inert medium. The dispersion or emulsification process was facilitated by the addition of about 1% by weight of a nonionic surfactant (Duponol-Me). Since the dispersing medium, water, and the aniline-containing solution are mutually immiscible, the emulsification step in effect created minute, substantially spherical beads of the aniline-toluene diisocyanate-polyol solution dispersed throughout the water.

The next step was to vigorously stir the dispersion and simultaneously add about 50 ml of ethylene diamine. This is a primary amine which dissolves in the water and reacts very quickly with the isocyanate at the surface of the beads to form a polyurea shell which completely surrounds and seals each bead. At this point, it should be noted that the reaction between the primary amine and the isocyanate occurs only at the interface between the primary amine-water solution and the aniline-toluene diisocyanate-polyol solution which is dispersed therein. Therefore, the reaction does not consume all the amine or all the isocyanate, because once the wall has formed the primary amine is no longer in contact with the isocyanate and, therefore, the reaction stops. Typically, the outer wall forms within a minute.

Urea functionalities are present on the inner surface of the outer wall and are thereby presented inwardly toward the slowly reacting polyol-diisocyanate solution in which the aniline is dissolved. The urea functionality contains an active hydrogen group which reacts with the isocyanate to form a biuret linkage which effectively bonds the slowly polymerizing polyol-diisocyanate solution to the inner surface of the outer wall. Therefore, as this polymerization reaction continues, the urethane is formed against the inner surface of the outer wall. At this point, it is to be noted that the aniline compound is precipitating from the polymerizing polyol-diisocyanate solution. This order of events is the result of selecting the components of the initial "monomer solvent" so that they react slowly and allow the outer shell to be formed before they polymerize to a point which may cause the aniline to precipitate.

These results were substantiated by a direct microscopic examination of the microcapsules immediately after the outer polyurea shell had been formed and at various times afterwards as the inner wall was forming. This examination was conducted by rupturing the shells and then examining the rubble under a microscope. The first observation clearly indicated that a single-walled microcapsule had been formed. However, as the observations continued, the dual-walled structure appeared. From this it was evident that the polyol-diisocyanate solution had polymerized and formed the second wall against the inner surface of the outer wall and caused the aniline compound to precipitate and migrate towards the center of the microcapsule.

The dual-walled structure indicated that the inner wall was bonded to the outer wall. Without this bond the "monomer solvent" would probably form a ball and exude the active agent rather than form an inner wall. This process had formed a substantially leakproof, hard microcapsule which would be very suitable for isolating various highly reactive materials.

The encapsulated aniline was then blended into an acrylic monomer and the capsules were ruptured as the monomer was applied as a coating. The curing characteristics of the coating clearly indicated that the aniline was present and active.

Encapsulation of Heterogeneous Catalyst and Ferromagnetic Material Within a Semipermeable Membrane

M.J. Marquisee and W.W. Prichard; U.S. Patent 3,954,666; May 4, 1976; assigned to E.I. DuPont de Nemours and Company are concerned with the encapsulation within a semipermeable membrane of a heterogeneous catalyst and a ferromagnetic material. Optionally, a cell stabilizing agent may be present. The resulting capsules are stable when suspended in an aqueous or nonaqueous phase, the catalyst is active for effecting a desired catalytic reaction, and the capsules can be captured and released from the solvent phase by means of a magnetic field.

The term "heterogeneous catalyst" is used to refer to catalysts which are insoluble in the reaction medium in which they function as catalysts. These catalysts are generally solids. Suitable heterogeneous catalysts include any insoluble catalyst which functions at temperatures below the melting point of the capsule walls. Catalysts employed for hydrogenation, e.g., nickel, palladium, platinum, ruthenium and rhodium; catalysts suitable for olefin isomerization, e.g., platinum, palladium and rhodium; oxidation catalysts, e.g., platinum and cobalt oxides; catalysts suitable for hydrosilylation of olefins such as palladium; and ion exchange resins including acidic types containing active groups such as carboxylic or sulfonic acid groups, for example, styrene-acrylic acid resins; and basic types, for example, those containing tertiary amine groups, may be successfully encapsulated. The preferred catalysts are those suitable for hydrogenation of olefins. The heterogeneous catalyst is encapsulated by being suspended in the phase that will end up inside the capsule.

By ferromagnetic material is meant any substance which is attracted by a magnet. Although any ferromagnetic powder with a particle size less than 1 micron is suitable, acicular iron, Fe_3O_4, iron powder, Alnico, nickel, cobalt, and CrO_2 are preferred. Ferromagnetic powders of particle size less than about 0.25 micron are preferred. The semipermeable microcapsules are preferably prepared by interfacial polycondensation. Polyamides prepared by interfacial polycondensation of an amine with an acid chloride are preferred.

An amine is reacted with an acid chloride by interfacial polycondensation. Suitable amines include any aliphatic or aromatic amine capable of undergoing interfacial polycondensation. Preferred are such aliphatic amines or their salts as hexamethylenediamine, ethylenediamine, piperazine, 2,5-dimethylpiperazine, 3-aminopentamethylenediamine, diethylenetriamine, 1,10-decamethylenediamine, polyethyleneimine, and aromatic amines or their salts such as m-phenylenediamine, p-phenylenediamine, 1,2,4-triaminobenzene, 1,2,4,5-tetraaminobenzene, and 4,4'-diamino-2,2'-biphenyldisulfonic acid. The amine components are normally employed as a 0.4 to 2.0 molar aqueous solution.

Acid chlorides include both aromatic and aliphatic acid chlorides capable of undergoing interfacial polycondensation. Preferred are acid chlorides obtained from such aliphatic acids as adipic acid, sebacic acid and dodecanedioic acid, and aromatic acids such as phthalic acid, isophthalic acid, terephthalic acid, trimesic acid, trimellitic acid, naphthalenedicarboxylic acids, bis(4-carboxyphenyl)methane, and bis(4-carboxycyclohexyl)methane.

The acid chloride components are normally employed as a 0.001 to 1.0 molar solution in the non-water-miscible organic solvent. Suitable solvents include aliphatic, cycloaliphatic and aromatic hydrocarbons and halogen-substituted hydrocarbons and include cyclohexane, chloroform, 1,1,2-trichloro-1,2,2-trifluoroethane, mineral oil, benzene, toluene and chlorobenzene.

The microcapsules can be water-filled, solvent-filled, or silica-gel-filled. The type of microcapsule chosen will depend upon the reaction medium in which the microcapsule is to be used. In the case of water-filled microcapsules, a cell stabilizing agent is preferably present. One type of cell stabilizing agent is an osmoticum, that is, a material which is soluble in the medium within the cell and is too large to migrate out of the semipermeable membrane. These osmotica function by causing osmotic pressure to build up within the microcapsule. Suitable osmotica include synthetic and natural polymers as well as other materials. Preferably the osmoticum is nonproteinaceous. By silica gel is meant a jelly to amorphous solid which is basically $SiO_2{\cdot}nH_2O$ and which can contain small amounts of other ingredients such as, e.g., Na_2O.

In the general procedure for preparing the microcapsules by interfacial polycondensation, the finely divided heterogeneous catalyst and the ferromagnetic material are dispersed in a small volume of an aqueous solution containing a suitable amine or amine salt which can participate in the formation of a polyamide, and optionally a cell stabilizing agent. A suitable organic solvent or solvent mixture containing a surface active agent is added to the aqueous suspension and the mixture is emulsified. The vigor of emulsification and the concentration of surface active agent in the organic solvent will largely determine the diameter of the microcapsule. After the desired droplet size is achieved, additional organic solvent containing a suitable acid chloride which can participate in the formation of the polyamide is added. Interfacial polymerization is allowed to proceed until the reaction is completed, normally for about 1 to 30 minutes. When the microcapsule is to be solvent-filled, the heterogeneous catalyst and ferromagnetic material are usually dispersed in the organic solution of the acid chloride.

The capsules can be harvested by sedimentation in a gravitational, centrifugal or magnetic field. The supernatant liquid is discarded and the remaining capsules are dispersed in a concentrated (20 to 100%) solution of a water-soluble detergent. Water-soluble nonionic detergents such as sorbitan monolaurate may be utilized. The capsule-detergent dispersion is diluted with water or a water-miscible organic solvent and the microcapsules are isolated by sedimentation. The resulting capsules are washed by repeated suspension in and sedimentation from fresh portions of water, a suitable aqueous solution, or an organic solvent.

The microcapsules generally have sizes of about 0.5 to 300 microns. Since the size of the microcapsules can be controlled during their preparation, the specific size prepared will depend upon the intended use of the microcapsule. Preferably, the microcapsules have sizes of about 1 to 200 microns.

Example 1: (a) A mixture of 0.15 g of platinum oxide and 0.3 g of finely divided iron particles was homogenized, by sonication, in 10 ml of chlorobenzene. This was mixed with a solution of 1.0 g of sebacyl chloride plus 0.2 g of trimesoyl chloride in 15 ml of chlorobenzene. An equal volume (25 ml) of a 0.5% aqueous solution of polyvinyl alcohol (Elvanol 50-42) was added and the mixture was emulsified by rapid stirring for 1 minute. A 15-ml portion of a solution made from 24.3 g of 1,6-hexamethylenediamine and 20 g of sodium carbonate in 130 ml of water was then added and stirring was continued for 15 minutes.

The solvent-filled capsules formed were spherical and each appeared to contain solid particles of iron and platinum oxide. The capsules were isolated by retaining them on the bottom of the glass vessel with a strong magnet while decanting the supernatant aqueous phase. They were washed with ethanol in this way and finally isolated from alcohol suspension by immersion of an electromagnet in the liquid and removal of the capsules containing the ferromagnetic iron particles. The packed volume of capsules, held in the bottom of a glass vessel while the supernatant alcohol was sucked off, was 40 ml.

(b) These were transferred to a Parr hydrogenation vessel, 10 g of styrene was added, the vessel was evacuated and pressured with 40 psi of hydrogen and shaken vigorously. A rapid uptake of hydrogen was noted, and hydrogen uptake ceased after 50 minutes. The product was analyzed by gas chromatography [⅛" x 5 ft column of 5% polyethylene glycol (Carbowax 20 M) on 60 to 80 mesh diatomite support, programmed from 40°C at 10°/min]. A large ethylbenzene peak was observed, and styrene was not detected.

The capsules were held in the bottom of the hydrogenation vessel while the supernatant was decanted. The capsules were washed with alcohol, and then 10 g of styrene was added and the hydrogenation restarted. Hydrogen uptake was rapid, but somewhat slower than in the original test. 50% of the styrene was reduced in 2 hours and 10 minutes.

Example 2: (a) A mixture of 0.1 g of platinum oxide, 0.5 g of iron powder, 0.1 ml of N,N,N',N'-tetramethylethylenediamine, 0.3 ml of 3-amino-1,5-pentamethylenediamine and 10 ml of aqueous colloidal sol containing 30% of SiO_2 (Ludox SM-30 colloidal silica) was homogenized by sonication for 1 minute. This suspension was emulsified by vigorous stirring with 30 ml of a 1:4 by volume chloroform-cyclohexane solution containing 0.3 g of sorbitan trioleate (Span 85) for 1 minute. A solution of 0.35 g of trimesoyl chloride in 30 ml of 1:4 chloroform-cyclohexane was added and stirring was continued for 15 minutes. The silica gel-filled capsules formed were recovered by centrifugation, and the packed lower layer of capsules was suspended in 10 ml of a 50% solution of sorbitan monolaurate (Tween 20) in water.

The capsules were again centrifuged, taken up in 30 ml of 85% alcohol, centrifuged, taken up in 30 ml of absolute ethanol, centrifuged and taken up in 30 ml of diethyl ether. The capsules were removed from the ether suspension with an electromagnet and dried at 100°C. The semipermeable microcapsules were obtained as a free-flowing black powder, weight 3.74 g.

(b) A 1-g aliquot of the dry capsules was used for hydrogenation of 20 g of styrene in 25 ml of ethanol. After 3 hours, hydrogenation was complete as indicated by the absence of a styrene peak by gas chromatographic analysis. The capsules were centrifuged, washed with ethanol and isolated magnetically from alcoholic suspension. They were resuspended in 20 g of styrene and 25 ml of ethanol and shaken with hydrogen. In 1.75 hours, reduction was 64.5% complete. The capsules were reisolated in the same manner and reused again. A 93% reduction was effected in 3.75 hours. Thus, the catalyst was still active after three reductions.

Spherical Alumina-Containing Particles as Carriers for Bulk or Bed Catalysts

The process of *H. Fischer, H. Schindler, W. Kuhrt and G. Weidenbach; U.S. Patent 4,013,587; March 22, 1977; assigned to Kali-Chemie AG, Germany* relates to the manufacture of spherical, surface-rich and pore-rich particles from activated alumina which may also contain silica and/or catalytically active metals and/or metal oxides. These particles are distinguished by good mechanical and thermal stability and are suitable as carriers for bulk or bed catalysts.

In the process, mechanically and thermally stable surface- and pore-rich spherical particles may be prepared from activated alumina or activated alumina and silica in an almost quantitative yield. If consideration is given only to the carrier and if it may contain silica, in light of the intended application, one proceeds as follows:

A concentrated aluminum oxide hydrosol of a pH value in the range of 3 to 5 is prepared by dissolving aluminum metal in hydrochloric acid and/or aluminum chloride in aqueous solution or by dissolving commercially available aluminum hydroxychloride in water, the concentration of which is adjusted so that the Al_2O_3 derived from the sol amounts to 15 to 35% by weight, preferably to 20 to 30% by weight of the mass of the calcined particles.

To the hydrosol is added with stirring alumina hydrate and/or activated alumina, preferably of an average particle diameter of maximally 10 microns, in an amount so that the Al_2O_3 content amounts to 65 to 85% by weight, preferably 70 to 80% by weight of the calcined particles.

In certain cases as proportional substitute of the aluminum oxide containing filler there is added to the hydrosol a quantity of pyrogenic silica such that the SiO_2 content of the calcined particles amounts to 10 to 40% by weight. To the mixture obtained there is added a soft to medium-hard wood flour, preferably freshly ground to a finer particle size in a quantity of 5 to 35% by weight, preferably 10 to 25% by weight relative to the mass of the calcined particles. This hydrosol which contains filler and wood flour is mixed with a concentrated aqueous solution of hexamethylene tetramine.

The mixture consisting of hydrosol, gel-forming agent, wood flour, and filler is sprayed or allowed to drop into a column filled with mineral oil of a temperature of 60° to 100°C. The gel particles are allowed to remain at the temperature of precipitation for a period of time from 4 to 16 hours; thereafter the gel particles are aged for 2 to 8 hours in aqueous ammonia solution, washed with water, dried at 100° to 150°C, or preferably at from about 120° to 200°C, preheated to 250° to 400°C and calcined at a temperature of 600° to 1000°C.

The process is particularly suitable for the manufacture of Cu/Cr catalysts for exhaust gases of automobiles. These products meet the more stringent requirements of a catalyst for exhaust gases of automobiles with regard to their mechanical properties as well as also their catalytic activity. Showing uniform size, symmetrical form and a smooth surface, these catalysts provide a homogenous and dense packing when formed into a bed. This results not only in a symmetric distribution of the interstitial spaces, a feature of importance for even flow through the catalyst bed, but this also substantially prevents the abrasion of individual particles, since the particles do not have the opportunity to move against each other or against the wall of the reaction container.

These catalysts are also distinguished by a high degree of resistance to abrasion and breaking, features which are even maintained after prolonged usage at elevated temperatures and which are not diminished by rapidly occurring and constantly recurring variations in temperature.

According to a preferred modification of the process, mechanically and thermally stable spherical particles with good catalytic activity may be obtained from activated alumina, copper and chromium oxide in nearly quantitative yield by:

(1) preparing a concentrated aluminum oxide hydrosol having a pH value of 3 to 5 by dissolving aluminum metal in hydrochloric acid or dissolving commercially available aluminum hydroxychloride in water, the concentration of which is adjusted so that the aluminum oxide derived from the sol amounts to 15 to 35% by weight, preferably 20 to 30% by weight of the calcined particles;

(2) mixing the hydrosol under stirring conditions with copper(II) oxide and chromium(III) oxide of a particle size of 5 to 100 μ in a quantity such that the content of the particles in copper(II) oxide and in chromium(III) oxide subsequent to their calcination amounts to 3 to 15% by weight each, preferably 7 to 10% by weight each (instead of the oxides, corresponding quantities of copper and chromium salts may also be coprecipitated as long as they are decomposed at the calcination temperature of the beads to form the oxides and without leaving other solid residues);

(3) by thereafter adding with stirring to the hydrosol such a quantity of activated alumina and/or alumina hydrate of an average particle diameter of maximally 10 μ that the content of the particles in Al_2O_3 amounts to 35 to 79% by weight, preferably 50 to 66% by weight relative to the weight of the final catalyst;

(4) adding to the hydrosol wood flour or starch of a particle size of maximally 100 μ of carbon black or carbon powder of a particle size of maximally 100 μ in a quantity of 3 to 30% by weight, preferably 5 to 20% by weight relative to the mass of the calcined particles;

(5) intensely mixing the suspension obtained with concentrated aqueous solution of hexamethylenetetramine;

(6) spraying and/or allowing the solution to drop and/or to flow into a column filled with mineral oil of a temperature of 60° to 100°C; and

(7) allowing the gel particles to remain in the oil for 4 to 16 hours at the temperature of the precipitation and by aging the particles subsequently for 2 to 8 hours in aqueous ammonia solution at a temperature of 60° to 100°C, by washing the particles with water, drying them at 120° to 200°C and by calcining them in two steps, initially at 300° to 400°C and subsequently at 600° to 1000°C.

The catalysts prepared in this fashion consist subsequent to their calcination at temperatures above 600°C only of a mixture of the oxides of aluminum, copper, and chromium, whereby 3 to 15% by weight each consists of copper(II) oxide and chromium(III) oxide and 15 to 35% by weight consists of aluminum oxide derived from the aluminum oxide hydrosol. The remainder is aluminum oxide derived from the coprecipitated alumina or its hydrate.

Example 1: To 5 liters of an aluminum oxide hydrosol prepared by treating aluminum shot with hydrochloric acid and containing 500 g of aluminum corresponding to 945 g of Al_2O_3, are added with stirring 4.73 kg of finely ground gibbsite, which has been partially dehydrated at 250°C and shows an average particle size of 2 μ and an alumina content of 80% by weight, corresponding to 3.785 kg Al_2O_3, as well as 250 g of soft wood flour which has been ground for 16 hours in a ball mill.

To the suspension is added at room temperature and under intensive mixing a concentrated aqueous solution of hexamethylenetetramine containing 400 g of hexamethylenetetramine. The mixture is allowed to drop into a 2 m long column filled with mineral oil heated to 90° to 95°C. The resulting spherical gel particles are withdrawn in batches from the bottom of the column, and they are allowed to age for 10 hours in mineral oil at 95°C and subsequently for 6 hours in 0.5% aqueous ammonia solution, before being washed in running water, being dried at 120°C and heated for one hour each at 350° and 800°C.

Following calcination, the resulting product is liberated from fines as well as broken or decomposed particles by prolonged sieving with intensive shaking of a sieve with an open mesh width of 2 mm. In the course of this treatment, those particles which, although already showing cracks, did as yet not break, are destroyed and thus are also removed from the useable product. The remaining material represents a yield of 96%.

Example 2: To 5 liters of an aluminum oxide hydrosol of a pH value of 4 which contains 500 g of aluminum corresponding to 945 g Al_2O_3 are added successively and with intensive stirring 3.02 kg of a pseudoboehmite of an average particle diameter of 3 μ and an alumina content of 75% by weight, corresponding to 2.265 kg Al_2O_3, 272 g of finely ground chromium(III) oxide, 295 g of finely ground copper(II) oxide powder (particle size of the oxides between 5 and 100 μ), 570 g of soft wood flour (54% smaller than 45 μ, remainder up to 100 μ) ground in a ball mill, as well as a concentrated aqueous solution of hexamethylenetetramine having a content of 400 g of hexamethylenetetramine. The mixture is allowed to drop into a 2 m long column filled with mineral oil heated to 90° to 95°C.

The resulting gel particles are removed in batches from the bottom of the column; they are then allowed to age for 12 hours at 90°C in mineral oil and subsequently for 4 hours at 90°C in 0.5% aqueous ammonia solution. After washing in running water, the particles are dried at 140°C before being heated for one hour at 350°C and subsequently at 700°C. The final product of catalyst contains 7.8% by weight CuO and 7.2% by weight of Cr_2O_3.

Hollow Ceramic-Coated Spheroid Catalyst Carriers

The process of *J. Stenzel and A. Hinz; U.S. Patent 4,077,908; March 7, 1978; assigned to Hoechst AG, Germany* relates to the production of a carrier material consisting of solid hollow and spheroidic particles supporting catalysts used in the decontamination of motor exhaust gas.

The process comprises placing spheroidal particles of material being oxidizable and/or low-melting and/or soluble in organic solvents onto a pelletizing table; distributing pulverulent ceramic material thereover and simultaneously spraying a 1% aqueous cellulose ether solution, thereby causing deposition of the pulverulent ceramic material on the spheroidal particles; drying the resulting pellets at temperatures within the range 20° and 95°C, preferably 40° and 85°C; freeing the pellets from the material being oxidizable and/or low-melting and/or soluble in organic solvents; and calcining the pellets at temperatures within the range 1000° and 1500°C.

Preferably, the spheroidal particles which are placed on the pelletizing table consist of sawdust, or a granular plastic material such as polyethylene or polystyrene. The spheroidal particles have a diameter within the range 1 and 5 mm, preferably 2 and 4 mm. Aluminum hydroxide, hydrous aluminum silicate or mixtures thereof can be used as the ceramic material.

The spheroidal hollow particles have a wall thickness of at least 1 mm and are, therefore, very strong. The diameter of the spheroidal hollow particles is within the range 2 and 10 mm. Loosely aggregated hollow spheroids offer as little resistance to flowing gas as solid spheroids, but they have lower bulk density and an enlarged inner surface area.

Example 1: Spheroidal particles having a diameter within the range 2 and 4 mm, prepared from agglomerated sawdust, were placed onto a pelletizing table (1 m in diameter; inclined at an angle of 30°; 12 rpm). A mixture of hydrargillite (α-aluminum hydroxide) and 5 wt % of bentonite (hydrous aluminum silicate) was distributed thereover and a 1% aqueous methylcellulose solution was simultaneously sprayed thereon, whereby the ceramic mixture was caused to deposit on the sawdust particles. The resulting pellets were sieved to remove all fractions having a diameter within the range 5 and 7 mm which were dried for 12 hours at 80°C. Following this, they were heated at increasing temperatures (50°C per hour) to 500°C and finally calcined for 10 hours at 1420°C.

The hollow spheroids so made had a diameter within the range 3.5 and 5 mm, a wall thickness within the range 1.2 and 2 mm, a strength within the range 0.5 and 2.5 kg/mm of spheroid diameter, an apparent density of 0.58 g/cc and an inner surface area of 2.0 m^2/g.

Example 2: (a) Spheroidal expandable polystyrene sieve fractions having a diameter within the range 0.2 and 0.1 mm were allowed to expand for 30 minutes at 135°C in a drying cabinet.

The spheroids so expanded to about fifty times their initial volume were sieved and the sieve fraction having a diameter within the range 1.0 and 1.5 mm was placed on the pelletizing table described in Example 1. Fine particulate, partially dehydrated reactive aluminum hydroxide (Alcoa A 16) was poured on by means of a chute and a 1% aqueous solution of methylcellulose and a dispersant [1% of Dolapix CA (Zechimmer and Schwarz)] was simultaneously sprayed on, whereby the pulverulent ceramic material was caused to deposit on the plastic spheroids so as to form a shell around them. The resulting pellets were dried for 12 hours at 80°C, heated at increasing temperatures (50°C per hour to 500°C) and finally calcined for 10 hours at 1250°C.

The resulting hollow spheroids had a strength within the range 1.0 and 3.5 kg/mm of spheroid diameter, an inner surface area of 2.5 m^2/g, a wall thickness within the range 1 and 2 mm, and an apparent density of 0.65 g/cc.

(b) The carrier material produced as described was used to support a catalyst for the removal of nitrogen oxides from motor exhaust gas.

ADHESIVES

Delayed-Tack Adhesives Containing Core-Shell Polymer Particles

N.K. Henderson and E. Thomson; U.S. Patent 4,091,162; May 23, 1978; assigned to Smith & McLaurin Limited, Great Britain provide a delayed-tack adhesive composition comprising particles which have a soft and tacky polymer core surrounded by a hard and nontacky polymer shell in admixture with a solid modifier, such as a solid plasticizer.

The delayed-tack adhesive composition can be prepared by a method comprising forming in a liquid a dispersion of particles of the soft and tacky polymer, forming around each of the particles a shell of the hard and nontacky polymer, providing in the dispersion particles of the plasticizer and removing the liquid at a temperature below the melting point of the plasticizer.

The hard and nontacky polymer shell makes the particles resistant to blocking when incorporated in the unactivated adhesive composition. On activation the plasticizer dissolves the shell and releases the core polymer, whereby the advantages which are derived from the use of a soft and tacky polymer are obtained.

A typical delayed-tack composition in dispersion is in the form of a latex containing polymeric particles, the centers or cores which consist predominantly of molecules of a polymer which is soft and tacky. An example of such a soft, tacky polymer is poly(2-ethylhexyl acrylate). The outer layers or shells of the particles consist predominantly of molecules of a polymer which is hard and nonblocking. An example of such a polymer is polystyrene.

Apart from 2-ethylhexyl acrylate, examples of monomers from which homopolymers or copolymers can be prepared for use as soft and tacky polymer cores are those from which addition polymers can be made, as e.g., C_3-C_{10} alkyl acrylates, C_5-C_{10} methacrylates, ethylene, propylene, butylene, butadiene, chloroprene, isoprene, and vinyl esters of saturated tertiary monocarboxylic acids (e.g., Versatic acid). In addition, soft and tacky polymers can be obtained from many monomers if the molecular weight is sufficiently low. To obtain a soft and tacky core, therefore, it is advantageous to include in the dispersion a molecular weight moderator to produce a low molecular weight polymer when the core is formed in the dispersion by polymerization of the monomers.

Apart from styrene, examples of monomers which can be used by themselves or as comonomers to give hard and nontacky polymer shells are those from which addition polymers can be made, as for example, C_1-C_3 alkyl methacrylates, acrylonitrile, methacrylonitrile, vinyl chloride, vinylidene chloride, and vinyl acetate. Obviously, it is essential that the shell polymer should be sufficiently hard and nontacky to be nonblocking, and this can be achieved by making the shell of a high-molecular weight polymer.

As the plasticizer in the composition, any of those used in conventional delayed-tack compositions can be used, the most common of these being dicyclohexyl phthalate. The production of a core-shell polymer latex involves the setting up of polymerization reaction conditions such that initially a latex with particles of a soft and tacky polymer are formed and then a hard and nontacky polymer is polymerized onto these particles.

Example 1: Preparation of Core-Shell Polymer – An example of a polymerization reaction which was found to give a suitable core-shell polymer dispersion is given below.

	Parts by Weight
Initial charge	
Water	200
Sodium bicarbonate	0.65
Lankropol KMA*	5.25
Monomer 1	
2-Ethylhexyl acrylate	89
Styrene	5
Monomer 2	
2-Ethylhexyl acrylate	25
Styrene	25
Acrylic acid	2

(continued)

	Parts by Weight
Monomer 3	
2-Ethylhexyl acrylate	2
Styrene	50
Acrylic acid	2
Initiator/emulsifier solution 1	
Water	50
Lankropol KMA*	23.2
Potassium persulfate	0.4
Initiator/emulsifier solution 2	
Water	30
Potassium persulfate	0.2
Ethylan HA**	2.0

*A sodium dialkyl sulfosuccinamate in 60% aqueous solution
**Nonylphenol polyglycol ether

The production procedure is as follows:

(1) The initial charge is heated to 85°C while stirring.

(2) 10% of the initiator/emulsifier solution 1 is added.

(3) Monomer 1 is added dropwise over a period of 2 hours. The rate is controlled so that the monomer reacts instantaneously, i.e., the reaction rate is controlled by the rate of monomer addition.

(4) The remainder of the initiator/emulsifier solution 1 is added simultaneously with monomer 1 at a rate such that the total amount is added over a period of 3¼ hours, i.e., the total time for the addition of monomers 1 and 2.

(5) The temperature is lowered to 70° to 75°C and monomer 2 is added over a period of 1¼ hours, again so that the monomer reacts immediately.

(6) After the addition of monomer 2 is complete, the temperature is increased to 80° to 85°C for 30 minutes.

(7) The temperature is lowered to 70° to 75°C. Monomer 3 and initiator/emulsifier solution 2 are added over a period of 1¼ hours, such that monomer 3 reacts immediately.

(8) After all monomer 3 has been added, the temperature is increased to 80° to 85°C and the reaction is continued for 1 hour.

The reaction product is a stable polymer latex of 43% solids content, denoted polymer latex A. In this, the polymer prepared from monomer 1 forms particle cores which have around them outermost shells of polymers prepared from monomer 3. An intermediate layer of polymer prepared from monomer 2 may be present in some of the particles.

Example 2: Use in Delayed-Tack Formulation –

Ingredients	Parts by Weight
(1) Water	41.2
(2) Dicyclohexyl phthalate (modifier)	40.2
(3) Poly-pale Ester 10	9.6
(4) Polymer latex A	38.0

Components (1), (2) and (3) were ground in a ball mill or pebble mill with a dispersing agent until a suitable particle size was obtained and then component (4) was added. The resulting aqueous dispersion was coated on normal label base paper in a manner known in the art and dried at a temperature below the melting point of the dicyclohexyl phthalate. In this way the adhesive was not activated. The dry coating weight was 25 g/m^2.

The paper with the delayed-tack adhesive composition coating was compared with a conventional delayed-tack label paper specially formulated for low temperature performance. The conventional deep-freeze labels gave poor to fair adhesion with no fiber tear, whereas the adhesive labels prepared by the method of this example gave 20 to 100% fiber tear.

A self-adhesive paper specially formulated for low temperature work gave approximately 50% fiber tear under the same test conditions. To test that the adhesive formulations had suitable blocking resistance properties before activation, samples of the coated paper were held in a press, adhesive side against nonadhesive side, at a pressure of 30 psi for 2 hours at 30°C and examined after cooling. There was no cling between the samples and it was concluded, therefore, that under normal conditions of storage no blocking would occur.

Example 3: Pressure-Sensitive Adhesive – An example of a polymerization reaction which has been found to give a suitable core-shell pressure-sensitive polymer is given below:

	Parts by Weight
Initial charge	
Water	200
Sodium bicarbonate	0.65
Lankropol KMA	5.25
Monomer 1	
Isobutyl methacrylate	94
Monomer 2	
2-Ethylhexyl acrylate	25
Styrene	25
Acrylic acid	2
Monomer 3	
2-Ethylhexyl acrylate	50
Styrene	2
Acrylic acid	2
Initiator/emulsifier solution 1	
Water	50
Lankropol KMA	23.2
Potassium persulfate	0.4
Initiator/emulsifier solution 2	
Water	30
Potassium persulfate	0.2
Ethylan HA	2.0

The production procedure is similar to that given for the preparation of polymer A, previously described. The reaction product is a stable polymer latex of 43% solids content which forms a pressure-sensitive adhesive composition.

Envelope Manufacture Using Microencapsulated Glue

In the manufacture of envelopes from an envelope sheet, two kinds of glue are normally used. For the bottom and side portions which are permanently sealed together, a back gum containing from about 60 to 70% of solids is used. On the envelope flap, a remoistenable seal gum is applied. In the process of manufacture normally used, the first step is to apply the remoistenable seal gum to the portion of the envelope sheet, which will later become the lid of the envelope. This is done, for example, by collating a number of envelope sheets so that approximately 9⁄16 inch of the lid portion of each envelope sheet is exposed. The glue, in liquid suspension, can then be conveniently rolled on. The coated envelope sheet is then dried.

The coated envelope sheet is then scored in the places where folds are desired and back gum is applied to the portion of the envelope sheet where the bottom flap and the side flaps will be sealed. The back gum is also applied in liquid suspension or solution. The bottom and sides are then immediately folded up to finish the envelope.

One of the disadvantages of this process is that once the back gum is applied, the bottom and side flaps must be immediately folded up and sealed. For reasons of storage and handling, it would be desirable to be able to apply the back gum without immediately folding the bottom and side flaps.

H.R. Lillibridge; U.S. Patent 4,134,322; January 16, 1979; assigned to Champion International Corporation provides an improvement in the process for manufacturing envelopes whereby the back gum is microencapsulated. A suspension of the microcapsules is applied to the appropriate area on the envelope sheet prior to the drying of the seal gum. Both adhesives are dried at the same time and the envelope sheet can be collated without first having to fold the bottom and sides. When it is desired to finish the manufacturing process, the bottom and sides are folded and appropriate pressure is applied. The microcapsules on the bottom are ruptured thereby spreading the gum and causing adhesion.

It would also be advantageous to apply the seal gum in the form of microcapsules to the flap as this would permit the end user to seal the envelope without moisture. This feature would be of particular advantage to large mailers using inserting machines.

The encapsulating material for the back gum should be of a hydrophobic nature; i.e., it should be water-insoluble. The encapsulating material can be a thermoplastic resin containing nonionizable groups, examples of which are polyvinyl chloride, polystyrene, polyvinyl acetate, vinyl chloride-vinylidene chloride copolymers, cellulose acetate and ethylcellulose. The critical feature in choosing the encapsulating material, in addition to water insolubility, is the rupture point of the capsule. It is important that the capsule shall be able to contain the back gum up to the point of pressure employed in the folding and sealing step.

It is also important that the melting point of the encapsulating material be sufficiently high so that it will not melt during ordinary storage conditions; thus, the melting point of the encapsulating material should be about 50°C. The rupture point for the capsule should be below about 50 psi; i.e., between 5 to 50 psi. The microcapsules have been more fully described in U.S. Patent 3,875,074.

The process is described with reference to Figure 8.1. An envelope sheet has main body portion **11**, lid portion **12**, side flaps **13** and **13a** and bottom flap **14**. Along the edge of lid portion **15**, which in an ordinary envelope for business correspondence is about 3⁄16 inch wide, there is applied a seal gum. The seal gum can be a vinyl-dextrin blend preparation.

Along the edge portion **16** and **16a** of bottom flap **14**, there is applied a microencapsulated suspension of back gum. The back gum can be any of the conventionally and readily available gums as used in the envelope trade. The width of this edge is, for an ordinary business envelope, typically about 3⁄16 inch, but this width can vary widely. It is important that the microcapsule suspension be applied only to the area of bottom flap **14** in which adhesion to side flaps **13** and **13a** is desired. The microencapsulated gum should not be applied to any portions of bottom flap **14** which will contact main body **11** directly.

Figure 8.1: Envelope Manufacture Using Microencapsulated Glue

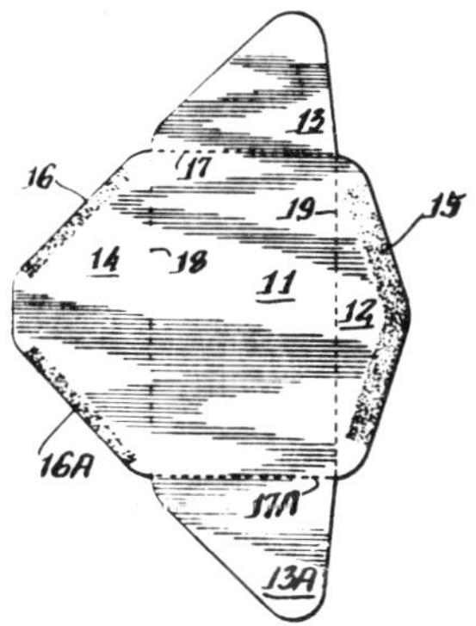

Source: U.S. Patent 4,134,322

Both the seal gum applied to portion **15** and the microencapsulated back gum applied to portions **16** and **16a** can be applied simultaneously or one can be applied after the other. After both have been applied, the envelope sheet is dried until the carrier or solvent for the seal gum and the microencapsulated back gum have evaporated.

Envelope sheets so treated may be stored in collated arrangement without running the risk of having the sheets adhere to each other. Either before or after such storage, the envelope sheet is scored along lines **17, 17a, 18** and **19** for folding.

When it is desired to assemble the envelope, side flaps **13** and **13a** are folded in along lines **17** and **17a** respectively. Then bottom flap **14** is folded along line **18** so that edges **16** and **16a**, which are coated with the microcapsules containing back gum contact edge portions **20** and **20a**, respectively, of side flaps **13** and **13a**. Pressure in the range of about 5 to 50 psi is then applied to the contact areas of edges **16** and **20** and on edges **16a** and **20a**. The pressure causes the microcapsules to rupture, thereby releasing the back gum and adhering bottom flap **14** to side flaps **13** and **13a**.

The microencapsulated glue can be applied to the seal (lid) of the envelope, permitting the end user to seal without the application of moisture.

ELECTROSTATOGRAPHY

Encapsulation of Toner Particles by Phase Separation

Electrostatography is perhaps best exemplified by the process of xerography as described in U.S. Patent 2,297,691. In this process, a photoconductor is first given a uniform electrostatic charge over its surface and is then exposed to an image of activating electromagnetic radiation which selectively dissipates the charge in illuminated areas of the photoconductor while charge in the nonilluminated areas is retained thereby forming a latent electrostatic image. This latent electrostatic image is then developed or made visible by the deposition of finely divided, electroscopic marking material referred to as toner on the surface of the photoconductor, which marking material conforms to the pattern of the latent electrostatic image. The visible image may then be utilized in a number of diverse ways.

For example, the image may be viewed in situ on the photoconductive insulator, fixed in place on the photoconductive insulator or transferred to a second surface such as a sheet of paper and fixed in place thereon as desired depending upon whether the photoconductive insulating material is reusable as is the case with amorphous selenium photoconductive insulators or nonreusable as is the case with particulate zinc oxide binder film-type xerographic plates.

The commercial xerographic development technique most widely used today is the technique known as cascade development which is described in U.S. Patent 2,618,552. This development technique is carried out by rolling or cascading across the latent electrostatic image-bearing surface, a developing mixture composed of relatively large carrier particles, each having a multiplicity of electrostatically adhering fine marking particles, known as toner particles, on its surface.

As this mixture cascades or rolls across the image bearing surface, the toner particles are electrostatically deposited on the charged portions of the image and not on the uncharged background areas of the image. In addition, toner particles accidently falling on these nonimage areas are physically removed therefrom by the electrostatic attraction of carrier particles which pass in close proximity to these unbound toner particles. The result of this development process is an excellent background-free copy of the electrostatic image made up of the toner particles electrostatically clinging to the image surface.

The common feature of electrostatographic systems is that they employ the lines of force from an electric field to control the deposition of finely divided marking material or toner on a surface, thus forming an image with the toner particles.

R.E. Wellman and R.W. Brown; U.S. Patent 4,016,099; April 5, 1977; assigned to Xerox Corporation provide an encapsulation process which enables the preparation of toner particles suitable for electrostatographic applications.

This is a liquid phase encapsulation process in which the wall phase is caused to deposit about the core phase by drowning of the dispersion of the core phase in the wall phase in a liquid which is miscible with the solvent for the wall material and which causes the wall material to phase-separate. This liquid is also generally a nonsolvent for the core material. It has been found in this process that the problem of agglomeration during phase separation and hardening of the wall material can be avoided or substantially reduced by drowning the dispersion of the core phase in the wall phase in a large excess of a nonsolvent liquid. Although generally it is only necessary that the core phase undergo phase separation prior to drowning of the resulting dispersion in the nonsolvent liquid, there are instances wherein it is advantageous to partially or completely effect phase separation of the wall material prior to the drowning step.

Several methods for effecting phase separation within the dispersions, emulsions or solutions obtained can be employed. For example, in an instance wherein the core and wall materials are dissolved in at least one relatively volatile solvent, phase separation can be effected by evaporation of the solvent. As the solvent is removed by evaporation, the concentration of the core and wall materials is progressively increased whereby substantially all of the core material preferentially phase-separates as a solvent-poor phase. Once phase separation of the core material is obtained, the resulting dispersion of the core material in the wall solution can be drowned or dispersed in a large excess of a liquid which is miscible with the solvent for the wall material and which will effect phase separation of the wall material whereupon the wall material deposits about the core material and the resulting encapsulated particles undergo hardening as a dilute dispersion in the nonsolvent liquid.

The encapsulated particles can be easily recovered from the nonsolvent liquid as, for example, by filtration. In this instance, as the concentration of the dissolved materials increases, the single phase system becomes increasingly unstable with respect to a two phase system comprised of a solvent-poor core phase and a solvent-rich wall phase.

After phase separation of the core material occurs, the wall phase becomes more concentrated as solvent is continuously removed. It is important for the dispersion of core material in the wall material solution to be drowned in the nonsolvent liquid while the viscosity of the dispersion is sufficiently low to permit ready dispersion of the dispersion of core material in the wall material solution in the nonsolvent liquid prior to completion of phase separation of the wall material from the solvent.

Alternatively, a solution of core and wall material in a common solvent can be emulsified, and the core phase separated by addition of a nonsolvent for the core. Thereafter, the resulting mixture can be drowned in a nonsolvent for the wall material to effect phase-separation of the wall material and encapsulation of the core material therewith as described above.

In still another variation, a solution of core and wall material in a common solvent can be emulsified together with concentration-dependent nonsolvent for the core and wall which is less volatile than the solvent and miscible therewith. Upon vaporization of the solvent, the nonsolvent becomes more concentrated effecting phase separation of the core. Thereafter, the dispersion of the core in the wall material is drowned in a nonsolvent liquid as described above to effect encapsulation of the core by the wall material in a dilute environment.

In a further modification, an insoluble core material can be dispersed in a solution of wall material and the resulting dispersion can be directly drowned in a liquid nonsolvent for the wall material effecting phase separation of the wall material and deposition thereof about the core material.

Any suitable polymeric material can be employed as the wall material for the encapsulated product of the process. Any organic polymer including homopolymers and copolymers can be suitably employed as either the core or wall material. The selection of a particular polymer for either the wall or core material is dictated by the properties desired in the ultimate encapsulated product.

In the preparation of electrostatographic toners, wall material resins containing a relatively high percentage of a styrene resin are preferred because better image quality is achieved. The styrene resin may be a homopolymer of styrene or styrene homologues or copolymers of styrene with other monomers containing a single methylene group attached to a carbon atom by a double bond.

It is considered important in the process that the core dispersion in the wall material solution be drowned and dispersed in sufficient nonsolvent liquid to preclude agglomeration of the encapsulated particles during the period of phase separation of the wall material from the solvent, since during this period the wall material is tacky and can give rise to the problems of agglomeration which are sought to be avoided herein. Since the encapsulated particles form a dilute dispersed phase within a continuous nonsolvent phase, the wall material is allowed to harden in a dilute environment which essentially precludes the occurrence of agglomeration. Volume ratios ranging from 4:1 to 8:1 or above are preferred.

The ratio of core and wall materials to the solvent system generally can be any practical dilution. Thus, the dissolved solids content of the solution may range from 0.5 to 50.0% by weight based on the solution, but this can also vary, one general limitation being phase separation of the core material and another being practicality of the solute concentration.

The ratio of wall material to core material may be between 99 parts by weight of wall material to 1 part by weight of core material and 1 part by weight of wall material to 99 parts by weight of core material. However, the preferred range is between a ratio of 7 parts by weight of wall material to 1 part by weight of core material and 1 part by weight of wall material to 7 parts by weight of core material as encapsulated particles having the best surface characteristics are obtained.

Once the solution or dispersion of core and wall materials is prepared or simultaneously with the preparation thereof, a colorant can be admixed therewith if a colored toner particle is desired.

The amount of colorant added for toner preparation can range from about 3 to 20 wt % based on the total weight of the colored encapsulated particle. If the colorant is a dye, substantially smaller quantities of colorant can be used. Preferably, prior to dispersion of the colorant in the solvent, dispersing aids can be added to the solvent such as surfactants, and dispersants to assist in effecting a uniform dispersion.

The encapsulated toner compositions obtained in accordance with the process can be admixed with solid or nonsolvent liquid vehicles therefor to form electrostatographic developer compositions. In general, successful results have been obtained with from 10 to 200 parts by weight of either solid or liquid vehicle to 1 part by weight of toner. Preferably, the vehicle to toner ratio ranges from 50:1 to 150:1. In such preferred compositions, the vehicle acts effectively to remove any toner particles which might tend to adhere to a nonimage area and the toner itself forms dense readily transferable and fusible images.

Example 1: To a Waring blender are charged 40 ml of acetone, 15 g of a 50/50 copolymer of docosyl acrylate and styrene and 15 g of a 75/25 copolymer of styrene and n-butyl methacrylate. The ingredients in the blender are heated to 45° to 50°C with no agitation. After the ingredients reach the desired temperature, they are then stirred within the Waring blender at high speed. Thereafter, 3.0 g of Monarch 74 carbon black are added to the mixture with stirring. The temperature is then lowered by the addition of 210 ml of acetone. The resulting mixture is then divided into portions and each portion is drowned in a large excess of ice water contained in a Waring blender. Thereafter, the contents of the blender are separated by filtration. The resulting encapsulated particles are evaluated on a Kofler Hot Bench and are found to have a stick point of 65°C.

Thus, the encapsulated particles behave essentially as the styrene/n-butyl methacrylate copolymer indicating that the core of the docosyl acrylate/styrene copolymer is completely encapsulated. There is no observable agglomeration. 27.1 grams of encapsulated material are recovered as the filter cake.

Example 2: 50 ml of a 10% solution of polystyrene in toluene and 50 ml of a 10% solution of poly(hexamethylene sebacate) in toluene are mixed together in a beaker equipped with a magnetic stirrer. Thereafter, 1.0 g of Monarch 74 carbon black is dispersed in this solution employing magnetic stirring. The solution is cooled to −10°C with continuous magnetic stirring at which point the poly(hexamethylene sebacate) has phase separated. The resulting dispersion is then drowned in a large excess of n-butanol in a Waring blender with continuous high speed agitation. About 200 ml of methanol are added during the drowning operation. Thereafter, the contents of the Waring blender are separated by filtration and the filter cake comprising encapsulated particles is dispersed in methanol with magnetic stirring and allowed to wash for about 1 hour. Thereafter the encapsulated particles are recovered by filtration and air dried. The encapsulated particles appear to be well encapsulated and pressure fixable and exhibit a stick point on the Kofler Hot Bench of about 95°C.

Example 3: This example illustrates the use of mutual incompatibility of polymers in a solvent to effect phase separation. 1.75 g of a hydroxy-terminated polybutadiene are dissolved in 50 ml of a 10% solution of polystyrene in methyl ethyl ketone in a beaker equipped with a magnetic stirrer. The solution is heated to 75°C at which temperature it appears as a clear, colorless solution. The solution is then heated with magnetic stirring and boiled down to a total volume of about 20 ml. At this point, the solution appears cloudy and viscous. The resulting hot dispersion is then drowned in 300 ml of methanol in a blender operating at low speed. The resulting dispersion is separated by filtration and the recovered encapsulated particles are dried. The stick point of the encapsulated particles is about 95°C indicating encapsulation of the core with a wall of polystyrene.

Encapsulation of Toner Particles by Polymerization and Coacervation

R.W. Brown; U.S. Patent 4,097,404; June 27, 1978; assigned to Xerox Corporation provides a method of encapsulating toners by polymerization and coacervation resulting in a copolymer encapsulated in an incompatible shell polymer. Thus, toner particles are prepared by mixing a solute polymer in a solvent monomer after which polymerization of the solvent monomer is initiated resulting in a polymer from the solvent monomer which phase-separates from the solvent monomer to form a solvent-poor phase which eventually comprises the capsule core. The solvent-rich phase then provides the material for the capsule wall.

The dispersion polymerization of a solvent monomer to form the capsule core and the subsequent coating of this core with a solute polymer to complete the encapsulation is effected by employing two incompatible polymers with the polymer from the monomer solution phase-separating from its monomer solution to form the solvent-poor phase and eventually the capsule core. When coacervation occurs in such systems, the solvent-poor phase forms the core material; the solvent-rich phase is found to deposit as the wall material. Thus, for example, n-butylmethacrylate may be employed as the monomer solution which phase-separates when polymerized to form the solvent-poor phase and eventually the capsule core and a 65/35 styrene/n-butylmethacrylate copolymer may be employed as a solute polymer which during the aforementioned polymerization becomes the solvent-rich phase and is then deposited as the wall material.

Encapsulation is accomplished during the heterogeneous liquid-phase polymerization where, e.g., a polymer A is dissolved in monomer B, and the materials are selected such that polymer A and polymer B are incompatible and phase-separating during the polymerization with polymer A forming a solvent-rich phase and polymer B forming a solvent-poor phase. When polymerization is completed, the polymer B will have coalesced as a capsule core and polymer A will deposit over the coalesced polymer B and form the capsule wall.

Colorants are normally dispersed in the starting monomer solution if the product is intended to be colored toner particles. Conventional suspension and dispersion polymerization techniques may be employed, and the continuous phase employed may either be aqueous or nonaqueous liquid materials.

The following three parameters generally control the combination of monomer and polymer A which may be employed in order that the polymerized monomer forms the core and the polymer the encapsulating wall: (1) polymer A is incompatible with polymer B; (2) polymer A is soluble in monomer B; and (3) polymer B will separate as the solvent-poor phase eventually resulting in the capsule core.

The polymer which eventually forms the capsule wall or polymer A may be any suitable polymer. Basically any organic polymeric material including homopolymers and copolymers may be employed as polymer A, subject to the following conditions: (a) a suitable monomer or monomers may be found in which it is soluble, the polymer of which it is incompatible with; and (b) it phase-separates as the solvent-rich phase during polymerization of the solvent monomer.

Polymer A, in addition, should be a solid as it will eventually deposit as the capsule wall and it should not contain unsaturation which can be activated at the reaction conditions for the solvent monomer. In addition, it is necessary that polymer A be insoluble or have a very limited solubility in the continuous liquid phase. Typical polymers include: olefin polymers, halo-olefin polymers, aliphatic vinyl and vinylidene polymers, aromatic vinyl polymers, heterocyclic vinyl polymers, acrylic and methacrylic polymers, polyethers, polysulfides and polysulfones; aliphatic and aromatic polyesters; aliphatic and aromatic polyamides; polyureas; polyurethanes; natural and modified natural polymers; and combinations of the above.

Any suitable monomer may be employed in the system which eventually forms polymer B or the capsule core. Monomer B which forms polymer B must be a mono- or polyethylenically unsaturated compound capable of undergoing free-radical or addition polymerization such as is normally employed in suspension or dispersion polymerization processes. The monomer should be liquid at the reaction conditions to act as a solvent for polymer A and to provide the necessary mobility for complete phase-separation and coalescence of the two polymer phases.

The monomer and the polymer formed from it, polymer B, should be insoluble or have very limited solubility in a continuous liquid phase and polymer B must be incompatible with polymer A. Polymer B should be capable of phase-separating from the solvent monomer as the solvent-poor phase and eventually coalesce to form the capsule core. Typical monomers include: acrylic acid and esters thereof, methacrylic acid and esters thereof, acrylonitrile, vinyl and vinylidene halides, vinyl esters, vinyl ethers, styrene and substituted styrenes, and combinations of the foregoing among others.

Oil-soluble initiators are normally employed. These include compounds such as organic peroxides, organic hydroperoxides, N-nitrosoacylanilides, triphenylmethylazobenzene, and aliphatic azobisnitriles. The continuous phase of the polymerization system most commonly employed is water, but organic liquids may also be employed. The continuous phase generally contains a suspending or granulating agent. Any suitable oil-soluble surfactants which aid the dispersion of the colorant in the system may be employed.

Example 1: The following reagents are employed in the amounts indicated as hereinafter described.

Monomer phase (218.5 g used)	
N-butylmethacrylate	140.0 g
MA-140 styrene-butylmethacrylate copolymer)	60.0 g
AIBN (azobisisobutyronitrile)	8.0 g
Triton N-101 (nonylphenylpolyethoxyethanol)	2.0 g
Molacco-H carbon black	10.0 g
Aqueous phase	
Polyvinyl alcohol	36.0 g
Water	900 ml

The polyvinyl alcohol is dissolved in water and placed in the reaction kettle under a constant argon sparge. The MA-140 and Triton N-101 are dissolved in the monomer. This monomer solution is divided into two portions with approximately ⅓ of the solution being used to dissolve the AIBN, which is found not to completely dissolve. The carbon black is dried at 100°C in vacuum for 1 hour and dispersed in the other ⅔ of the solution on the Polytron mixer for 15 minutes. The carbon black dispersion is allowed to set undisturbed for 2 hours. The two monomer portions are then recombined by stirring on the Polytron mixer for about 2 minutes. The monomer phase is dispersed in the aqueous phase at 800 rpm for about 15 minutes. The temperature is then raised and held constant at about 75°C by means of a large water bath and at the same time the stirring rate is decreased to 300 rpm.

This condition is maintained for 1½ hours at which time the polymerization is substantially completed. The reaction mixture is then cooled to 25°C with stirring. The resulting polymer particles are then separated from the reaction mixture by filtration. The encapsulated toner so produced is applied employing a conventional cascade development system to a latent electrostatic image after which the visible image is fixed by application of pressure resulting in a sharp, clear reproduction of the original employed.

Example 2: The following materials are employed as hereinafterdescribed to produce an encapsulated toner.

Monomer phase (107 g used)	
N-butylmethacrylate	120.0 g
MA-140	80.0 g
AIBN	4.8 g
Triton N-101	2.0 g
Molacco-H carbon black	10.0 g
Aqueous phase	
Polyvinyl alcohol	36.0 g
Water	900 ml

The procedure employed in Example 1 is again repeated with the exception that the monomer phase is dispersed in the aqueous phase at 800 rpm for 5 minutes and the polymerization is continued for 1½ hours. The carbon black dispersion in this run is found to be better than in Example 1. The particle sizes are found to vary between 1 and 15 μ. The conversion rate in this synthesis is found to be 28.6% at a quarter hour and 100% at one-half hour, with the polymerization appearing to be essentially completed after 25 minutes. The encapsulated toner particles are separated from the reaction mixture and employed in a xerographic imaging process as in Example 1.

Encapsulated Water Paper for Electrostatographic Reproduction on Both Sides

Many theories as to the mechanism by which papers conduct electricity have been advanced but there is no generally accepted theory. It is, however, known that the electrical conductivity of the paper is dependent on its moisture content and upon the distribution of the moisture through the fiber structure, and that the conductivity is extremely sensitive to changes in the moisture content of the paper.

The problems encountered relating to paper dryness are especially noticeable in situations where copies are made in the duplex mode, i.e., where images are produced on both sides of the paper. Copying in the duplex mode causes problems in terms of low paper conductivity because the first fusing step drys the paper and renders it relatively nonconductive before it is subjected to the second copying procedure. This may occur even when the paper contains a hydrated salt since the salt will tend to lose its water of hydration at the temperature encountered during the first fusing step.

L.E. Geer; U.S. Patent 4,020,210; April 26, 1977; assigned to Xerox Corporation has developed a paper sheet adapted for the electrostatographic reproduction of images on both sides thereof. The electrostatographic image is formed by the deposition of toner particles onto the sheet in imagewise configuration and fusing the toner into the sheet by the application of heat and pressure thereto. The sheet bears a surface sizing material having dispersed therein a multiplicity of microcapsules which microcapsules comprise water or a hydrated salt encased in an impervious capsule wall of a solid material capable of being ruptured by the heat and pressure applied to the sheet during the fusing of the image formed on the first side thereof.

The microcapsules employed in the process comprise a nucleus and a wall material. The nucleus, which typically accounts for 70 to 90% by weight of the microcapsule, is either free water or a water-containing, i.e., hydrated, salt. Both organic and inorganic hydrates can be employed provided that the salt selected is inert to paper. Preferred salts are those which release their water of hydration at a relatively low temperature, since temperatures above about 400°F at the paper-fuser interface will tend to scorch the paper. Thus, hydrates which give up their water of hydration at temperatures no greater than about 300°F are particularly desirable.

Typical hydrated salts which may be employed include lithium chloride monohydrate, calcium chloride hexahydrate, zinc nitrate hexahydrate, potassium carbonate dihydrate, copper sulfate pentahydrate, magnesium sulfate heptahydrate, zinc sulfate heptahydrate, sodium tetraborate decahydrate, sodium sulfite heptahydrate, sodium sulfate decahydrate, barium hydroxide octahydrate, magnesium acetate tetrahydrate and magnesium nitrate hexahydrate. The heptahydrates of magnesium sulfate and zinc sulfate and the decahydrate of sodium tetraborate are particularly useful.

Any substance which can be deposited around the nucleus and will rupture upon being subjected to the heat and pressure of the fusing operation can be considered a candidate wall material. Suitable wall materials include gelatin, ethylcellulose, poly(methyl methacrylate), starches, carboxymethylcellulose, rosin, paraffin, tristearin, poly(vinyl alcohol), polyethylene, polypropylene, polystyrene, polyacrylamides, polyethers, polyesters, polyamides, polybutadiene, polyisoprene, silicones, epoxies and polyurethanes. Of course, when uncombined water is the core material, the wall must be of a water-insoluble material.

The size of the microcapsules to be incorporated into the paper sheet will vary over a range of from about 5 to 80 μ in diameter with a diameter range of from 20 to 30 μ being preferred. The microcapsules are added to the base paper sheet in combination with a surface size. Typically the particles are combined with a binder material and applied to the paper surface in the conventional fashion. In addition to the binder and microcapsules, the sizing formulation will normally contain a surface coating such as, e.g., a coating clay. Typically, the coating material will be present in a weight ratio of from 10:1 to 3:1 of the binder material. Typically, sufficient microcapsules are included in the paper to provide sufficient water upon its release to provide about 2% water by weight of the paper. Since some of the released water may be vaporized during the first fusing, sufficient microcapsules to provide a water concentration of up to about 6% or more may be incorporated into the paper.

Example: A surface size composition is prepared by mixing starch and 25 μ diameter microcapsules containing magnesium sulfate heptahydrate encapsulated in a 2 μ thick wall of gelatin in an aqueous dispersion. In addition to the starch and microcapsules, a standard coating clay is provided in an amount such that the ratio of clay to starch is 7:1 on a weight basis.

A typical bond paper substrate is selected which comprises a 100% chemically bleached mixed hardwood/softwood paper. The sizing material is applied to both sides of the paper sheet with an air-knife/trailing blade coating device and dried. Sufficient sizing material is applied to provide water in an amount of 6 weight percent of the paper sheet upon release of 6 molecules of water per molecule of the hydrated salt. The coated paper is imaged in the normal xerographic mode and the toner fused into the paper by the application of heat and pressure. The fuser roll provides sufficient heat to raise the paper surface temperature to about 350°F and simultaneously applies sufficient pressure to rupture the microcapsules. The gelatin capsule wall is ruptured by the fusing operation and water molecules of the hydrate are thermally liberated.

Sufficient released water is absorbed and retained by the paper fibers to maintain at least about 2 weight percent water in the paper sheet after the fusing operation. The paper is again subjected to the xerographic operation on its reverse side. Problems related to dehydration of the paper, such as curl and toner disturbances, are significantly reduced by use of the paper of the process as compared to the use of ordinary paper.

Coated Carrier Particles for Toners

The process of *E.S. Baltazzi and P. Datta; U.S. Patent 4,055,684; October 25, 1977; assigned to Addressograph Multigraph Corporation* relates to carriers for use in developer formulations which charge electroscopic powders triboelectrically. These carriers are useful in electrophotographic processes for developing latent electrostatic images in which a colored toner adhered to the surface of a carrier particle is caused to be attracted from the carrier particle to develop a latent electrostatic image.

It was found that carrier particles consisting of a solid matrix coated with a dispersion of an ion-exchange resin in a polymeric binder can be used in developer mixes in order to provide a means for controlling the triboelectric charge induced in an electroscopic powder mixed therewith. Use of the carriers permits matching the carrier to the desired electroscopic powder or toner in order to impart the requisite triboelectric properties thereto. This results in a wide latitude of toner formulations being useful rather than requiring, as heretofore, that toners be specially formulated to have the triboelectric properties required for the particular positive or negative development involved in the electrophotographic process. Ion-exchange resins can be selected to charge whichever toner is chosen positively or negatively as desired.

In addition to the advantageous triboelectric properties possessed by these carriers, their use results in developer mixes which are longer-lived and less susceptible to toner filming than previously available developer mixes.

The ion-exchange resin (both anionic and cationic) to be used is dried and finely ground and then dispersed in a polymeric binder. The sizes of the ion-exchange resin particles which are used in the dispersion are preferably in the micron to submicron range. The binder is a polymeric material which may be characterized as a low surface energy thermoplastic polymer. Use of such a binder increases the developer mix life and prevents toner filming and bias shorting.

Some materials which are especially adapted for this purpose are polycarbonate resins, acrylic resins, novolak resins, heat curable silicone rubbers, fluorinated polymers and other low surface energy polymers. As carrier matrix materials it is possible to use a wide variety of substances, e.g., glass beads, ceramic beads, grains of sand or metallic particles. Nonmetallic matrix materials are useful for use in cascade development systems. Where a magnetic brush developing system is used it is necessary that the matrix be magnetic. For this purpose various irons and steels have been used, e.g., spherical steel beads and irregularly-shaped iron powders.

Example 1: A quantity of 1,000 g of Dowex MSC-1 cation-exchange resin was dried in a fluidized bed dryer at 100°C for 1 hour, pulverized in a jet mill and sifted through a 325 mesh screen. A 20 g quantity of resulting powdered cation-exchange resin was dispersed in 400 g of a 5% solution of a copolymer of vinylidene fluoride and tetrafluoroethylene (Kynar-7201) in a 1:1 mixture of methylethylketone and acetone to give a pigment to binder ratio of 1:1. This mixture was then placed in a blender and blended for 30 minutes after which it was diluted with the methylethylketone-acetone mixture mentioned above to give a 5% total solids concentration in the resulting dispersion.

A 4 kg quantity of 175 μ average particle size spherical steel beads was loaded into a fluidized bed coating apparatus. Air was introduced at 15 cfm and the frequency of the apparatus was adjusted to 6,000 rpm. The ion-exchange dispersion described above was pumped through an atomizing spray nozzle. The entire dispersion was applied in about 40 spray cycles repeated at 5 minute intervals. The resulting coated steel beads were then dried in a fluidized bed oven at 100°C for 2 hours.

Example 2: A quantity of 1,500 g of the coated carrier particles of Example 1 were mixed with 22.5 g of a toner containing polymers prepared from styrene and acrylic monomers, polyvinylbutyral and carbon black. The resulting developer mix was poured into the toning unit of an electrostatic copying machine (Addressograph Multigraph Model 2000). Copies of a photographic transparency were made using zinc oxide-coated paper. The optical density of the copies obtained was determined by means of a Macbeth Densitometer. The copies were found to have an optical density of 1.4. The copy density was maintained for up to 60,000 copies.

Example 3: A quantity of 1,500 g of the coated carrier particles of Example 1 were mixed with 22.5 g of a toner containing polyamide resin, maleic-modified rosin, polyketone resin, polyethylene, lithium stearate, carbon black and a positive-orienting dye. The resulting developer was poured into the toning unit of an electrostatic copying machine (Addressograph Multigraph Model 2000). Copies of a photographic transparency were made using zinc oxide-coated paper. The optical density of the image produced was 1.5 with no degradation of density observed in up to 50,000 copies.

Example 4: A quantity of 500 g of Dowex MSC-1 cation-exchange resin was pulverized with a jet mill and sifted through a 325 mesh screen. A 40 g quantity of the powdered cation-exchange resin was then dispersed in 400 g of a 5% solution of polycarbonate resin in chloroform (Lexan-140). The pigment to binder ratio was 2:1. The resulting formulation was placed in a blender, blended for 30 minutes and then diluted to obtain 5% total solids in the resulting dispersion. The resulting dispersion was used to coat 4 kg of iron powder having a particle size range of 75 to 200 μ. A quantity of 400 g of the coated iron powder was mixed with 10 g of the toner of Example 2. Zinc oxide-coated paper was charged negatively, exposed through a photographic transparency and toned with a hand-held magnetic brush. Copies without any background were obtained.

Example 5: A quantity of 500 g of Dowex MSA-1 anion-exchange resin was pulverized with a jet mill and sifted through a 325 mesh screen. A 20 g quantity of the powdered anion-exchange resin was then dispersed in 400 g of a 5% solution of externally catalyzed silicone (General Electric Silicone 4191) in a 1:1 mixture of tetrahydrofuran and acetone. The pigment to binder ratio was 1:1. The resulting dispersion was placed in a blender, blended for 30 minutes and then diluted to obtain a 5% total solids dispersion.

A quantity of 0.8 g of catalyst (General Electric Catalyst 4192-C) was added to the resulting dispersion in a concentration of 4% by weight of silicone. The dispersion was then used to coat a 4 kg quantity of 150 μ average particle size spherical steel beads using a fluidized bed coating apparatus as described in Example 1. The coating resulting from this treatment constituted 1.5% of the weight of the coated steel beads. The coating thickness was 1 to 2 μ.

Example 6: A quantity of 150 g of the coated carrier particles of Example 5 was mixed with 3.7 g of the toner of Example 3. Paper coated with 1,4-diphenyl-1,4-di(4-phenyl)phenylbutatriene sensitized with 9-(dicyanomethylene)-2,4,7-trinitrofluorene was charged positively with a corona using a potential of 5,000 volts, exposed through a photographic transparency and toned with a hand-held magnetic brush using the resulting developer mix. Positive copies displaying a copy density of 1.5 were obtained. The surface charge on toner was found to be -2.5×10^{-10} coulomb per square centimeter.

Example 7: The procedure of Example 1 was followed except that irregularly-shaped iron powder having a particle size range of 75 to 200 μ was used.

Example 8: A quantity of 4 kg of the coated carrier particles of Example 7 was mixed with 75 g of the toner of Example 3. The resulting developer mix was poured into the developer unit of an electrostatic copier (Addressograph Multigraph Model 5000). Copies having a copy density of 1.1 were obtained. The surface charge was determined to be 4.4×10^{-10} coulomb per square centimeter. No degradation of image density was observed even under extreme humidity conditions within the range of relative humidities of 10 to 75%.

CELLULOSE MICROCAPSULES HAVING ADSORBING CAPACITY

Precursor Microcapsules Subjected to Ester Hydrolysis

The process of *M. Morishita, Y. Yokokawa, T. Nishikawa, M. Mishiro, S. Ohashi,*

M. Fukushima, Y. Inaba, and T. Matsuda; U.S. Patent 4,118,336; October 3, 1978; assigned to Toyo Jozo Company, Ltd., and Asahi Kasei Kogyo Kabushiki Kaisha, both of Japan relates to a cellulose microcapsule having adsorbing capacity consisting of outer semipermeable barrier layer of cellulose and adsorbent powders dispersed within inner cellulose gel matrix. The process for producing cellulose microcapsules comprises subjecting a precursor microcapsule having adsorbing capacity, consisting of outer semipermeable barrier layer of cellulose ester derivative and adsorbent powders dispersed within inner gel matrix of cellulose ester derivative, to ester hydrolysis.

As the cellulose ester derivative, any cellulose ester derivative may be used so far as it can be used for wall films of the microcapsules. Examples of such cellulose ester derivative include fatty acid esters of cellulose such as cellulose monoacetate, cellulose diacetate, cellulose triacetate, cellulose propionate and cellulose butyrate, mixed fatty acid esters of cellulose such as cellulose acetate propionate and cellulose acetate butyrate, inorganic acid esters of cellulose such as cellulose nitrate, cellulose sulfate and cellulose phosphate, and aromatic acid esters such as cellulose benzoate.

As the adsorbent, any material may be used so far as it has an adsorption capacity that is not deactivated in adsorption capacity by ester hydrolysis. Examples of such adsorbents include powders of activated charcoal, bone black, silica gel, silica-alumina gel, zeolite, bentonite, ion-exchange resins and metal chelate resins.

The microcapsules having wall films composed of a cellulose ester derivative, containing adsorbents and having selective adsorbing ability, which are used in the process, are those having wall films composed of a cellulose ester derivative and containing an adsorbent as the core substance of each microcapsule, which are obtained by, e.g., a coating method according to curing-in-liquid procedure, a coating method according to phase separation procedure, a drying-in-liquid method, etc.

One example of the method is as follows: A method is featured in which an adsorbent is dispersed in a solution of a cellulose ester derivative in a hydrophilic solvent, the resulting dispersion is further dispersed in the form of the droplets in a vehicle, which is poorly miscible with the solvent for the cellulose ester derivative, and then a solvent, which is a nonsolvent for the cellulose ester derivative, is miscible with the solvent for the derivative, and is miscible or poorly miscible with the vehicle, is added to the dispersion, to obtain microcapsules having wall films composed of a cellulose ester derivative, containing adsorbents and having selective adsorbing ability.

In the abovementioned method, the cellulose ester derivative, which is a wall material for the adsorbent, is properly selected and first dissolved in a hydrophilic solvent. As this solvent, any solvent may be used so far as it can dissolve the cellulose ester derivative and is poorly miscible, i.e., is entirely immiscible or is miscible in an amount of at most about 15%, with the vehicle mentioned later, and is not required to be limited to a solvent low in boiling point and high in vapor pressure. Examples of the solvent include acetone, methanol, ethanol, isopropanol, dimethylsulfoxide, N,N-dimethylformamide, water, acidic water and basic water.

Another method is as follows: Microcapsules having wall films composed of a cellulose ester derivative, containing adsorbents and having selective adsorbing ability are prepared by dispersing the adsorbents in a solution of a cellulose ester derivative in a hydrophilic solvent, the derivative being able to form a semipermeable film in an aqueous medium, and then contacting the resulting dispersion with an aqueous medium.

The cellulose ester derivative capable of forming a semipermeable film in an aqueous medium, which derivative is a wall material for the adsorbent, is properly selected and first dissolved in a hydrophilic solvent. As this hydrophilic solvent, any solvent may be used so far as it does not deteriorate the adsorption capacity of the adsorbent, is miscible with the aqueous medium, and can dissolve the cellulose ester derivative. Such solvents include N,N-dimethylformamide, dimethylsulfoxide, N,N-dimethylacetamide, acetone and alcohol.

A further technique is as follows: microcapsules having wall films composed of a cellulose ester derivative, containing adsorbents and having selective adsorbing ability is prepared by dissolving a cellulose ester derivative in a solvent, which is poorly miscible with water, has lower boiling point than that of water and has higher vapor pressure than that of water, dispersing an adsorbent into the thus-formed solution, dispersing the resulting dispersion to the form of droplets in a separately prepared aqueous solution containing a surfactant or a protective colloid, and then removing the solvent.

The cellulose derivative, which is a wall material for the adsorbent, is properly selected and first dissolved in a solvent. As this solvent, any solvent may be used so far as it can dissolve the cellulose ester derivative, is poorly miscible, i.e., immiscible or miscible by at most about 15% (v/v), with water, has lower boiling point than that of water and higher vapor pressure than that of water. Examples of such solvent include ethyl ether, isopropyl ether, methylene chloride, ethylene chloride, chloroform, carbon tetrachloride, benzene, cyclohexane, n-hexane, methyl acetate and ethyl acetate; preferably, methylene chloride, ethylene chloride, chloroform, carbon tetrachloride, benzene and ethyl acetate.

Still another method is as follows: Microcapsules having wall films composed of a cellulose ester derivative, containing adsorbent and having selective adsorbing ability is prepared by dissolving a cellulose ester derivative in an organic solvent, which is poorly miscible with the vehicle mentioned later, is miscible with water, and has lower boiling point than that of water, adding to the thus-formed solution such an amount of water that the cellulose ester derivative is not deposited, dispersing an adsorbent into the solution, dispersing the resulting dispersion into a liquid paraffin or silicone oil used as a vehicle, and then removing the organic solvent. In this method, the cellulose ester derivative, which is a wall material for the adsorbent, is properly selected and dissolved in an organic solvent.

As the solvent, any organic solvent may be used so far as it is poorly miscible with the vehicle such as liquid paraffin or silicone oil, is miscible with water, and has lower boiling point than that of water. Examples of such organic solvent include acetone, methylethylketone, methanol, ethanol and propanol. Particularly preferable organic solvent is acetone or methanol which easily dissolves the cellulose ester derivative even when it is in a hydrated state, and is lower in boiling point than water.

The microcapsules prepared according to the methods as mentioned above are subjected to ester hydrolysis to convert cellulose derivatives into cellulose. The ester hydrolysis should be conducted without disintegrating or dissolving the microcapsules. That is, the ester hydrolysis is carried out in a manner such that the microcapsules are dispersed in an aqueous acid or alkali solution, which has been properly controlled in concentration so as to be sufficient and necessary for the removal of ester residues of the cellulose ester derivative used in the microcapsules, and so as not to disintegrate or dissolve the microcapsules.

Examples of the acid used in the ester hydrolysis include sulfuric, hydrochloric and phosphoric acids, while examples of the alkali include sodium hydroxide, potassium hydroxide, ammonia and triethylamine. The ester hydrolysis is carried out at a temperature which is usually from 50° to 80°C, preferably 60° to 70°C for from 30 to 120 minutes, preferably 30 to 60 minutes. When an aqueous acid solution is used, its concentration is preferably from 0.5 to 5 N; when an aqueous alkali solution is used, its concentration is from 0.2 to 2 N. If necessary, a catalyst may also be used. The degree of ester hydrolysis is usually 95% or more, preferably 98% or more.

The cellulose microcapsules so prepared have an outer diameter from about 100 to 5,000 μ and have an outer barrier layer of continuous solid phase cellulose which is 0.5 to 5 μ in thickness and contains micropores of from about 10 to 80 A in diameter, adsorbent powders being dispersed within cellulose gel matrix inside of the outer barrier layer. The microcapsules have a void volume equal to at least 25% of the total volume thereof. They are not deactivated in adsorption capacity and molecular sieving effect by deesterification and far more excellent in acid resistance, alkali resistance and solvent resistance than those before deesterification.

Accordingly, they can stably display their various abilities over long periods of time even in acidic solutions, alkali solutions and organic solvent solutions, and thus can be put into various uses such as, e.g., extraction and purification of antibiotics from fermentation liquids, extraction and purification of nucleic acids from the cells of microorganisms, extraction of natural dyes, recovery of valuable substances from waste liquors, decolorization, and treatment of waste liquors by removal of organic compounds.

Example 1: In a solution of 100 g of cellulose diacetate (Asahi Chemical Co.) in 1.2 liters of N,N-dimethylformamide (DMF) was homogeneously dispersed 100 g of an activated charcoal (Carborafin). The resulting dispersion was dropped to the form of droplets into water by use of an atomizer cup (diameter 50 mm) to obtain microcapsules encapsulated with cellulose diacetate, containing activated charcoal (size of microcapsules: 0.2 to 1.5 mm in diameter).

800 g of the thus-prepared microcapsules containing activated charcoal were sufficiently washed with deionized water, charged into 6,200 ml of an 0.25 N aqueous sodium hydroxide solution and then stirred at 70°±2°C for 1 hour to saponify the wall films of the microcapsules. Subsequently, the microcapsules were sufficiently washed with water until the pH of the wash water became 7.0 or less to obtain cellulose microcapsules containing activated charcoal. The acetylation degree of the cellulose of the microcapsules before saponification was 54.1%, but less than 0.4% after saponification.

Example 2: In a solution of 40 g of cellulose diacetate (acetylation degree:

54.5%) in a mixed solvent comprising 1 liter of methylene chloride and 400 ml of acetone was dispersed 40 g of Carboraffin. The resulting dispersion was added with stirring at room temperature to 6 liters of an aqueous solution containing 30 g of sodium laurylbenzene sulfonate dissolved therein, and the stirring was further continued, whereby the solvent was evaporated to form a precipitate.

The precipitate was recovered by filtration, washed with water and then dried to obtain microcapsules encapsulated with cellulose diacetate of 0.25 to 1.5 mm in particle size containing activated charcoal. 70 g of the thus-obtained microcapsules were sufficiently wetted with 400 ml of deionized water, charged into 2,100 ml of a 0.25 N aqueous sodium hydroxide solution kept at 75°C and saponified with stirring at 70°C for 1 hour. Subsequently, the microcapsules were sufficiently washed with water until the pH of the wash water became 8.0 or less to obtain cellulose microcapsules containing activated charcoal (acetylation degree of the cellulose: less than 0.4%).

Example 3: In a solution of 5 g of cellulose diacetate in 60 ml of dimethylsulfoxide (DMSO) was homogeneously dispersed 10 g of activated charcoal powders (Kyoryoku Shirasagi). The resulting dispersion was dispersed to the form of fine droplets into 300 ml of liquid paraffin of Japanese Pharmacopoeia (19 cp at 25°C) under propeller stirring, and the stirring was further continued for several minutes to make the dispersed state of the system stable. Subsequently, 100 ml of a mixture of water and acetone (4:1) was added as a nonsolvent at a rate of 5 ml per minute to the above liquid paraffin solution in the dispersed state to form microcapsules encapsulated with cellulose diacetate of 500 to 1,000 μ in particle size containing activated charcoal.

The thus-formed microcapsules were recovered by filtration using a filter cloth, sufficiently washed with n-hexane and then dried. 10 g of the microcapsules were sufficiently wetted with 100 ml of boiling water for 30 minutes, thereafter allowed to drain, charged into 500 ml of a 0.25 N aqueous sodium hydroxide solution kept at 75°C and saponified with stirring at 70°±2°C. Subsequently, the microcapsules were washed with water and dried to obtain cellulose microcapsules containing activated charcoal which had not been changed in shape from the microcapsules before saponification.

Example 4: In a solution of 150 g of cellulose diacetate in 3.5 liters of acetone containing 13% of water was dispersed 225 g of Kyoryoku Shirasagi. The resulting dispersion was poured with stirring into 9 liters of liquid paraffin of Japanese Pharmacopoeia containing 0.5% of Ranex and dispersed to the form of droplets of 600 to 1,500 μ in size. The stirring was further continued for 4 hours, whereby the acetone was evaporated to rigid microcapsules encapsulated with cellulose diacetate of 600 to 1,500 μ in particle size containing activated charcoal.

Subsequently, the microcapsules were washed several times with n-hexane and then dried to obtain 380 g of the microcapsules. 100 g of the above microcapsules were sufficiently swelled for 30 minutes with 1,000 ml of boiling water, charged into 5,000 ml of a 0.25 N aqueous sodium hydroxide solution and saponified with stirring at 70°±2°C. Thereafter, the microcapsules were washed with water and then dried to obtain cellulose microcapsules containing activated charcoal.

Example 5: Evaluation – The cellulose microcapsules containing adsorbent powders which were obtained in Examples 1 and 2 (hereinafter referred to as test samples 1 and 2) were examined for adsorption capacity. As controls, there were used activated charcoal powders (Carboraffin, control sample 1), commercially available granular carbons (Aldoster-B 1-L, control sample 2; and Aldoster-P 5-L, control sample 3), and the cellulose ester derivative microcapsules containing adsorbent powders which were used as starting materials, in Examples 1 and 2 (hereinafter referred to as control samples 4 and 5).

The amount of adsorbent powders used was 1 g in each case. The measurement of adsorption capacity was carried out in such a manner that each of the abovementioned samples was added to 100 ml of a 0.01% aqueous methylene blue solution ($OD_{595\ m\mu}$ + 5.0); the resulting mixture was stirred, allowed to stand for 24 hours and then filtered, and the filtrate was measured in $OD_{595\ m\mu}$ value to evaluate the adsorption capacity of each sample for methylene blue. The adsorption capacities of the cellulose microcapsules containing adsorbent powders which were obtained in Examples 1 and 2 were scarcely lower than the adsorption capacity of the conventional activated charcoal powders (control sample 1), were superior to those of the commercially available granular carbons (control samples 2 and 3), and were equal to those of the microcapsules before saponification (control samples 4 and 5).

Cellulose Precipitated Around Droplets of Dispersion

M. Morishita, M. Fukushima, T. Sasagawa, Y. Inaba, Y. Yokokawa, S. Araragi, N. Yoshida, and H. Uchiyama; U.S. Patent 4,123,381; October 31, 1978; assigned to Toyo Jozo Company, Ltd., and Asahi Kasei Kogyo Kabushiki Kaisha, both of Japan here provide a direct process for producing cellulose microcapsules having adsorbing capacity, consisting of outer semipermeable barrier layer of cellulose and adsorbent powders dispersed within inner cellulose gel matrix. The method comprises dispersing adsorbents in a solution of cellulose dissolved in a solvent which is not adversely affected by the adsorbing capacity of adsorbents and capable of dissolving cellulose, then forming the resulting dispersion into droplets and finally effecting precipitation of cellulose on the droplets.

Cellulose is first dissolved in a solvent which is not adversely affected by the adsorbing capacity of adsorbents and capable of dissolving cellulose. It is not necessarily required to use cellulose of high purity. Inexpensive pulp, ground pulp and regenerated cellulose may preferably be employed. As solvents which are not adversely affected by the adsorbing capacity of adsorbent powders and capable of dissolving cellulose, xanthate solution, and cuprammonium solution are preferred for industrial application.

The concentration of the solution to be used is not limited, so long as it can dissolve cellulose. There may be utilized, e.g., an aqueous alkaline solution of so-called viscose prepared by adding 10 to 50% of carbon disulfide to alkali cellulose; copper tetraammine hydroxide (cuprammonium) solution containing 2 to 7% (w/v) of copper, 5 to 15% of ammonia and 5 to 15% of cellulose. Generally, the appropriate concentration of cellulose is about 1.5 to 15% [w/v (at 20°C, 200 to 2,000 cp)] and preferably about 1.7 to 13% (at 20°C, 280 to 1,800 cp).

There may also be used such cellulose solution as cellulose xanthate solution (viscose) or cellulose cuprammonium solution which are obtained in the method for producing viscose rayon or cuprammonium rayon in a suitably diluted concentration. Subsequently, the adsorbent powders are dispersed in the above solution. As adsorbents, there may be utilized material having adsorbing capacity, e.g., those mentioned above in U.S. Patent 4,118,336. The amount of adsorbent is normally about 90% (w/w) or less, preferably about 40 to 60%, based on cellulose microcapsules obtained.

This solution having cellulose dissolved therein to which the adsorbent powders are added, is sufficiently mixed to form a uniform dispersion, which is then formed into droplets by a so-called orifice method wherein the solution is formed into droplets by using a tube or turnplate having single or plural orifices of 1 to 10 mm in diameter. Alternatively, it may be performed by a dispersion method wherein the solution is dispersed to the form of droplets in a vehicle such as liquid paraffin or silicone oil, which is poorly miscible with the solvent used, does not precipitate cellulose and has a viscosity suitable for forming liquid droplets. The amount of the vehicle used in the dispersion method is about 5 to 30 times the amount of the solution to be dispersed.

Then, these liquid droplets are subjected to precipitation of cellulose by decrease or loss of solubility of cellulose in the solvent by dilution or modification of the solvent. Modification of the solvent may be performed, e.g., by dropwise addition of droplets in an aqueous solution containing solvent modifying acid compounds such as hydrochloric acid or sulfuric acid, simultaneously causing dilution of the solvent. Alternatively, it may be performed in the dispersion method, by similarly incorporating an aqueous solution of acid compounds in the dispersion of the solution in a vehicle, simultaneously causing dilution of the solvent. Furthermore, in the dispersion method, the dispersion may be subjected to reduced pressure or heating to separate or remove cellulose solubilizing components therefrom.

The cellulose microcapsules of the process have an outer diameter from about 100 to 5,000 μ and have an outer barrier layer of continuous solid phase cellulose which is 0.5 to 5 μ in thickness and contains micropores of from about 10 to 80 A in diameter, adsorbent powders being dispersed within cellulose gel matrix inside of the outer barrier layer.

The cellulose microcapsules containing adsorbent powders may be used for various purposes, e.g., treatment of waste liquors such as removal and recovery of organic compounds, which are coloring components, from colored waste liquors in dye industry, caramel industry, beverage industry wherein coloring agents are used and fermentation industry wherein syrup is used; removal or recovery of proteins from waste liquors containing organic compounds such as proteins in food industry for processing fish or meat and pharmaceutical industry; decolorization of alcoholic beverages; and adsorption and recovery of medicines in pharmaceutical industry.

Example 1: A viscose dope obtained by a known process (composition: cellulose 8.5%, sodium hydroxide 6.5%, carbon disulfide on the basis of cellulose 35%, viscosity 700 cp, at 20°C) was diluted with 4 N sodium hydroxide solution to adjust the cellulose content to 6.4%. In 240 ml of the thus-prepared viscose dope were uniformly dispersed 24 g of activated charcoal (Kyoryoku Shirasagi). Then, the resulting dispersion was added dropwise from an atomizer cup having 18 orifices of 5 mm in diameter to 10 liters of 3.6 N aqueous hydrochloric acid solution to obtain cellulose microcapsules of 1 to 5 mm in diameter containing activated charcoal powders.

Example 2: A viscose dope was diluted with 2 N sodium hydroxide solution to adjust the cellulose content to 5.1%. In 200 ml of the thus-prepared viscose solution were uniformly dispersed 25 g of activated charcoal (Carboraffin). The resulting dispersion was dispersed under propeller stirring to the form of fine droplets into 600 ml of liquid paraffin of Japanese Pharmacopoeia (19 cp, at 25°C). Stirring was further continued to stabilize the dispersed state. Then, 200 ml of 3.6 N aqueous hydrochloric acid solution were added to the dispersion at the rate of 8 ml per minute to form microcapsules of 0.5 to 1.2 mm in diameter containing activated charcoal.

Then, the microcapsules were filtered with a filter cloth, sufficiently washed with n-hexane, petroleum ether and acetone in this order, and further washed with water to obtain cellulose microcapsules containing activated charcoal powders.

Example 3: Evaluation – The cellulose microcapsules obtained in Examples 1 and 2 were tested for their acid resistance, alkali resistance, solvent resistance and adsorption capacity, and compared to commercial adsorbents. The test results show that cellulose microcapsules of this process are excellent in acid resistance, alkali resistance and solvent resistance. Furthermore, the adsorbing capacity of the cellulose microcapsules is similar to that of powdery activated charcoal and is deteriorated little by the microencapsulation process. The cellulose microcapsules are superior in adsorbing capacity to commercially available granular activated charcoal.

THERMOPLASTIC EXPANDABLE MICROSPHERES

Use of Citric Acid with Polymerizable Monomeric Composition

Expansible thermoplastic polymer particles containing volatile fluid foaming agent are know and described in U.S. Patent 3,615,972. Such particles are popularly known as expandable microspheres and consist of a synthetic resinous thermoplastic shell containing a single symmetrical encapsulated volatile fluid foaming agent therein as a distinct and separate liquid phase. When such expandable microspheres are heated to a temperature sufficient to heat plastify or soften the thermoplastic resinous shell the particles expand to form monocellular gas-filled spheres.

Such expandable microspheres have a wide variety of applications in paper, coatings, as lightweight fillers and the like. In employing the polymerization procedure set forth in U.S. Patent 3,615,972, as part of the suspending system there is employed an aqueous solution of a copolymer prepared from the combination of diethanolamine and adipic acid in equimolar proportions. Substantial difficulty has been encountered in maintaining desired quality control of the amine/acid copolymer. Variations in the properties of the amine/acid copolymer result in batch-to-batch variation of expandable microspheres prepared employing the copolymer.

These difficulties are overcome by an improvement developed by *W.E. Cohrs; R.E. Gunderman, and W.A. Crozier; U.S. Patent 4,016,110; April 5, 1977; assigned to*

The Dow Chemical Company in a method comprising suspending in water a colloidal silica dispersing agent, a polymerizable monomeric composition and a volatile liquid expanding agent, dispersing the volatile liquid expanding agent and monomeric composition within the water as a plurality of droplets, polymerizing the monomeric material to form a plurality of particles, the particles having a thermoplastic resinous shell of generally spherical configuration, the particles generally symmetrically encapsulating a single liquid occlusion as a distinct and separate liquid phase within the particle, the particles being generally impenetrable to the liquid raising agent.

The improvement comprises employing from about 0.2 to 1 part by weight of citric acid per 100 parts by weight of monomeric composition in the substantial absence of a polymer of equimolar parts of adipic acid and diethanolamine. The citric acid used may be hydrous or anhydrous or may be employed in the form of an aqueous solution; or alternately, it may be dispersed within the monomer. The weight proportions as hereinbefore set forth apply to the citric acid monohydrate. Generally it is desirable to add citric acid to the aqueous phase. However, if desired it may be incorporated within the oil of monomer blowing agent phase and is quickly extracted therefrom by the aqueous phase during initial mixing of the reactants.

Example: Styrene/acrylonitrile/divinylbenzene microspheres are prepared in the following manner: a water phase is prepared by admixing colloidal silica, potassium dichromate and sodium chloride in the quantities set forth in the table.

	Run 1	Run 2
Components, g		
Deionized water	3,144	3,144
Colloidal silica, 30 wt % aqueous dispersion	180	180
Copolymer of diethanol amine and adipic acid	–	12
Citric acid	3	–
Potassium dichromate	1.2	1.2
Sodium chloride	24	24
pH adjusted to	no adjustment	4.0
Styrene	720	720
Acrylonitrile	480	480
Divinylbenzene	1	1
Neopentane	480	480
Lauroyl peroxide	4.8	4.8
Properties of product		
Yield, %	89	89
Conversion, %	90	90
Encapsulation, %	95	97
Bulk density, g/cc	1.0	0.9
Particle size spread, μ	1-22	2-17
Particle size average, μ	10	10

For purposes of illustration, a comparative polymerization is made employing the amine/acid copolymer hereinbefore referred to. In the case of Run 2 containing the amine/acid copolymer, the pH is adjusted to about 4 employing hydrochloric acid. A reactor is then cooled to about 20°C; the aqueous phase is then added to the reactor and the reactor agitated. The reactor is evacuated, purged with nitrogen, again evacuated and the polymerizable or monomer phase added. The contents of the reactor are agitated as violently as possible for a period of about 20 minutes. The contents of the reactor are then pumped from the reactor to a mechanical homogenizer. The discharge from the homogenizer is returned to the reactor until the desired degree of dispersion is obtained.

The conduits from the reactor to the homogenizer and return line are gas purged and the liquid contents thereof are returned to the reactor. The reactor is agitated at a speed of about 100 rpm and maintained at a temperature of 60°C for a period of 23 hours. At the end of the 23 hour period, the contents of the reactor are cooled to 23°C and the product discharged.

Repeated polymerization using the composition as shown in Run 1 provides substantially improved consistency of results over that employed using the formulation of Run 2. Similar beneficial results are obtained when employing the monomeric compositions set forth in U.S. Patent 3,615,972.

Vinylidene Chloride, Acrylonitrile and a Small Amount of Additional Copolymerizable Monomer

Substantial difficulty has been encountered in the preparation of relatively large quantities of expandable microspheres employing vinylidene chloride as a major monomeric component and acrylonitrile as a minor component in that the rate of reaction is such that during at least one period during the reaction the amount of heat or peak exotherm that is required to be removed from the reaction mixture is greater than the amount that can be conveniently removed by means of most conventional agitated jacketed batch reaction vessels. Thus, the vinylidene chloride polymer expandable microspheres can readily be prepared in small quantities. However, equipment limitations with regard to heat transfer prevent a convenient scaling up or increasing of the batch size.

This difficulty is overcome by an improvement developed by *J.L. Garner; U.S. Patent 4,075,138; February 1, 1978; assigned to The Dow Chemical Company* in the preparation of synthetic resinous thermoplastic microspheres employing from 60 to 90 parts by weight of vinylidene chloride and from 40 to 10 parts by weight of acrylonitrile. The method comprises preparing an oil phase containing the polymerizable component and a liquid blowing agent which volatilizes at a temperature below the heat softening point of the polymer prepared from the monomer mixture, dispersing the oil phase in the water phase, the water phase containing a dispersion stabilizer, the oil phase being dispersed as a plurality of droplets having diameters from about 1 to 50 μ, initiating polymerization of the monomer in the droplets to form a plurality of hollow polymer particles having symmetrically encapsulated therein a volatile fluid foaming agent.

The improvement comprises employing from about 3 to 12 parts by weight of a copolymerizable monomer having a propagation constant of from about 2 to 15,000 liters per mol second and $(r_1/r_2) > 1$ wherein r_1 is the reactivity ratio for the copolymerizable monomer and r_2 is the reactivity ratio for acrylonitrile, the copolymerizable monomer being selected from the group consisting of methacrylonitrile, methyl methacrylate, styrene, 1,3-butadiene and mixtures thereof. The definition of r_1/r_2 is described in *Polymer Handbook* by Brandrup and Immergut, II-141, Third Edition, 1967, Interscience Publishers, with the further limitation that the vinylidene chloride/acrylonitrile/volatile fluid foaming agent and the copolymerizable monomer are mutually soluble at a temperature between about 20° to 90°C.

The polymerizable monomers, blowing agents and optionally a suitable free radical initiator are incorporated into an oil phase; a water phase is prepared employing suitable suspending agents. The process is described at great length in U.S. Patent 3,615,972. The water and oil phases are mixed employing violent agitation sufficient to disperse the oil phase in the water phase and to form droplets having diameters from about 1 to 50 μ. The resulting reaction mixture is then polymerized in a generally oxygen-free reaction vessel at temperatures from about 20° to 90°C (preferably 40° to 65°C). The vinylidene chloride and acrylonitrile of commercial purity are satisfactory. The third monomeric component beneficially has one or more of methacrylonitrile, methyl methacrylate, styrene, 1,3-butadiene and mixtures thereof.

A wide variety of the fluid foaming agents are readily employed as described in U.S. Patent 3,615,972. These fluid foaming agents are soluble in the monomeric mixture and generally insoluble in the resultant polymer. Particularly advantageous blowing agents include butane, isobutane, neopentane and mixtures thereof. Generally such blowing agents are incorporated in the microspheres in a proportion of from about 10 to 30 weight percent, based on the total weight of the microspheres.

Example: A plurality of polymerization runs are carried out, each using the following basic recipe:

Ingredients	Parts by Weight
Oil phase	
Vinylidene chloride	560
Acrylonitrile	200
Divinylbenzene (as a 55% solution in diethylbenzene)	5.5
Isobutane	89
sec-Butyl peroxydicarbonate	4
Water phase	
Deionized water	1,322
Ludox HS*	110
Potassium dichromate	0.4
Diethanolamine-adipic acid equimolar copolymer**	5.5
Sodium chloride	25
HCl (aqueous) to pH 4	

*30% aqueous dispersion of colloidal silica.

**60 wt % aqueous solution. The copolymer has a viscosity of about 100 cp at 25°C when a 10 wt % solution in water is measured.

The oil phase and the water phase are then mixed employing high speed violent agitation with an impeller blade rotating at about 10,000 rpm. The reaction mixture is then transferred to an agitated, nitrogen-purged, jacketed reaction vessel instrumented to permit the determination of the polymerization exotherm. A plurality of polymerizations are carried out adding the indicated quantities of additional monomer. The reactor is heated to 50°C and maintained at that temperature for about 20 hours.

When the foregoing recipe containing only vinylidene chloride and acrylonitrile as monomers is polymerized, a maximum exotherm in excess of 1,030 calories per minute is obtained. When 19 parts by weight methacrylonitrile are added, the maximum exotherm is 710 calories per minute, and when 38 parts by weight methacrylonitrile are added the maximum exotherm is 420 calories per minute; with 38 parts by weight methyl methacrylate, the maximum exotherm is 360 calories per minute. The reaction time of the polymerization does not appear to significantly increase, but the maximum heat evolved per unit time or peak exotherm is significantly more uniform permitting polymerization in large vessels which need not be designed for a high heat transfer characteristic in order to retain the reaction mixture at the desired temperature.

Similar beneficial and advantageous results are obtained when the methacrylonitrile of the foregoing illustration is replaced with styrene, 1,3-butadiene and mixtures thereof.

Incorporation of Thermoplastic Expandable Microspheres in Heat Plastifiable Matrix

W.E. Cohrs and R.E. Gunderman; U.S. Patent 4,108,806; August 22, 1978; assigned to The Dow Chemical Company have developed a process for the incorporation of expandable thermoplastic synthetic resinous monocellular microspheres having a thermoplastic resinous shell, a volatile fluid foaming agent therein within a heat plastifiable matrix material.

The steps of the method comprise admixing the microspheres and matrix forming material, heat plastifying the matrix material and mechanically working the mixture to form a matrix about the microspheres without causing expansion thereof, subsequently passing the mixture into a zone of lower pressure wherein the microspheres expand to form a plurality of hollow, generally monocellular particles within the matrix and cooling the mixture below the heat plastifying temperature.

Also described is an extruded body comprising a continuous heat plastifiable matrix having therein a plurality of synthetic resinous microspheres, the microspheres being monocellular and having a resin shell having encapsulated therein as a distinct and separate phase a volatile fluid expanding agent.

The expandable microspheres may be used in admixture with various matrix materials including synthetic resins, tars, waxes and the like. The only critical requirement for the matrix material is that it be heat plastifiable and at its heat plastification temperature it does not act as a rapid solvent for the microspheres to cause the destruction thereof by solvent action or heat plastify at a temperature sufficiently high that the microspheres are destroyed by thermal degradation.

Various synthetic resins beneficially are admixed with expandable microspheres and extruded to provide a foamed product, or alternately, by reducing the temperature of the extruder adjacent the die, the solid resinous matrix is extruded which contains the unexpanded microspheres. Such an unexpanded product may then be heated at a later time to cause expansion at ambient pressure. Beneficially when employing synthetic resinous matrices, it is generally desirable to provide the resin in a finely divided form to facilitate admixture with the microspheres. The finely divided (passing 50 mesh screen U.S. Sieve Size) particulate resin is particularly advantageous when a screw extruder or screw injection molding machine is employed, and neither of these devices provides a high level of mixing of the heat plastified resin within the apparatus.

Desirably, when a heat plastifiable matrix is employed for the preparation of the microsphere-containing product, a wide variety of additives may be utilized including dyes, pigments, fillers and plasticizers. Particularly advantageous are glass reinforcing fibers.

The use of expandable microspheres provides synthetic resinous foam having a generally uniform small cell size and permits blowing agent retention in cases where such retention would not occur for a desirable length of time without the expandable microspheres, e.g., polyolefins such as polyethylene are readily processed by conventional techniques to provide an expandable granule but such granules have a useful life which is much too short for most commercial applications. In contrast, by employing expandable microspheres a molding granule is readily prepared which has a shelf life in excess of 6 months.

Example 1: A plurality of blends of resin and an expandable microsphere having a polymer shell of about 60% styrene, 40 weight percent acrylonitrile having encapsulated therein a distinct and separate droplet of isobutane (about 20% by weight of the microspheres) and 10 parts by weight of the microspheres are employed with 80 parts by weight of resin and the resulting mixture extruded from a screw extruder under the various conditions set forth below. In the table the polymer matrices are: (I) blend of 90 weight percent high density polyethylene with 10 weight percent copolymer of about 80 weight percent ethylene with 20 weight percent vinyl acetate; (II) copolymer of about 80 weight percent ethylene with 20 weight percent vinyl acetate; (III) ABS resin (Tybrene); and (IV) butadiene rubber (Tufprene).

	. Foam Composition. .			. . . . Extrusion Conditions.								
Run No.	Polymer Matrix	Weight Percent	Weight Percent MS*	. Temperatures, °C . Zone 1	Zone 2	Die	Screw Speed (rpm)	Die Press (psig)	Screen Pak	Slot Die	No Die	Foam Density (pcf)
1	I	80	10	200	400	350	20	900	x	–	–	59.1
2	I	80	10	200	350	305	20	1,000	x	–	–	38.1
3	I	80	10	200	300	270	20	1,200	x	–	–	26.4**
3A	I	80	10	200	300	270	20	1,200	x	–	–	38.3
4	I	80	10	200	275	250	20	2,700	x	–	–	24.6
5	I	80	10	200	275	250	25	3,500	x	–	–	19.9
6	I	285	260	20	1,200	x	–	–	24.3	–	–	–
7	I	285	260	200	280	250	20	3,200	x	–	–	21.4
8	I	285	260	200	280	250	55	900	–	x	–	19.3
9	I	285	260	200	280	250	55	0	–	–	x	28.5
1	II	90	10	200	280	260	45	500	x	–	–	30.5
2	II	90	10	200	265	250	60	900	x	–	–	19.9
3	II	90	10	200	265	250	83	900	x	–	–	16.7
4	II	90	10	200	265	250	20	200	x	–	–	17.4
5	II	90	10	200	265	250	60	900	x	–	–	23.7
1	III	90	10	400	400	350	20	200	x	–	–	59.6
2	III	90	10	210	400	350	47	200	x	–	–	48.6
1	IV	90	10	200	300	270	20	800	x	–	–	19.75
2	IV	90	10	200	360	285	20	200	x	–	–	42.2
3	IV	90	10	200	350	305	72	500	x	–	–	36.7
4	IV	90	10	200	400	325	20	150	x	–	–	50.9**
4A	IV	90	10	200	400	325	20	150	x	–	–	63.75
5	IV	90	10	200	400	325	72	500	x	–	–	46.4**
5A	IV	90	10	200	400	325	72	500	x	–	–	53.6

*MS is microspheres.

**Water cooled.

The densities of the resultant products are measured. In each case, the product is a uniform, fine-celled foam showing no evidence of rat holes or other significant imperfections.

Example 2: The product extruded from the first run is divided into a plurality of pellets measuring about ⅛" x ⅛" x ¼" and placed in a hollow metal mold which in turn is placed in a circulating air oven having a temperature of about 150°C for a period of about 30 minutes. The mold is subsequently removed from the air oven and cooled to ambient temperature. On opening the mold and removing the contents the particles are found to have foamed to fill the mold and form a unitary reproduction of the internal configuration of the mold.

Example 3: The procedure of Example 1 is repeated using a mixture of 60 parts by weight of a polyvinyl chloride plastisol grade resin (Geon 121), 40 parts by weight of di-(2-ethylhexyl)phthalate and 6 parts by weight of expandable microspheres having a shell of 75 parts by weight vinylidene chloride, 25 parts by weight acrylonitrile and containing about 20 weight percent neopentane. The mixture is extruded at a temperature of about 130°C. The product obtained is a fine-celled rubbery foam.

PAPER COATINGS

Use of Encapsulated Accelerator and Cross-Linking Agent for Controlled Cure

The process of *M.J. Shaw; U.S. Patent 4,091,130; May 23, 1978; assigned to Allied Paper Incorporated* relates to improvements in a method for coating paper with a coating formulation which comprises a reactive polymer, having reactive carboxyl, hydroxyl or amido groups, an aminoplast cross-linking agent and a curing accelerator catalyst, wherein the coating formulation is applied to the paper, dried and calendered. The improvement comprises obtaining a controlled cure by encapsulating either the accelerator catalyst or cross-linking agent, or both, in microcapsules. The pressure applied to the paper in the calendering step is sufficient to cause rupture of the microcapsules thereby releasing the coating component or components encapsulated. Thus, rapid cure is controlled in a manner similar to the use of water boxes heretofore employed. The process is applicable to the application to paper of all coatings, including pigmented coatings, barrier coatings and top coatings.

In addition to providing a controlled cure, the process offers the advantage of greater versatility in the coating step with regard to formulations, conditions of coating and application. It permits the use of a wider class of aminoplasts than heretofore available, for instance those in which the pot life is too short or which are too viscous for use in conventional application equipment.

A particularly preferred system is a formulation in which the reactive polymer is a compound selected from the group consisting of starch, protein, casein and synthetic carboxylated polymers, the cross-linking agent being an aldehyde or an aldehyde amine resin and the catalyst being an acid catalyst. Preferably, the coating components are water-soluble or dispersible.

In the forming of the microcapsules, for encapsulating either the cross-linking agent or the catalyst, a wide variety of procedures are available and known.

One illustrative method of making minute or microscopic capsules of film-forming hydrophilic polymeric material containing an acid catalyst comprises making an aqueous sol of a hydrophilic polymeric material, e.g., gelatin, and emulsifying therein a water-immiscible organic liquid, in which the acid catalyst is suspended until the required microscopic drop size is obtained, and diluting the emulsion with water or an acidified aqueous solution in such amount as to cause the hydrophilic polymeric material to deposit around each microscopic drop of acid. All of the steps are carried out at a temperature above the gelation or solidification point of the polymeric material.

In the case of gelatin, the temperature during these steps is maintained at 50°C or above. Gelation or solidification of the encapsulating material is then achieved by cooling to a temperature below the gelation or solidification point of the material. If this latter step is performed rapidly, as by rapid cooling, the pore size of the resulting capsules will be small. Whereas the particle size of the capsules is not particularly critical, a preferred range of particle size is 0.5 to 30 μ depending upon the particular coating and calendering equipment employed.

Typical pigment-containing formulations for a web offset paper coating are:

	Broad Range	Preferred Range
	..........(%)...........	
Reactive polymer based on pigment	5-50	10-25
Aminoplast based on polymer	2-20	5-10
Accelerator acid based on aminoplast	0.1-10	0.2-2

These ranges can, of course, vary depending upon application. For a coated printing paper, a typical pigment-containing formulation would be 14% binder based on pigment, 5% aminoplast based on binder, and 0.25% encapsulated accelerator based on aminoplast. For a barrier coating or pigment coating, a typical formulation comprises 30% binder based on pigment, 10% aminoplast based on binder and 1% encapsulated accelerator acid based on aminoplast.

Example: A sheet of 40 pounds per ream of bleached kraft paper is coated to provide a pigmented coat in a conventional blade coater with the following composition:

Ingredients	Parts by Weight
Pigment clay, No. 1 coating clay	1,000
Latex Dow 620 (50% solids), butadiene-styrene copolymer modified to contain acrylic groups	200
Starch	50
Urea-formaldehyde curing resin (dry)	7.5
Acid accelerator [encapsulated (dry)]	0.5

The acid accelerator is encapsulated by any known procedures, for instance, that disclosed in U.S. Patent 3,886,084. The paper picks up approximately 10 pounds per ream of coating material. The coated paper is dried to coalesce the latex binder and then is calendered in a roll calender having a calender pressure of about 250 psi. Following calendering, cure takes place within minutes to yield a water-resistant, smooth coating surface.

Opaque Microcapsular Release Paper for Pressure-Sensitive Adhesives

The process of *A.E. Vassiliades and D.N. Vincent; U.S. Patent 4,075,389; February 21, 1978; assigned to Champion International Corporation* relates to a microcapsular release system for use in conjunction with pressure sensitive adhesives, particularly to an opaque release coating sheet comprising air-containing microcapsules.

Surprisingly, it was found that a coating composition comprising a major amount of air-containing microcapsules as the primary release agent and a relatively minor amount of a secondary release agent, such as a silicone, a methoxysilane, a stearato chromic chloride, polyethylene, and the like, provides a release paper having easily controllable release properties. Since the air-containing microcapsules are opacifying agents as well as release agents, the release paper can be made from rather inexpensive substrates, such as unbleached kraft paper and still provide a release paper having an exceptionally high opacity and whiteness. If desired, various colors can be imparted to the paper by simply staining the walls of the microcapsular moiety with suitable dyes.

The air-containing microcapsular release agents have an average particle diameter below about 2 μ, preferably between 0.25 and 1 μ. The release properties of the release coatings may be controlled and the desired properties provided by: varying the amount of release agent; varying the type of secondary release agent; employing various microcapsular wall materials; and adding the secondary release agent at different points in the process.

The secondary release agent may be: (a) added to the emulsion prior to encapsulation; (b) added to a dispersion of preformed precursor microcapsules; (c) added to a dispersion of activated, air-containing microcapsular release agents; (d) added to the emulsion with the encapsulating agent, e.g., urea-formaldehyde; or (e) added in any combination of methods (a), (b), (c) and (d). The production of air-containing microcapsules in this manner is described in detail in U.S. Patent 3,585,149.

The process for providing the precursor microcapsules may be described briefly as a simple admixing of at least four ingredients. These ingredients are: a water-immiscible oily material; an amphiphilic emulsifying agent; at least one solution comprising a polymeric resin, the solution selected from the group consisting of:

(1) solutions comprising a hydrophobic, thermoplastic resin as the solute, the resin not having appreciable solubility in the oily material, and a water- and oil-miscible organic liquid as the solvent, the thermoplastic resin being capable of being separated in solid particle form from solution upon dilution with water;

(2) solutions comprising a partially condensed thermosetting resin as the solute and water as the solvent, the resin condensate being capable of being separated in solid particle form from solution upon dilution with water, and

(3) mixtures of (1) and (2); and,

water in a quantity sufficient to cause the separation of at least one of the polymeric resins from solution.

The sequence of the admixing must be such that encapsulation of the emulsion by at least one of the synthetic resins in the admixture by dilution and ultimate separation from solution in solid particle form about a nucleus of oil in water upon dilution with water occurs no sooner than simultaneously with the formation of the emulsion.

The water-immiscible oily material forms the core of the precursor microcapsules and is driven from the microcapsules and replaced by air upon activation. Especially preferred lipophilic nucleus materials include mineral spirits, benzene, xylene, toluene, styrene, turpentine, and oils having a like volatility.

Exemplary of the amphiphilic emulsifying agents which can be used in the process are: naturally-occurring, lyophilic colloids including gums, proteins and polysaccharides, such as gum arabic, gum tragacanth, agar, gelatin, and starch; and synthetic materials such as hydroxyethylcellulose, methylcellulose, polyvinyl alcohol, polyvinylpyrrolidone, and copolymers of methyl vinyl ether and maleic anhydride.

The preferred thermoplastic resins are those containing nonionizable groups, since the extent to which a resin ionizes has an ultimate effect on the resin's hydrophilic-hydrophobic properties. Resins such as polyvinyl chloride and polystyrene are nonionizable, and are, therefore, preferred.

The partially condensed, thermosetting resins which may be used must also be of a hydrophobic nature in their solid, infusible state. These resins comprise that broad class of compositions defined as formaldehyde condensation products. The preferred formaldehyde condensation products are partially-condensed melamine-formaldehyde, phenol-formaldehyde and urea-formaldehyde resins.

Example 1: 50 g of mineral spirits are emulsified with a mixture of 112.5 g of 20% by weight of a benzylated starch emulsifier solution in water and 6 g of a 28.6% by weight solution of a chromium complex of a stearic acid in isopropanol. The foregoing ingredients are emulsified in a Waring blender until the average particle size of the emulsion droplets is about 1 μ. Next, 10 g of an aqueous B-stage urea-formaldehyde condensate (60.8% by weight solids) are slowly added to the emulsion with continued agitation.

A paper substrate is coated with the resulting microcapsular release coating and is dried at a temperature of about 170°C for a period of time sufficient to drive the mineral spirits core material from the microcapsules and replace the oil with air. The resulting paper has excellent release properties and water-resistance. The TAPPI opacity of the release paper is 92.5 percentage points which is equivalent to a 21.0 unit increase over the opacity of the original uncoated paper. The release paper has a coat weight of only 4.6 pounds per ream.

Example 2: 56 parts by weight of a high viscosity polyvinyl alcohol (Denka EP-130) are dissolved into 644 parts by weight of water to provide a homogenous solution. Next, 112 parts by weight of an aliphatic hydrocarbon oil having a boiling range of 160° to 180°C are dispersed in the polyvinyl alcohol solution by emulsification.

Emulisification is continued until the oil droplets have an average diameter of about 0.5 μ. Next 21 parts by weight of a solution containing 7 parts water and

14 parts of a modified melamine-formaldehyde resin are added to the emulsion at a temperature of 40°C. The emulsion is continuously agitated for a period of about 10 minutes, and then 7 parts by weight of a silicone-polyglycol copolymer are added with continued agitation until the secondary release agent is uniformly distributed throughout the emulsion.

The resulting release composition is applied to a paper substrate at a concentration of 4.5 lb/3,000 ft^2 of paper. The resulting release paper is dried for 30 minutes at a temperature of 60°C to drive off the oil.

In order to test the release properties of the coated release paper, a commercial cellophane tape is coated with a rubber-based pressure-sensitive adhesive and is applied to the coated release paper. The resulting laminate has a release value of 20 grams per inch when tested on a Keil Tester.

A cellulose acetate tape coated with an acrylic pressure-sensitive adhesive is applied to a second sample of the release paper. The resulting laminate has a release value of 75 grams per inch when tested on a Keil Tester.

Example 3: 140 parts by weight of a monofunctionally-substituted starch (Emulsicote 87) are dispersed in 560 parts by weight of water at a temperature of 40°C. The resulting suspension is heated to a temperature of 80°C with continuous stirring for a total time of 1 hour. Next, 140 parts by weight of an aliphatic hydrocarbon having a boiling point range of 160° to 180°C are dispersed by emulsification in the starch solution which had been cooled to a temperature of 40°C.

The emulsification is continued until the size of the oil droplets reaches an average diameter of about 0.5 μ. Next, 67 parts by weight of a mixture containing 20 parts by weight water and 40 parts by weight of a modified melamine-formaldehyde resin are added to the emulsion with continued agitation. Finally, 18.9 parts by weight of a glycol polysiloxane are admixed with the microcapsular dispersion.

The resulting capsule-containing release composition is applied to a paper substrate to form a release paper at a concentration of 4.0 lb/300 ft^2 of the paper. The coated paper is then dried for a period of 30 minutes at a temperature of 60°C. A cellophane tape having a rubber-based pressure-sensitive adhesive is applied to the release paper and tested on a Keil Tester. The resulting laminate has a release value of 12 grams per inch.

A cellulose acetate tape that is coated with an acrylic pressure-sensitive adhesive is applied to a second sample of the release paper and the release properties of the resulting laminate are tested on a Keil Tester. This laminate has a release value of 45 grams per inch.

OPACIFIERS

Aldehyde Condensation Product Polymerized Using Amphiphilic Acid Catalyst

D.N. Vincent and R. Golden; U.S. Patent 4,087,581; May 2, 1978; assigned to Champion International Corporation found that opaque, substantially spherical microparticles are provided by a process which comprises forming a prepolymer of urea and formaldehyde and admixing an aqueous solution of the prepolymer with an oily material containing an emulsifying agent. A water-in-oil emulsion is thereby formed and an amphiphilic acid catalyst is admixed with the emulsion causing the prepolymer to polymerize. The resultant particles are admixed with an aqueous liquid, such as water, under conditions of brisk agitation while heating the particles to remove residual oily material. Optionally, the particles may be separated from the aqueous liquid.

Suitable water-immiscible oily materials include any organic solvent capable of acting as the continuous phase of a water-in-oil emulsion. The preferred solvents are those having a relatively low cost and a low toxicity, such as mineral spirits or xylene. The emulsifying agent is admixed with the oily material in amounts sufficient to provide preferably between about 0.02 and 0.08 part per part of oily material.

The preferred emulsifying agents are the ethylene oxide-propylene oxide block copolymeric condensation products (Pluronic and Tetronic). A suitable inorganic opacifying pigment, preferably TiO_2, may be provided in the emulsion.

The inorganic opacifying pigment becomes incorporated in the polymeric structure at a point depending upon its position during the polymerization step, e.g., at the particle-solvent interface or homogeneously distributed throughout the polymer phase.

The ratio of the internal, aqueous phase to the external, water-immiscible solvent phase is preferably in the range of between about 1 and 2 parts by weight of the internal phase per part by weight of the external phase. Although it is possible to utilize a higher ratio of internal to external phase, it is preferred to use an approximately 2:1 ratio.

Suitable polymerization catalysts are those polymerization catalysts that are soluble in the continuous oily phase, but which have a significant affinity for the internal, or water phase, such as anhydrous hydrochloric acid, SO_2, SO_3, BF_3, BF_3 etherate, titanium tetrachloride, phosphoric acid, phosphorus pentachloride, silicon tetrachloride, phosphorus trichloride, sulfuryl chloride, organic carboxylic acids and alkyl acid phosphates. The acid catalyst is employed in amounts necessary to bring the final pH of the prepolymer phase to a pH of between about 1 and 2.

The catalyst is added at about ambient temperatures under mild agitation, preferably in the temperature range of 10° to 25°C. The polymerization reaction is exothermic, resulting in a temperature rise, so that the polymerization reaction occurs at temperatures preferably in the range of between 40° and 50°C.

Example 1: 90 g of urea are added to a solution of 165 g of 37% aqueous formaldehyde and 45 g of water, adjusted to pH 9.3 with NaOH and heated for 1 hour at 65° to yield a prepolymer solution containing about 50% solids. Using a Waring blender, 140 g of this prepolymer solution are emulsified in a solution of 6 g of a polyethylene oxide-polypropylene oxide block copolymer (Pluronic L 122) emulsifier dissolved in 100 g of toluene to produce a low viscosity water-in-oil emulsion.

The emulsion then is treated with 4 ml of a 33% by weight solution of titanium tetrachloride in toluene, resulting in an exothermic reaction which raises the temperature from about 28° to 50°C. After stirring for 2 hours, the resulting solvent dispersion consists of water droplets and solid polymer particles dispersed in the oil phase, with little or no tendency for coagulation of the polymer particles. This is separated into a clear supernatant phase, containing the oily solvent and some of the emulsifying agent, and a heavier phase, the inverted sludge, containing about 40% solids and about 20% oily solvent. The phase separation is accomplished by centrifugation. The inverted sludge is redispersed in about 200 g of water and is subjected to high-shear agitation while heating to steam distill off the oily solvent as a mixture with a portion of the excess water.

The resulting product is free of toluene and consists of an aqueous dispersion of 0.25 to 2 μ polymer particles, which have fused together into substantially spherical agglomerates (super-particles) 1 to 5 μ in diameter. The super-particles are made basic with ammonia and blended with a carboxylated styrene-butadiene rubber latex paper coating adhesive [Dow 620 SBR (10 parts by weight latex solids to 100 parts polymer solids)] and coated on a paper substrate.

The Kubelka-Munk scatter coefficient of the paper coating is measured using a Huygen Model 2100 digital opacimeter and computational methods described in the literature. A scatter coefficient of approximately 4,000 cm^2/g is obtained. Formulated and coated under the same conditions, a water-dispersible paper-coating grade of anatase TiO_2 gives coatings with a scatter coefficient of 3,800 to 4,000 cm^2/g.

Example 2: 200 g of a prepolymer solution prepared by heating 165 g of 37% aqueous formaldehyde, 45 g of water, 89 g of urea and 1 g of melamine, adjusted to pH 9.3 with sodium hydroxide, at 70°C for 1 hour are emulsified in a solution of 6 g of a polyethylene oxide-polypropylene oxide block copolymer attached to a central amine-functional group (Tetronic 1502) which acts as an emulsifying agent, dissolved in 100 g of xylene. 0.06 meq of sulfur dioxide (as a 4 N solution in xylene) are added to the water-in-oil emulsion, resulting in a temperature rise from about 28° to 48°C. After 1 hour the resulting solvent dispersion is centrifuged, the inverted sludge phase is mixed with water and steam distilled under high-shear agitation. The product is free of residual xylene, and a coating on paper, prepared as described in Example 1, has a scatter coefficient of about 4,500 cm^2/g.

Example 3: Paper handsheets were prepared using microcapsular opacifiers prepared as described in Example 1 and anatase titanium dioxide as fillers, added to the furnish to enhance opacity and brightness.

Three samples of a 300 g air-dry mixture of 50% pine and 50% hardwood pulps, each, were disintegrated in a dynapulper and were refined in a valley beater to a CFS of 250 to 350. After each batch was pressed and shredded individually, the three batches were combined and the composite was shredded until a 10.0 g sample gave a CFS of 275 to 325. Moisture of the composite was obtained by dispersing several 10.0 g samples in 100 ml of distilled water under a Hamilton Beach dispersator for 2 to 3 minutes, forming pads in a Buchner funnel, drying the pads on a hot plate, and calculating the percentage moisture. This result was used to calculate bone dry weights of fiber for paper furnish formulations.

Nine handsheets were prepared for each of the filler pigment samples (three at 5, 10, and 15% as bone dry weight, respectively) by weighing out 3.0 g bone dry samples of fiber into plastic bottles, adding the appropriate weight of filler (0.1, 0.30, and 0.45 g bone dry) as necessary, diluting with distilled water to 110 ml total volume, dispersing under the Hamilton Beach dispersator for 3 minutes, and forming in a Noble and Wood sheet mold, with the following results:

. . . Opacifiers, %. . . .		GE Brightness F/W	TAPPI Opacity
–	–	78.9/79.7	76.6
TiO_2	5	81.4/82.2	81.1
TiO_2	10	82.9/83.6	84.5
TiO_2	15	84.1/85.4	87.1
Microcapsule (Ex. 1)	5	81.5/82.2	80.5
Microcapsule (Ex. 1)	10	83.7/85.2	84.6
Microcapsule (Ex. 1)	15	84.5/86.1	86.6

The microcapsular opacifiers compared favorably with anatase titanium dioxide in this application.

Vesiculated Silica Microspheres

The process of *L.S. Sandell; U.S. Patent 4,011,096; March 8, 1977; assigned to E.I. DuPont de Nemours and Co.* provides vesiculated silica microspheres containing from 0 to 90% by weight of pigment based on the total weight of the microspheres, the microspheres having an average diameter from 0.5 to 50 μ, the maximum diameter of the vesicles being less than 50 μ and the volume of the vesicles being from 5 to 95% of the microspheres. The vesiculated silica microspheres are substantially spheroidal and, preferably, have a substantially smooth, continuous surface. The average diameter of the microspheres is preferably less than 50 μ, e.g., when used as a paper filler, and less than 25 μ, e.g., when used as an opacifying agent in paint.

The microspheres contain at least one and preferably a plurality of vesicles. The vesicles exist primarily in the form of discrete, substantially spheroidal bubbles which are distributed throughout the silica microsphere and defined by the continuous silica component of the microsphere. The average diameter of the vesicles can range from 0.1 μ to less than 50 μ, and preferably from 0.1 to 1.0 μ. The total volume of the vesicles is preferably from 10 to 80% of the total volume of the microsphere. The vesicles are preferably completely enclosed within the microsphere, i.e., are encased in a substantially continuous shell.

The vesiculated silica microspheres are prepared by the steps of:

(a) forming an oil-in-water emulsion by contacting a siliceous aqueous phase with a first oil phase, the siliceous aqueous phase composed of water and at least one silicon compound selected from the group consisting of colloidal silica and alkali metal silicates; the first oil phase composed of at least one water-immiscible hydrocarbon selected from the group consisting of liquid and low melting aliphatic and aromatic hydrocarbons, distributed in at least one of the phases is at least one oil-in-water emulsifying agent;

(b) forming an oil-in-water-in-oil emulsion by contacting the oil-in-water emulsion formed in (a) with a second oil phase, the second oil phase composed of a nonionic water-in-oil emulsifying agent and at least one water-immiscible hydrocarbon selected from the group consisting of aliphatic, aromatic and chlorinated hydrocarbons;

(c) adding an acid to the oil-in-water-in-oil emulsion formed in (b), the acid being added in an amount from 0.5 to 2.0 times the amount of the acid needed to react stoichiometrically with the total amount of base present in the siliceous aqueous phase of (a) to gel the siliceous aqueous phase and form a slurry of vesiculated silica microspheres; and

(d) separating the vesiculated silica microspheres from the slurry formed in (c). To insure that the microspheres are freed from any residual oil from the second oil phase on the surface of the microspheres, the separated microspheres of (d) can be

(e) dispersed in an aqueous or alcoholic solution of a hydrophilic surfactant,

(f) separated from the solution of surfactant, and

(g) washed with water or alcohol.

By dispersing the microspheres in an aqueous or alcoholic solution of hydrophilic surfactant in accordance with (e), any residual oil on the surface of the microspheres is dispersed in the surfactant solution which is then separated from the microspheres in step (f) by conventional techniques such as filtration. Washing the microspheres with water or alcohol in accordance with (g) insures the removal of any residual surfactant or salts formed during processing which may remain on the surface of the microspheres.

For optimum effectiveness as an opacifying agent the vesiculated silica microspheres should be activated, i.e., the first oil phase present within the vesicles should be removed leaving the vesicles essentially gaseous. Prior to use in a coating composition or filler, the microspheres can be activated rapidly by heating or slowly by allowing the microspheres to dry at room temperature for a sufficient length of time. The activation can be considered complete when the microspheres appear substantially opaque on microscopic examination.

The appearance of opacity in the activated microspheres indicates the presence of a majority of vesicles having a diameter of less than about 1 μ, and particularly in the range of 0.1 to 1.0 μ, which provides increased light scattering efficiency and, therefore, opacity. The activation process may occur after the microspheres are incorporated in an end use system, e.g., a paint vehicle or a fibrous substrate, by drying after application of the composition containing the microspheres to a substrate.

The microspheres of the process are particularly useful as high performance opacifying agents in surface coatings, such as latex paints. In such an application, it is desirable that the microspheres be pigmented, preferably with titanium dioxide. The microspheres may be added dry, or preferably as an aqueous wetcake to a preformulated aqueous latex emulsion. For example, from 30 to 70% by volume of microspheres, based on the total volume of solids in the paint composition, may be mixed with a typical starting paint or masterbatch emulsion formulated at about 34 PVC (pigment volume concentration) and containing about 3 lb/gal (0.36 kg/liter) of TiO_2 with little or no extender.

The microspheres are also useful as an opacifying agent and filler for fibrous substrates such as paper. In the paper industry, fillers such as TiO_2, clay or calcium carbonate are added to the paper furnish prior to formation of the fibrous web on the papermaking machine. Since these fillers generally contain particles of less than 1 μ in diameter, a substantial portion of the filler passes through the fibrous web and remains in the white water. The microspheres of the process have higher retention than the common fillers because of their larger particle size and at the same time provide high opacity.

Example 1: 1 volume of a 38% by weight solution of sodium silicate (ratio of SiO_2 to Na_2O = 3.25) is diluted with 4 volumes of water. A siliceous aqueous phase is then prepared by mixing 2.5 ml of an octylphenoxy polyethoxyethanol [a nonionic oil-in-water emulsifying agent (Triton X-405)] and 30 ml the previously prepared diluted solution of sodium silicate. A first oil phase is prepared by mixing 5 ml of an ethoxylated alcohol [a nonionic oil-in-water emulsifying agent (Merpol SH)] in 25 ml of cyclohexane in a 4 oz wide mouth jar. The first oil phase is then stirred by attaching the 4 oz wide mouth jar to a conventional mixing apparatus, i.e., a Chemapec Model E1 vibromixer fitted with a 45 mm stirrer disc.

The oil-in-water emulsion is prepared by slowly adding the above prepared siliceous aqueous phase to the first oil phase with stirring. After complete addition of the siliceous aqueous phase, stirring is continued for 5 minutes. A brilliant white oil-in-water emulsion is formed containing oil droplets having an approximate average diameter of less than 2 μ.

To form an oil-in-water-in-oil emulsion, 10 ml of the above prepared oil-in-water emulsion is mixed with 30 ml of a second oil phase consisting of 2 volumes of cyclohexane, 3 volumes of carbon tetrachloride and 0.5 volume of sorbitan monooleate [a nonionic water-in-oil emulsifying agent (Span 80)] in a 4 oz wide mouth jar. The mixture is stirred for 1 minute by the conventional mixing apparatus described above.

While stirring is continued, a mixture consisting of 30 ml of the second oil phase described above and 0.25 ml of glacial acetic acid are added to the oil-in-water-in-oil emulsion prepared above to form an oil slurry of the silica microspheres. Stirring is continued for 4 minutes after addition is complete.

The silica microspheres are separated from the oil phase by centrifugation. The microspheres are then mixed with a 50% by volume aqueous solution of a hydrophilic fatty acid ester [a nonionic oil-in-water emulsifying agent (Tween 20)] and separated from the aqueous solution by centrifugation and the supernatant liquid discarded. The microspheres are then washed by repeated centrifugation in water to a specific resistance of at least 20,000 ohm-cm.

In the first wash water the microsphere suspension has a pH of 5.1. Examination of a drop of the aqueous suspension with a light microscope shows discrete spherical microspheres averaging about 10 μ in diameter. A drop of the aqueous suspension is placed on a glass slide and heated on a hot plate over low heat for a few minutes to remove the liquid entrained in the vesicles. The microspheres are examined under a microscope and found to be predominately opaque, indicating the presence of vesicles from 0.1 to 1 μ in diameter. Examination of the microspheres by scanning electron microscopy reveals uniform spheres with generally smooth surfaces and occasional small surface irregularities. A fractured sample of the microspheres shows vesicles with an average diameter of about 1 μ.

Example 2: The procedure of Example 1 is followed except that the first oil phase consists of 25 ml of a paraffin solvent [BP about 190°C (Exxon Low Odor Paraffinic Solvent)] and 4 ml of the oil-in-water emulsifying agent described in Example 1.

The resulting vesiculated silica microspheres have an average diameter of about 15 μ and become opaque upon heating indicating the presence of vesicles from 0.1 to 1 μ in diameter.

Example 3: The procedure of Example 1 is followed except that 3 g of titanium dioxide pigment (TiPure R-900), and 2.5 ml of the octylphenoxy polyethoxyethanol described in Example 1 are mixed with 30 ml of the diluted sodium silicate solution by ultrasonics and the first oil phase contains 4 ml of the oil-in-water emulsifying agent described in Example 1.

The resulting vesiculated silica microspheres containing TiO_2 have an average diameter of about 15 μ. The microspheres develop additional opacity upon heating. Under a scanning electron microscopy, the microspheres appear slightly irregular in shape and exhibit textured surfaces. A fractured sample of the microspheres shows entrained titanium dioxide particles and an average vesicle diameter of about 1 μ.

Example 4: The procedure of Example 1 is followed except that the first oil phase is prepared by dispersing 6 g of the titanium dioxide pigment described in Example 3 and 4 ml of the oil-in-water emulsifying agent described in Example 1 in 25 ml of the paraffinic solvent described in Example 2 and 2 ml of a lyophilic ethoxylated alcohol [a nonionic emulsifying agent (Merpol OA)].

The resulitng vesiculated silica microspheres containing TiO_2 are nonuniformly sized microspheres having an average diameter of about 50 μ.

Vesiculated Crosslinked Polyester Granules

It has been proposed that granules of vesiculated polymers with diameters of the order of 0.5 to 500 μ be used in paints as matting or texturing agents. By vesiculated granules is meant granules of polymer which comprise a plurality of internal cells or vesicles. Ideally, each vesicle is formed as a discrete entity within a mass of nonporous polymer, i.e., the polymer granule does not have a continuous porosity extended from one cell to another, but comprises a plurality of discrete isolated vesicles surrounded by a continuous wall of polymer. They may be present in a minor proportion of imperfect vesicles in which some of the polymer defining the wall of the vesicles has either not formed or has been broken away, allowing entry from one vesicle to its neighbor. Thus, it is a characteristic feature of granules having a vesiculated structure that while they may well be vapor-permeable, they are not normally permeable to liquids.

When vesiculated polymer granules in which the vesicles are vapor-filled are incorporated in a paint composition, they can, unlike extender pigments used hitherto as flatting agents in paint, contribute opacity to a dry film of the paint by reason of their vesiculated structure. In order to do this effectively it has been proposed that the granule diameter should be at least five times the mean vesicle diameter. Further gains in opacity may be made by pigmenting the granules.

R.H. Gunning, B.C. Henshaw and F.J. Lubbock; U.S. Patent 4,137,380; January 30, 1979; assigned to Dulux Australia Ltd., Australia have found that vesiculated granules of crosslinked polyester resin can be prepared in the form of an aqueous slurry, the granules of which are dimensionally stable.

In the process of preparing an aqueous slurry of dimensionally stable vesiculated crosslinked polyester resin granules:

(a) droplets of water are dispersed in a solution of a carboxylated unsaturated polyester resin which has an acid value of 10 to 45 mg KOH/g in ethylenically unsaturated monomer copolymerizable therewith and which has a solubility in water at 20°C of less than 5% by weight and in the presence of a water-soluble polyamine which contains at least 3 amine groups per molecule and which has a dissociation constant in water (pK_a value) of 8.5 to 10.5, at a concentration such that there are 0.3 to 1.4 amine groups present per polyester resin carboxyl group;

(b) the unsaturated polyester resin solution containing disperse particles of water is stably dispersed as globules in water in the presence of a dispersion stabilizer for the disperse globules; and

(c) addition polymerization is then initiated within the globules which are thereby converted to granules of crosslinked vesiculated polyester granules.

If it is required to pigment the vesicles or the polymer of the granules then the desired pigment must be predispersed in the abovedescribed water droplets and polyester resin solution respectively.

Example 1: The preparation of dimensionally stable vesiculated crosslinked polyester resin granules having a diameter of approximately 30 μ is as follows: A polyester resin made from phthalic anhydride, fumaric acid and propylene glycol (mol ratios 1:3:4.4) was dissolved in styrene to a concentration of 70% by weight. The solution had a Gardner-Holdt viscosity of Z_3. The acid value of the solid polyester was 22.0 mg KOH/g.

A colloid solution A was prepared by dissolving 1.8 parts of a fast dissolving grade of hydroxyethylcellulose in 326.2 parts of water and a colloid solution B was prepared by dissolving 7.5 parts of a poly(vinyl alcohol/vinyl acetate) in 92.5 parts of water. The poly(vinyl alcohol/vinyl acetate) was a partially hydrolyzed poly(vinyl acetate) of approximate average molecular weight 125,000, 87 to 89% hydrolyzed and with a viscosity (as a 4% weight aqueous solution at 20°C) of 35 to 45 cp.

The following ingredients were mixed using the polyester solution described above.

	Parts
Polyester resin solution	91.0
Styrene	45.5
Diethylenetriamine	0.9
Benzoyl peroxide (50% active constituent in plasticizer)	7.5

The resulting homogeneous liquid was added, with constant mechanical agitation, to a mixture of: 90.0 parts, colloid solution B; 328.0 parts, colloid solution A; and 0.3 parts, diethylenetriamine.

Globules of disperse resin solution formed and the mixture was stirred vigorously until the globule size was 30 μ maximum. The stirring rate was then reduced and the following mixture added: 100.0 parts, water; and 1.5 parts, diethylaniline.

The resulting polymerization reaction leading to crosslinking of the polyester resin was detected by the resultant exotherm. The granules which formed were of about 30 μ maximum diameter and were observed to contain aqueous vesicles of about 1 μ diameter. When examined by transmitted light under a microscope the granules appeared translucent and brown, but as they dried out they became opaque. The degree of vesiculation was estimated to be about 70% by volume and the shrinkage was less than 5%.

Example 2: The preparation of dimensionally stable vesiculated crosslinked polyester resin granules of 20 μ maximum diameter, in which the vesicles contained pigment particles, is as follows: An aqueous mill base was prepared by blending together the following ingredients with a mechanical stirrer: 208.0 parts, titanium dioxide pigment; 0.8 parts, sodium hexametaphosphate; and 104.0 parts, water.

A water-in-oil type emulsion was prepared by vigorously stirring a mixture of 170 parts of aqueous mill base and 0.9 parts of diethylenetriamine into a mixture of 91.0 parts of polyester resin solution (as in Example 1) and 45.5 parts of styrene, to which was then added 7.5 parts of a 50% by weight paste of benzoyl peroxide in a plasticizer liquid.

The emulsion was then immediately poured into a mixture of: 328.0 parts, colloid solution A; and 90.0 parts colloid solution B (as per Example 1) and stirred vigorously until the particle size of the disperse globules was about 20 μ maximum diameter. The stirring rate was then reduced and 1.5 parts of diethylaniline added.

The batch was allowed to exotherm as the disperse resin solution polymerized to crosslinked polyester resin granules, which had a vesicle content of approximately 70% by volume.

Examination of fractured granules with a scanning electron microscope confirmed the presence of pigment particles within the vesicles. The granules had a shrinkage of 4%.

Interfacial Reaction Between Thermosetting Condensation Product and Water-Soluble Polymers

M.P. Powell; U.S. Patent 4,089,834; May 16, 1978; assigned to Champion International Corporation found that microcapsular opacifiers may be produced having excellent water-resistance, controlled wall strength, uniformity of particle size and which yield surface finishes having excellent hiding power when employed in surface coatings, such as paint films and the like.

The process for the formulation of microcapsular precursor opacifiers comprises admixing: (a) a solution comprising an oil-soluble, partially condensed thermosetting condensation product in a water-immiscible oily material; and (b) an aqueous solution of a water-soluble polymeric material, thereby forming an emulsion, the thermosetting condensation product and the water-soluble polymeric material being capable of interaction to form a solid, crosslinked resinous material, and subjecting the emulsion to conditions whereby the polymeric materials react to form microcapsules having solid capsular walls about a nucleus of the oily material. The precursor capsules are then treated to expel the oily core material and replace it with air.

Surprisingly, it has been discovered that by providing an oil-soluble, thermosetting condensation product wall-forming material in an oil phase and admixing this oily solution with a water-soluble polymer in an aqueous phase, microcapsular opacifiers are produced having unexpectedly good water-resistance. By providing the thermosetting condensation product in the oil phase, its distribution is confined within the capsule and thus forms the inside of the capsule wall. In this manner, substantially all of this polymeric material is efficiently utilized.

The oil-soluble, partially condensed, thermosetting condensation products include A-stage or B-stage resins, i.e., resins not having reached the infusible or insoluble stage. However, the B-stage resins are especially preferred.

Exemplary of suitable oil-soluble resins are the condensation reaction products of formaldehyde with phenols, such as, hydroxybenzene (phenol), m-cresol and 3,5-xylenol; carbamides, such as ureas; triazines, such as melamine; amino and amido compounds, such as aniline, p-toluenesulfonamide, ethylene urea and guanidine; ketones, such as acetone and cyclohexanone; aromatic hydrocarbons, such as naphthalene; and heterocyclic compounds, such as thiophene. Under the influence of heat, these resins change irreversibly from a fusible and/or soluble material into an infusible and insoluble material.

The preferred formaldehyde condensation products employed are partially-condensed melamine-formaldehyde, phenol-formaldehyde and urea-formaldehyde resins. The B-stage melamine- and urea-formaldehyde resins are especially preferred.

The preferred oily materials are those oils having a fairly high vapor pressure (high volatility), so that they can be completely and easily expelled through the micropores of the solid-walled microcapsules over a wide range of temperatures, e.g., by the application of moderate amounts of heat, e.g., –32° to 180°C, preferably between about 0° to 100°C. It is especially preferred to employ oils which can be driven from the microcapsules at temperatures conventionally employed in the drying of paper webs or paper coatings, e.g., about 85°C. Preferred oils include mineral spirits, benzene, xylene, toluene, styrene monomer, turpentine, and oils having a like volatility.

The water-soluble polymeric material which reacts chemically with the partially condensed formaldehyde condensation product dissolved in the oil phase may be any suitable water-soluble polymer capable of reacting with the formaldehyde condensation polymer at the oil-water interface to form a solid microcapsular shell. Suitable water-soluble polymers which may be employed include thermoplastic resins, such as polyvinyl alcohol, methylcellulose, a styrene-maleic acid salt, e.g., the sodium or ammonium salt thereof, and the like. The preferred water-soluble polymer is a styrene-maleic acid ammonium salt.

In order to produce suitable opacifying agents, the microcapsules produced must have an average particle size of below about 1 μ, and preferably between about 0.25 and 0.8 μ.

Example 1: (a) 20 g of a 50% by weight melamine-formaldehyde solution in mineral spirits are diluted with 80 g of mineral spirits to a total weight of 100 g of solution. The melamine-formaldehyde solution is emulsified with 150 g of a 5% by weight aqueous solution of a copolymer of styrene-maleic acid ammonium salt. Emulsification is continued until particles of the desired size and uniformity, viz, below about 1 μ, are obtained.

Next, the emulsion is heated to a temperature of 50°C while under agitation for approximately 6 hours to induce an interfacial chemical reaction between the partially condensed formaldehyde condensation polymer and the styrene-maleic acid copolymer at the water-oil interface thereby forming microcapsules. A partial curing of the capsules is effected during the heating period. The extent of curing may be varied depending upon desired properties of the final product and its application.

(b) The microcapsular dispersion produced in (a) is activated to remove the oily core by injecting the dispersion by means of a fine air feed nozzle into a spray drying chamber heated to a temperature of about 100°C. Optionally, the activated microcapsules may be subjected to a subsequent drying treatment in a fluidized bed in order to provide additional crosslinking of the wall materials. The dried air-containing microcapsular product is collected, mixed with inorganic pigments, and the mixture is dispersed in an aqueous paint system.

The paint is applied to a substrate and the resulting paint film has excellent hiding power and resistance to water.

Example 2: (a) An aqueous solution of a 7% by weight styrene-maleic acid ammonium salt is prepared having a pH of 7.0 at 25°C. Meanwhile, a 20% by weight solution of a melamine-formaldehyde (50% by weight in xylene-butanol) in mineral spirits is prepared by simple dilution of the melamine-formaldehyde with the mineral spirits.

An oil-in-water emulsion is prepared in a high shear mixer by admixing 100 g of the melamine-formaldehyde in mineral spirits solution with 150 g of the aqueous styrene-maleic acid copolymer solution at a temperature of 25°C.

Next, 10 ml of a 5% by weight solution of sulfamic acid is added to the emulsion and dispersed well therein. The emulsion is then heated at a temperature of 40°C for a period of 2 hours to chemically react the styrene-maleic acid with the melamine-formaldehyde and form precursor microcapsules containing oil.

(b) Clay and a latex binder is added to the microcapsular dispersion of Example 2(a) to form an aqueous paint formulation. Next, the resulting paint system is coated onto a substrate and the paint film is dried at a temperature of about 100°C in order to drive the oily core material from the precursor capsules present in the paint film. The resulting paint has excellent water-resistance.

(c) The procedure of Example 2(b) is repeated with the exception that the paint film is permitted to dry at ambient temperature.

As in the case of the prior example, the film has good resistance to water.

VOID-CONTAINING MICROCAPSULES

From Thermoplastic or Thermosetting Resins

The process of *R.G. Temple; U.S. Patent 4,089,800; May 16, 1978; assigned to PPG Industries, Inc.* is capable of producing void-containing microcapsules having an average diameter of from about 0.1 to 250 μ. This involves preparing a solution containing an organic polymer, a good solvent for the polymer and an organic liquid nonsolvent which is miscible with the polymer solvent. The solution is then atomized into a bath containing a liquid which is miscible with the polymer solvent, but which is immiscible with the nonsolvent. The bath liquid extracts the good solvent from the polymer solution, causing gellation of the polymer particles around discrete droplets of the nonsolvent, which are simultaneously precipitated out of the solution, thereby forming microcapsules having encapsulated therein droplets of the organic liquid nonsolvent. The nonsolvent can then be removed from the microcapsules by evaporation to produce void-containing microcaplues. These find use as opacifiers.

The organic polymers employed may be of the thermoplastic or thermosetting type. Examples of thermoplastic resins which may be used include cellulose derivatives, acrylic resins, polyolefins, polyamides, and polycarbonates.

A preferred group of thermoplastic polymers are copolymers of acrylates, such as 2-ethylhexyl acrylate, and/or methacrylates, such as methyl methacrylate, with up to 50% of a comonomer, such as dibutyl maleate or fumarate, butyl glycidyl maleate or fumarate and glycidyl methacrylate. These thermoplastic polymers may be prepared in or dissolved in a solvent, such as benzene, toluene, butanol, acetone, xylene, or the like.

The thermosetting resins which may be used are curable to a crosslinked thermoset condition by the use of either heat and/or a curing catalyst.

The thermosetting resin is selected from the group consisting of alkyd resins, carboxylic acid-amide interpolymers, and interpolymers of hydroxyl esters of ethylenically-unsaturated acids with at least one other polymerizable ethylenically-unsaturated monomer.

The solvents or solvent combinations employed will vary somewhat, depending on the particular resin utilized. When thermoplastic polymers are utilized, methylene chloride and acetone have been found to be particularly useful. Some of the preferred nonsolvents include water, n-heptane, ethanol and VM&P naphtha.

The weight ratio of the nonsolvent to the solvent generally falls in the range of from about 1:1 to 1:100 in solution compositions. The preferred ratio is from about 1:1 to 1:20, and the most preferred range is from 1:6 to about 1:20.

The basic requirement for the bath into which the above-described solution is atomized is that it contain a liquid which is miscible with the good polymer solvent and immiscible with the nonsolvent so that it will extract the polymer solvent from the solution. As will be apparent, the bath liquid must not be a solvent for the polymer if microcapsules are to be produced. Thus, appropriate bath liquids can be selected on the basis of the known physical properties of liquids and polymers. A preferred bath liquid is water.

In producing void-containing microcapsules by the method, the liquid nonsolvent is removed as by evaporation. The method is also applicable to producing microcapsules in which the nonsolvent can perform a secondary function in addition to the formation of the microcapsule and remains entrapped in the polymeric microcapsule until performance of the additional function is desired. Thus, the nonsolvent can be encapsulated in the polymeric microcapsules and remain entrapped until the wall is ruptured, punctured or worn away, or until it diffuses through the wall. The polymer of the polymer wall may be selected in that it is biodegradable, and thus slowly releases the entrapped nonsolvent. Accordingly, in some instances the nonsolvent may be a solid, liquid or a gas, depending upon the function desired.

For example, the nonsolvent may be a medicament; food; vitamin; mineral; biocide, such as insecticides; chemical reactant, such as curing agents, catalysts, and the like; herbicide, fungicide, mildewcide, and the like, as well as perfumes, odorants, fertilizers, repellents, and the like.

In addition, various adjuvants may be incorporated in the microcapsules, e.g., conventional pigments may be incorporated.

The compositions employed may be atomized at a solids content of from 0.5 to 35% by weight, based on the weight of the total composition, or higher when desired. The solids content will depend on the nature of the atomization apparatus, the molecular weight of the polymer, the strength of the solvents employed, the viscosity of the polymer and the temperature at which the composition is atomized. A solids content of from about 2 to 20% by weight, based on weight of total composition, is preferred.

The viscosity of the composition to be atomized should be such as to permit the formation of individual particles rather than the formation of strings of polymer, which is indicative of high viscosity. For this reason, it is usually desirable that the molecular weight of the polymer be less than about 140,000, and preferably less than 100,000 and, most preferably, less than 90,000.

Example 1: A solution was prepared by dissolving 45 g of polymethyl methacrylate in 850 g of acetone, then 200 g of a nonsolvent, n-heptane, were added slowly while the solution was maintained under constant agitation. The solution was then sprayed at room temperature utilizing a siphon spray gun into a water bath maintained under agitation with a Cowles mixer. The nonsolvent was then evaporated to provide void-containing microcapsules having a particle size of from about 0.1 to 250 μ in diameter.

Example 2: In this example, Example 1 was repeated except that the solution contained 45 g polymethyl methacrylate, 900 g acetone solvent and 100 g n-heptane nonsolvent. The solution was sprayed into a water bath utilizing conditions similar to those of Example 1, and upon evaporation of the nonsolvent, void-containing microcapsules were produced.

Example 3: A solution consisting of 45 g of polymethyl methacrylate, 900 g of acetone (solvent) and 200 g of n-heptane (nonsolvent) was prepared as above. However, in this example, the solution was sprayed into the water bath utilizing a standard electrostatic spraying system operated at 20 to 40 kV and a distance of from 1 to 3 ft. As in the previous examples, the water extracted the polymer solvent from solution, causing the formation of microcapsules containing droplets of the nonsolvent. Drying of these microcapsules evaporated the nonsolvent to produce void-containing microcapsules.

In Situ Production of Void Microcapsules on a Substrate

S. Babil, J.A. Claar and R.G. Temple; U.S. Patent 4,064,294; December 20, 1977; assigned to PPG Industries, Inc. have also found that microcapsules can be produced in situ in a film formed from a water-based coating composition or, alternatively, during the manufacturing process of the water-based coating composition. A principal process involves the in situ production of void-containing microcapsules in a film formed from a water-based coating composition. This principal process involves as a first step the preparation of a polymer composition which may be a homogeneous solution containing a water-immiscible organic polymer, a water-immiscible lower volatility nonsolvent which is miscible with the solvent; or an emulsion containing as the continuous phase a water-immiscible organic polymer dissolved in a water-immiscible solvent for the polymer and, as the discontinuous phase, droplets of a lower volatility nonsolvent dispersed in the continuous phase.

The polymer composition is then emulsified under agitation and in the presence of a surfactant into the water-based coating composition. The coating composition containing this emulsified polymer composition is then applied to a substrate and the solvent is evaporated from the polymer composition to produce microcapsules containing discrete droplets of the nonsolvent. Subsequent drying of the water-based coating and evaporation of the nonsolvent produce a film having incorporated therein structured, closed cell, void-containing microcapsules with the voids serving to provide opacity and gloss control to the film. In an alternative to the principal process, microcapsules containing the nonsolvent are produced in situ in the water-based coating composition prior to forming a film therefrom.

The process is extremely versatile and flexible and, in addition to providing for the in situ production of void-containing microcapsules in a film or microcapsules containing nonsolvent in the water-based coating composition from which the film is formed permits the in situ production in the film of microcapsules in which pigments are entrapped in the voids or in the polymeric walls of the microcapsule or in which certain nonsolvents which serve a secondary function remain entrapped in the microcapsules until performance of the function is desired. Such nonsolvents include, for instance, medicaments, minerals, biocides, perfumes, chemical reactants, fertilizers, etc.

A wide variety of organic polymers may be utilized in preparing the abovementioned homogeneous solution with the sole criterion being that they are insoluble in water. Such polymers may be of either the thermoplastic or thermosetting resin types.

The thermoplastic resin is selected from the group consisting of an alkyl acrylate or methacrylate, polystyrene, copolymers of styrene and vinyl monomers, polyolefins, and polycarbonates. The thermosetting resin is selected from the group consisting of interpolymers of hydroxyesters of ethylenically-unsaturated acids with at least one other polymerizable, ethylenically-unsaturated monomer, alkyd resins, and carboxylic acid-amide interpolymers.

The solvents or solvent combinations employed herein will vary somewhat, depending on the particular resin utilized. When thermoplastic polymers are utilized, methylene chloride has been found to be a particularly useful solvent. Some of the preferred nonsolvents include n-heptane and VM&P naphtha. In the preparation of the solution, weight ratio of nonsolvent to solvent is described in U.S. Patent 4,089,800. The surfactant utilized may be an anionic surfactant, a nonionic surfactant, a cationic surfactant, an amphoteric surfactant or combinations thereof. The surfactant is generally present in an amount ranging from about 1 to 10% by weight, based on the polymer solids employed. The surfactant selection will depend upon the polymer, solvent and nonsolvent utilized.

For example, when water is emulsified in a polymer solution of methylene chloride, surfactants such as a sodium salt of a sulfate ester of an alkylphenoxy poly(ethyleneoxy)ethanol and dioctyl sodium sulfosuccinate have been successfully employed and are preferred.

Various water-based coating compositions may be utilized in practicing the porcess. Thus, any of the water-based coating compositions utilized or known in the coatings industry heretofore may be employed. For example, water-based coating compositions derived from aqueous polymer lattices (e.g., latex-based coatings or paints), water-soluble polymers, aqueous polymer emulsions and aqueous polymer dispersions are suitable. The preferred water-based coating compositions employed are those derived from polymer lattices.

The preferred coalescable polymers for use in lattices are acrylic polymers, i.e., polymers containing one or more acrylates or methacrylates, copolymers of vinyl acetate with a minor amount of a vinyl halide or an ester of an unsaturated acid, and copolymers of vinyl aromatic hydrocarbons with alkyl acrylates, dienes or other monomers.

Example 1: This illustrates the production of void-containing microcapsules in situ in a film in which a homogeneous solution is employed as the microcapsule precursor material.

A homogeneous solution was first prepared by admixing 60 g of polystyrene (molecular weight 70,000) with 200 g of methylene chloride (solvent) and 200 g of n-heptane (nonsolvent). This solution was then emulsified under agitation using a standard Cowles mixer into a standard acrylic latex in the presence of a surfactant. The acrylic latex utilized was a 50% total solids acrylic polymer latex derived from a monomer mixture containing 43% methyl methacrylate, 55% butyl acrylate and 2% methacrylic acid [AC388 (Rohm and Haas)]. The surfactant utilized was the sodium salt of an alkylphenoxy poly(ethyleneoxy)ethanol (Alipal CO433). A sample of latex containing this emulsified solution (i.e., microcapsule precursor) was then sprayed, utilizing a conventional spray gun, onto a metal Q-panel (Bonderite 100) and permitted to air-dry. Upon drying, the resultant film exhibited opacity indicating the presence of void-containing microcapsules.

An additional sample of this latex was then applied to a microscope slide and Polaroid photographs of the latex sample were taken during the air-drying process, utilizing light from below the slides to show the presence of microcapsules. The photographs, in sequence, showed the presence of the microcapsule precursors (i.e., droplets of emulsified solution), the formation of microcapsules containing droplets of nonsolvent upon evaporation of the solvent, and the formation of void-containing microcapsules upon evaporation of the nonsolvent.

As will be understood, the microcapsules photographed during their formation with bottom light appeared black in coloration due to the deflection of the light passing from below. Application of top light to the dried film showed opacity (i.e., whiteness), proving that the void-containing microcapsules formed by the process provide opacity.

Example 2: This illustrates the production of void-containing microcapsules in situ in a film in which an emulsion is employed as the microcapsule precursor material.

An emulsion was prepared by first dissolving 15 g of polystyrene (molecular weight 70,000) in 300 g of methylene chloride to form a continuous phase polymer solution. Into this polymer solution was then emulsified (using a Cowles mixer) a mixture of 45 g of water, 3 g of Alipal CO433 surfactant and 2 g GAF RE410 (free acid of a complex organic phosphate ester), thereby forming as the discontinuous phase droplets of water dispersed in the continuous polymer solution phase. This emulsion was then emulsified under agitation utilizing a Cowles mixer, into an acrylic latex composition. The acrylic latex composition consisted of 300 g of AC388 acrylic latex, 300 g of water and 2 g of Empapol PO-18 (potassium oleate) surfactant to form a latex composition containing as the microcapsule precursor the above described emulsion. This latex composition was then applied to a substrate as in Example 1 and also permitted to air-dry. The resultant film showed opacity, indicating the presence in the film of in situ produced microcapsules.

MICROSPHERES

Cell-Specific, Biocompatible Microspheres

Knowledge of the nature, number and distribution of specific receptors on cell surfaces is of central importance for an understanding of the molecular basis underlying such biological phenomena as cell-cell recognition in development, cell communication and regulation by hormones and chemical transmitters, and differences in normal and tumor cell surfaces. In previous studies, the localization of antigens and carbohydrate residues on the surface of cells, notably red blood cells and lymphocytes, has been determined by bonding antibodies or lectins to such macromolecules as ferritin, hemocyanin or peroxidase which have served as markers for transmission electron microscopy. With advances in high resolution scanning electron microscopy (SEM), however, the topographical distribution of molecular receptors on the surfaces of cell and tissue specimens can be readily determined by similar histochemical techniques using newly developed markers resolvable by SEM.

Recently commercially available polystyrene latex particles have been utilized as immunologic markers for use in the SEM technique. The surface of such polystyrene particles is hydrophobic and hence certain types of macromolecules such as antibodies are adsorbed on the surface under carefully controlled conditions. However, such particles stick nonspecifically to many surfaces and molecules and this seriously limits their broad application. Though these particles, while of the proper density for separating adsorbed or labelled membranes from other membranes, are uncharged and are not capable of any derivatization by ionic or covalent bonding of protein and other biological molecules, and are thus limited to use to generalized studies on phagocytosis.

The preparation of small, stable, spherical particles which are biocompatible, i.e., do not interact nonspecifically with cells or other biological components and which contain functional groups to which specific proteins and other biochemical molecules can be covalently bonded is disclosed in U.S. Patent 3,957,741.

The hydroxyl or amino groups can be activated by cyanogen bromide for covalent bonding of proteins and other chemicals containing amino groups to the polymeric latex. Methacrylic acid residues which impart a negative charge onto the particles are likely to prevent nonspecific binding to cell surfaces and to provide carboxyl groups to which a variety of biochemical molecules can be covalently bonded using the carbodiimide method. Crosslinking of the polymeric matrix is essential to maintain the stability and size of the particles in both aqueous solution and in organic solvents commonly used in the fixation and dehydration of biological specimens for electron or light microscopy.

The polymeric microspheres ranging in diameter from 300 to 2000 A have been successfully utilized as biocompatible immunochemical markers of red blood cells and lymphocytes in scanning electron and light microscopy. However, the density of the microspheres is so close to that of the cell membranes that isolation of the cell membranes or bound receptor sites is not possible.

Amine-, hydroxyl- and/or carboxyl-substituted microspheres are provided in accordance with the process of *S.-P.S. Yen, A. Rembaum and R.S. Molday; U.S. Patent 4,035,316; July 12, 1977; assigned to California Institute of Technology* having a density of at least 1.30 g/cc, preferably above 1.40 g/cc, or a density below 1.15 g/cc, preferably below 1.08 g/cc. The density of cellular organelles is of the order of about 1.20 g/cc. The beads of the process being considerably smaller than biological cells and being capable of binding a protein conjugate, can attach to specific receptor sites on the surface of the cell membrane and after fragmentation of the membrane can be recovered by sedimentation or centrifugation techniques.

The microspheres are synthesized by free radical initiated emulsion polymerization or high energy radiation induced copolymerization of a first ethylenically-unsaturated monomer containing a covalently bondable moiety such as hydroxyl, primary amine or carboxyl, and ethylenically-unsaturated comonomer having a density differing from the monomer by at least 15% and a crosslinking agent to form small, round microspheres at least 80% of which have a uniform diameter below 5 μ, and preferably below 1 μ, suitably 300 to 2000 A. The microspheres have a density above 1.3 or below 1.15 g/cc, are hydrophilic, hydrolytically stable, are biocompatible and have sufficient mechanical strength to be useful as an adsorbent in column or film chromotography, gel filtration and permeation separation and analysis. The microspheres are of well characterized structure and outstanding purity and the hydrophilic properties and size and mechanical properties can be systematically varied by selection of monomer and polymerization conditions.

The microspherical beads containing hydroxyl, carboxyl or amine groups can be covalently bonded to antibodies and other biological materials and are useful as specific cell markers for scanning electron microscopy. The particles are found to bind to hormones, toxins, lectins, and other molecules and have application in the detection and localization of a variety of cell surface receptors. Particles tagged with fluorescent dye or radioactive molecules serve as sensitive markers for fluorescent microscopy and as reagents for quantitiative study of cell surface components by covalently bonding lectins, antigens, hormones and other molecules to these spheres, and detection and localization of specific carbohydrate residues. Antibodies, hormone receptors and other specific cell surface components can also be determined.

These reagents also have application in highly sensitive radioimmune assays, as visual markers for fluorescent and transmission electron microscopy, for radioactive quantitation of specific cell surface receptors and as potential therapeutic reagents.

Technique for isolation of cell membranes and membrane receptors comprises the steps of covalently bonding an antibody or antigen molecule to the microspheres. The bonded microspheres are then to be added to cells to label and bind to specific conjugate receptor, antigen or antibody sites on the cell membrane. The labelled cells are then disrupted into fragments by nitrogen decompression, homogenization or other standard procedure. The membrane fragments are then centrifuged to equilibrium on linear density gradients.

The first covalently bondable monomer is suitably a primary amine, carboxyl, or hydroxyl substituted acrylic monomer and should comprise at least 10% by weight of the monomer mixture, generally from 20 to 60% thereof. Exemplary monomers are acrylamide, an hydroxy lower alkyl acrylate, an amino lower alkyl acrylate, acrylic acid, methacrylic acid or the like. Representative monomers may be selected from compounds of the formula:

$$R^1-\underset{\displaystyle\quad}{\overset{\overset{\displaystyle CH_2}{\|}}{C}}-\overset{\overset{\displaystyle O}{\|}}{C}-O-R^2-Z$$

where R^1 is H or lower alkyl of 1 to 8 carbon atoms, R^2 is alkylene of 1 to 12 carbon atoms, Z is OH or R^3-N-R^4 where R^3 and R^4 are H, lower alkyl or lower alkoxy. 2-hydroxyethyl methacrylate, 3-hydroxypropyl methacrylate, 2-dimethylaminoethyl methacrylate and 2-aminoethyl methacrylate are readily available commercially.

Minor amounts of 0.35%, suitably 10 to 25% by weight of the monomer mixture may comprise a compatible comonomer such as a lower alkyl methacrylate, acrylic or methacrylic acid, styrene or vinyl toluene.

The crosslinking agent is present in the monomer mixture in an amount from 1 to 10% and is a liquid polyunsaturated compound such as a diene or a triene capable of addition polymerization with the unsaturated group of monomer. Suitable compounds are low molecular weight liquid polyvinyl compounds such as ethylene glycol dimethacrylate (EGD), divinyl benzene, trimethylolpropane trimethacrylate and N,N'-methylene-bisacrylamide.

The commercial forms (95%) of hydroxyethyl methacrylate (HEMA) and hydroxypropyl methacrylate (HPMA) as supplied contain small amounts of methacrylic acid, hydroxyalkoxyalkyl methacrylate and dimethacrylates–ethylene dimethacrylate in HEMA and propylene dimethacrylate in HPMA. HPMA is generally a mixture in which the principal monomers comprise 68 to 75% of 2-hydroxypropyl and 25 to 32% of 1-methyl-2-hydroxyethyl methacrylate.

The density varying comonomer is present in the monomer mixture in an amount sufficient to raise or lower the density to the desired range. It is to be realized that the crosslinked microspheres have a greater density than the monomers. The acrylic monomers and comonomers generally have a density of about 0.9 to 1.0 g/cc and they form microspheres having a density of about 1.24 g/cc. If one-half of the hydroxyethyl methacrylate monomer is replaced with a monomer such as trifluoroethyl methacrylate which has a density of 1.16 g/cc, about 30% higher, the resulting microsphere would have a density of about 1.42. Representative density varying comonomers are provided in the following table.

Comonomer	Density, g/cc
Trifluoroethyl methacrylate (TFEM)	1.16
Pentafluorostyrene	1.412
Vinyl ethyl ketone	0.985
Vinyl ethyl ether	0.76
Vinyl iodide	–
Vinyl bromide	1.5
Hexafluoropropyl methacrylate	1.16
Methacryloxymethyl pentamethyl disiloxane	0.903
1,3-Bis(methacryloxymethyl)-disiloxane	0.996

Emulsion polymerization is conducted at temperatures from about 60° to 120°C with agitation in presence of an inert gas such as nitrogen or argon in the presence of an emulsifier and free radical inhibitor. The monomers, emulsifier and inhibitor are introduced into distilled water in a container. The container is immersed in a heated bath. In about 1 hour nearly quantitative yields are achieved. Emulsifier and other ionic impurities are removed from the latex suspension on a mixed bed ion-exchange column and the microsphere particles are then dried. The density of the particles is then determined by centrifugation at 100,000 *g* for 12 hours on a linear sucrose gradient. The diameter of the particles was measured by transmission and scanning electron microscopy.

The surface active emulsifying agent is preferably present in an amount below 10% by weight of the monomer mixture, typically from 2 to 5% thereof, to minimize the after treatment for removal of the agent from the microsphere suspension. Suitable agents are ionic materials such as sodium dodecyl sulfate (SDS), sodium lauryl sulfate, sodium stearate or nonionic materials such as polyethylene oxide lauryl ether.

The free radical initiator may be present in amounts from 0.01 to 3% by weight of the monomer mixture and may be a persulfate, peroxide, azo or redox material. Suitable materials are ammonium persulfate (AP), benzoyl peroxide, lauroyl peroxide, t-butyl hydroperoxide, t-butyl perbenzoate, cumene peroxide, azodiisobutyronitrile, azodiisobutyro-amide or mixtures thereof with reducing agents such as sodium bisulfite or sodium thiosulfate.

Example: (a) 0.9 g of 2-hydroxyethyl methacrylate (HEMA), 0.3 g of methacrylic acid (MAA), 1.5 g of hexafluoroisopropyl methacrylate and 0.3 g of bis-acrylamide were combined with distilled water to form a 3% total monomer solution. 0.12 g of SDS and 0.012 g of AP were added and the container inhibited with argon was placed in a tumbling container and inserted in a 98°C bath for 1 hour.

400 A diameter microspheres in 99% yield having a density of 1.46 g/cc were recovered. Density was determined by means of a cesium chloride density gradient.

(b) An aqueous suspension of the beads of (a) (20 to 55 mg/ml) is adjusted to pH 10.5 and is activated with CNBr (10 to 20 mg/ml of suspension) at 25°C. The pH of the reaction mixture is maintained at 10.5 with 1 N NaOH. After 10 to 15 minutes, the activated beads are added to an equal volume of 5 mM dansyl-ϵ-lysine or $[^3H]$-glycine in 0.2 M carbonate buffer at pH 10 and the suspension is stored for 12 hours at 4°C. Uncoupled reagents are removed by extensive dialysis against several changes of 0.1 M NaCl.

In related work *A. Rembaum, S.-P.S. Yen and W.J. Dreyer; U.S. Patent 4,138,383; February 6, 1979; assigned to California Institute of Technology* provide suspensions of microspheres having a selected uniform diameter below 3500 A. The crosslinked beads, being considerably smaller than the biological cells, can be custom synthesized to closely match the size of the receptor site. The beads when covalently bound to a protein conjugate can be utilized to label a specific receptor site on the cell membrane.

The uniformly small-sized microspheres are synthesized by the substantially instantaneous free radical initiated aqueous emulsion polymerization containing a very dilute total monomer content, suitably from 0.5 to 35% and preferably from 3 to about 20% by weight. The microspheres are hydrophilic, hydrolytically stable, are biocompatible and of sufficient mechanical strength for biological applications. The microspheres are of well characterized structure, of outstanding purity and the hydrophilic properties, size and mechanical properties can be systematically varied by selection of monomer and polymerization conditions.

The composition of the monomer mixture is essential to obtain beads of the desired characteristics. The monomers should be water-soluble under the conditions of polymerization such that oil droplets do not form as in conventional emulsion polymerization in order to form the fine, uniformly shaped beads.

The covalently bondable monomers utilized are freely water-soluble and should comprise from 25 to 50% by weight of the monomer mixture described above in U.S. Patent 4,035,316.

The crosslinking agent also as previously described is present in the monomer mixture in an amount from 5 to 20% by weight, preferably 6 to 12%. The commercial form (95%) of hydroxyethyl methacrylate (HEMA) and hydroxypropyl methacrylate (HPMA) as supplied has also been described above.

The monomer mixture should contain a large percentage, suitably from 40 to 70% of sparingly water-soluble monomers having hydrophobic characteristics since this is found to result in freely suspended individual beads. In absence of such monomers, the polymer is too water-soluble and the resultant product is a gel of aggregated soft particles. The crosslinking agent is sparingly soluble. Hydrophobic characteristics can be provided with monomers such as styrene, vinyl toluene or lower alkyl acrylates suitably methyl methacrylate or ethyl methacrylate.

The amount of free radical catalyst also influences the size of the beads for a given monomer concentration. As the amount of catalyst is increased the size of the beads decreases. However, the reaction at increased catalyst level becomes too fast to control causing uneven size distribution. The free radical catalyst is usually present in an amount from 0.003 to 0.1% by weight of the polymerization mixture. Representative free radical catalytic initiators are ammonium persulfate (AP); or other inorganic persulfate, benzoyl peroxide, t-butyl peroctoate, isopropyl percarbonate, cumene hydroperoxide, dicumyl peroxide, 1,3-bis(t-butylperoxyisopropyl)-benzene, methyl ethyl ketone peroxide, acetyl peroxide, di-t-butylperoxide, t-butyl hydroperoxide, azo compounds such as azodiisobutyronitrile and the like.

Also present in the polymerization mixture is a surface active agent such as sodium dodecyl sulfate (SDS), octylphenoxy polyethoxy ethanol, sodium lauryl sulfate, sodium stearate and others. Increasing levels of surface active agent results in smaller bead diameter. However, for biological analytical uses, the surfactant must be removed from the final bead suspension. Therefore, low levels in the range of 0.03 to 0.5 part by weight of the polymerization mixture are preferred.

The monomers are freshly vacuum distilled before polymerization to remove impurities and inhibitor, if present. The polymerization reaction is preferably conducted in the absence of oxygen, suitably in vacuum or in the presence of an inert gas such as argon. In order to assure uniformity of particle size and to foster uniform initiation throughout the polymerization mixture, the polymerization mixture is intimately stirred before initiation, e.g., by tumbling the polymerization container for about 5 minutes before subjecting the mixture to heat.

Initiation is defined as the step of creating a free radical followed by addition of the free radical to an unsaturated bond of the monomer. In the process, initiation should occur throughout the volume of the polymerization mixture within 10 to 60 seconds of applying heat to the mixture. In the particular embodiment the container is placed in a bath and hot water was added to the bath. The container is then immersed in the hot water and rotated for polymerization.

The temperature of the bath must be at or above the decomposition temperature of the free radical catalyst and suitably at a higher temperature. For example, in the case of ammonium persulfate, initiation at 60°C will be slow resulting in nonuniformly sized beads having diameters larger than desired. However, initiation at 100°C results in initiation and propagation at nearly quantitive yield of very small, uniformly shaped particles within about 1 hour and the size distribution is within ±10% of the average size. Mixing such as by tumbling should continue throughout the polymerization step.

A series of polymerization runs were conducted by adding the monomers, catalyst, ammonium persulfate (AP), and surfactant, sodium dodecyl sulfate (SDS), to 100 cc of distilled water. The polymerization mixture was added to a sealed tumbling container inhibited with argon and tumbled for 4 to 5 minutes before being inserted in a 98°C bath for 1 hour.

HEMA was distilled in the presence of 0.5% hydroquinone at 95°C, 1 mm Hg pressure; methyl methacrylate (MMA) was distilled at 60°C, 200 mm Hg pressure; methacrylic acid (MAA) was distilled at 60°C, 10 mm Hg pressure; and ethylene glycol dimethacrylate (EGD) was distilled at 98°C, 4 mm Hg pressure. The amounts of monomer, catalyst, surfactant and the results of the runs are presented in the following table.

Emulsion Copolymerization of Methacrylates
Percent Concentration (w/w)

Ex. No.	HEMA	MMA	MAA	EGD	Total Monomer	SDS	AP	Diameter A	Percent of Solid
1	0.9	1.59	0.3	0.21	3.0	0.120	0.013	300	*
2	2.0	3.44	0.66	0.45	6.49	0.110	0.012	600±90	*
3	2.1	3.71	0.7	0.49	7.0	0.110	0.012	750±100	*
4	3.3	5.83	1.1	0.77	11.0	0.108	0.011	–	*
5	4.5	7.95	1.5	1.05	15.0	0.097	0.011	1,400±110	*
6	4.8	8.48	1.6	1.12	16.0	0.097	0.010	1,550±120	*
7	7.5	13.25	2.5	1.75	25.0	0.092	0.010	2,300±170	3.2
8	9.0	15.90	3.0	2.1	30.0	0.086	0.009	2,900±150	5.0
9	10.5	18.55	3.5	2.45	35.0	0.079	0.008	3,400±120	6.5
10	3.0	5.30	1.0	0.70	10.0	0.1	0.01	1,000±60	*
11	4.5	7.55	1.5	1.05	15.0	0.1	0.01	1,400±90	*
12	6.0	10.60	2.0	1.40	20.0	0.1	0.01	2,000±100	*
13	7.5	13.25	2.5	1.75	25.0	0.1	0.01	2,200±100	2.2
14	9.0	15.90	3.0	2.10	30.0	0.1	0.01	2,700±110	3.9
15	10.5	18.55	3.5	2.45	35.0	0.1	0.01	3,300±100	4.9

*No solid.

Percent solid was the coagulum remaining after filtration of the latex through Whatman No. 1 filter paper. Emulsifier and other ionic impurities were removed from the latex suspension by chromatography on a mixed bed ion-exchange column consisting of Biorad AG 1X10 and AG 50WX12 resins.

The concentration of latex particles in solution was based on dry weight analysis. A known volume of solution was dried at 107°C to constant weight. The density of the latex particles was determined by centrifugation at 100,000 *g* for 12 hours on a linear sucrose gradient.

The carboxyl content of the copolymer latex was determined by potentiometric titration. The main components of the aqueous emulsion polymerization system were two water-soluble monomers (HEMA and MAA) and a water-insoluble monomer (MMA) resulting in a high concentration of hydroxyl and carboxyl groups on the surface of the spheres.

The actual composition of the polymerizing mixture, the yields and the diameters of particles determined by SEM are shown in the table. The diameter of these particles measured by transmission electron microscopy is approximately 200 A smaller than by SEM, presumably due to the gold coating used in the latter.

It can be approximately calculated that particles with a diameter of 600 A have 4,200 carboxyl groups per particle (based on potentiometric titration and a density of 1.24 g/cm^3) and that each carboxyl group corresponds to an area of 270 square angstroms.

The preparation of fluorescent or radioactive latex spheres is as follows: Tritiated glycine and dansyl-ε-lysine were coupled to copolymer latex spheres (600 A in diameter) by the cyanogen bromide procedure adapted from the method of Cuatrecasas, *Biol. Chem.*, 1970, 245:3059.

An aqueous suspension of latex spheres (20 to 55 mg/ml) adjusted to pH 10.5 was activated with CNBr (10 to 20 mg/ml of suspension) at 25°C. The pH of the reaction mixture was maintained at 10.5 with 1 N NaOH. After 10 to 15 minutes the activated spheres were added to an equal volume of 5 mM dansyl-ε-lysine or [^{3}H]-glycine (1 mCi/μmol) in 0.2 M carbonate buffer at pH 10 and the suspension was stirred for 12 hours at 4°C.

Uncoupled reagents were removed by extensive dialysis against several changes of 0.1 M NaCl.

The preparation of derivatized latex spheres is as follows: Diaminoheptane and ε-aminocaproic acid were bonded to latex spheres using the aqueous carbodiimide reaction.

10 mg of 1-ethyl-3-(3-dimethylaminopropyl)-carbodiimide (EDC) were added with stirring to 5 ml of latex (25 mg/ml) suspended in 0.01 M diaminoheptane or 0.01 M ε-aminocaproic acid at pH 6 to 7 and 4°C.

After stirring for 2 hours in the cold, the suspension was exhaustively dialyzed against 0.1 M NaCl.

Spherical Cellulose Beads for Chromatography

Cellulose and its derivatives are widely used as chromatographic materials and polymeric carriers. Cellulose is mostly used in a form of fibers and powder for this purpose. These forms make the packing of columns difficult and exhibit a high flow resistance during application. This fact limits their use to small analytical columns and they are unsuitable for some techniques, as for example, in gel permeation chromatography.

The method of *J. Peska, J. Stamberg and Z. Blace; U.S. Patent 4,055,510; October 25, 1977; assigned to Ceskoslovenska akademie ved, Czechoslovakia* relates to the manufacture of spherical cellulose particles in bead form which enables the control of the particle shape and porosity of the particles. Resulting cellulose sorbents are suitable carriers and materials for chromatography. The method consists in heating a viscose (an aqueous solution of sodium cellulose xanthate) suspension in a water-immiscible liquid to 30° to 100°C under stirring to form spherical droplets, and solidifying them, and in the subsequent acidic decomposition of the solid xanthate globules either directly by addition of an acid soluble in the dispersion medium, or additionally after isolation and eventual washing of the particles to achieve the required wet volume.

Liquids with the viscosity up to 100 cs are advantageously used as dispersion medium and surfactants and/or modifying reagents (e.g., epichlorohydrin), and may be added to the suspension.

Example 1: Technical viscose (100 grams containing 8.2% of cellulose and 6% NaOH, γ = 40) was dispersed in 400 ml of transformer oil (viscosity 26 cs) in a 1 liter sulfonating flask at the laboratory temperature and agitation by 460 rpm. The suspension was heated for 1.5 hours to 90°C under continuous stirring, filtered, and the solid was immediately washed with ethanol. The decomposition of cellulose xanthate was completed by stirring in a solution of 20 ml of acetic acid in 80 ml of ethanol for 1 hour. After thorough washing with benzene, ethanol and water and drying in vacuum, 32.8 ml of macroporous globules was obtained; the fraction of diameter 0.35 to 0.15 mm amounted to 85 volume percent.

Example 2: A suspension of 100 grams of viscose in a 5% solution of polystyrene in chlorobenzene (viscosity 7.74 cs) was heated with agitation at 300 rpm similarly as in Example 1, filtered and the solid was washed with methanol and decomposed by stirring in a 10% aqueous solution of sulfuric acid. After washing, 73 ml of the wet globular sorbent was obtained which was separated into fractions: 1-0.75 mm 42%, 0.75-0.63 mm 36%, 0.63-0.50 mm 5%, 0.50-40 mm 8.5% and 0.40-0.31 mm 1.5%.

Example 3: A suspension of 100 grams of viscose in 300 ml of chlorobenzene and 300 mg of technical sodium dodecyl benzene sulfonate (Mersolate, 50% of dry material, the average length of alkyl C_{12}) was heated in the same way as in Example 1. After cooling to 35°C, a solution of 50 ml of acetic acid in 50 ml of chlorobenzene was poured into the agitated suspension. After filtration and washing, 84 ml of the sorbent was obtained which had the following composition by wet screen analysis: 1-0.75 mm 9%, 0.75-0.63 mm 17%, 0.63-0.50 mm 13%, 0.50-0.40 mm 29% and 0.40-0.31 mm 6.5%.

Example 4: A suspension of 100 grams of viscose in 300 ml of transformer oil was heated as in Example 1, filtered, and the solid was washed with benzene, methanol and water. The decomposition was completed with 10% sulfuric acid for 1 hour at 35°C. After washing, 59.5 ml of beads was obtained which had the screen analysis: 0.25-0.16 mm 70%, 0.16-0.125 mm 12%, 0.125-0.09 mm 10% and 0.09-0.08 mm 1%.

Refractory Metal Oxide Microspheres

The process of *A.J. Noothout and O. Votocek; U.S. Patent 4,011,289; March 8, 1977; assigned to Reactor Centrum Nederland, Netherlands* relates to a method of manufacturing microglobules by forming a dispersion of droplets of an inorganic phase in an organic phase which is immiscible with water, such that the droplets of the inorganic phase solidify. The solidified droplets are subsequently separated from the organic phase, washed, dried, and optionally subjected to further heat treatment. The watery phase contains inorganic hydrated oxides or components from which they can form and, if required, finely divided carbon. The organic phase is immiscible with water; it has a temperature ranging from 50° to 150°C and contains, if required, ammonia or an ammonia-releasing agent.

It was found that internal voids and cavities in microglobules can be avoided by including a surface active agent (SAS) in the organic phase and with judicious selection of the concentration of the surface active agent, the viscosity of the organic phase, the temperature of the organic phase and the viscosity of the aqueous phase and thus microspheres or microglobules of uniform configuration and free or substantially free of voids are produced.

The minimal SAS concentration as used herein is a concentration at which the microglobules that are being formed and solidifying just fail to adhere to each other. Generally speaking, the minimum amount is about 0.04% by volume. When a certain maximum concentration is exceeded, such as about 2.0 volume percent, a deviation from the globular shape appears. The preferred range is from 0.5 to about 2.0% by volume. The process is particularly suited to the production of small microglobules having a diameter ranging from about 5 to 250 microns.

A relatively high viscosity organic liquid is necessary for obtaining good microglobules without cavities and dents. Thus, the viscosity of the organic liquid at the working temperature must be at least 0.5 cp and may range up to at most about 10 cp, also taken at the working temperature.

The optimum and maximum concentration of surface active substance may be determined experimentally. It was found that this concentration is a function of the respective viscosities of the watery phase, the organic phase and the SAS itself and that the concentration of the surface active substance decreases with an increase in the viscosity of both the aqueous phase and the organic liquid. It is assumed that the SAS is a liquid; the viscosities of these three substances limit the maximum SAS concentration. The maximum SAS concentration is an important factor in process control.

Along with the solid globules that are segregated, SAS is continuously entrained outside the organic phase. If, as a result of this entrainment the SAS concentration drops below the minimum value, the globules begin to adhere to each other.

In practice, therefore, the procedure is implemented near the maximum emulsifier concentration, and the relation, which is to be determined experimentally, is particularly important. The water phase optionally contains one or more of the above ammonia-releasing agents. If it is desired to prepare globules of refractory metal oxides, the inorganic phase may consist of metal-hydroxide sols, watery metal-salt solutions, anion-deficient metal-salt solutions or mixtures of these liquids.

Suitable metal cations are selected from the group of: Fe^{+2}, Fe^{+3}, Al^{+3}, Be^{+2}, $(ZrO)^{+2}$, $(HfO)^{+2}$, $(TiO)^{+2}$, Sc^{+3}, Y^{+3}, trivalent rare-earth cations, U^{+4}, $(UO_2)^{+2}$, Th^{+4}, Pu^{+4}, $(PuO_2)^{+2}$ and actinide cations which may have higher atomic numbers than Pu. The anions of such metals may be any one of Cl^-, NO_3^-, $SO_4^=$, formate or acetate. One may also use silicon dioxide sols, separately or mixed with the abovementioned liquids.

A suitable method of manufacturing microglobules consists in spraying by means of sprayers of a watery phase with a viscosity ⩾12 cp at 0°C over an organic phase having a preassigned SAS concentration. It should be noted that the maximum emulsifier concentration in the organic phase at this relatively low viscosity of the inorganic phase is restricted only by the viscosities of SAS and organic phase. The following table lists examples of combinations of organic liquids and various SAS compositions. Other similar combinations are also useful.

System	Organic Liquid Viscosity (cp) 20°C	90°C	SAS Viscosity at 20°C (cp)	SAS Concentration* (% by vol)
Liquid paraffin + Span 80	136	8.5	95-1,100	0.5-0.6
Dobane + Span 80	11.0	1.7	95-1,100	0.9
Dobane + Span 85	11.0	1.7	170-230	2.0
Dobane + Atlox 3386	11.0	1.7	2,000-5,000	0.5

*At which deformation begins

The liquid paraffin used is a substantially aliphatic hydrocarbon liquid fraction of petroleum. Dobane PT-12 (Shell Netherland) is generally a mixture of alkyl-aryl-substituted hydrocarbons and is characterized as one or more alkyl-substituted benzenes having in the side chain an average of about 12 carbons.

Example: Dispersion in Air by Spraying – For the dispersion in air, stainless steel sprayers manufactured by Lechler were used. In order to attain an average droplet diameter of 300 microns, the type SZO 0.8/60 (0.8 mm bore, 60° spray angle) and SZO 1.2/90 (1.2 mm bore, 90° spray angle) were selected.

An aqueous nitrate-deficient uranyl nitrate solution, 1 part by volume of formula $UO_2(NO_3)_{1.6}(OH)_{0.4}$, of 2.85 molar concentration was mixed, while cooling was being applied, with 1.2 parts by volume of a cooled watery solution which was 3 molar with respect to both hexamethylenetetramine and urea. The solution was sprayed in the cooled state. The average diameter of the product could be adjusted within certain limits by means of the spraying pressure used. For example a spraying pressure of 1.05 to 1.1 atmospheres yielded particles having an average diameter of 100 microns after sintering to virtually the theoretical density. A screen analysis indicated that the particle-size distribution in the sintered product is aptly described as a log-normal distribution.

The reproducibility of the spraying method is good, as the following table indicates. The table summarizes the results of screen analysis of four successively prepared batches using a bath size of about 140 grams of UO_2 per batch. The output amounted to 286 ml/hour at a pressure of 1.1 atmospheres.

Screen Size	..... Percent by Weight of UO_2 Globules......			
(μ)	1	2	3	4
+175	4.3	3.3	4.2	5.2
150-175	8.0	5.0	6.5	6.8
125-150	11.9	11.8	10.7	12.4
105-125	23.3	23.2	24.5	23.8
90-105	12.8	12.8	12.4	13.0
75-90	12.5	13.4	12.7	13.6
-75	27.3	30.4	28.9	25.2

Electrically Conductive Thermoplastic Wax Composition Containing Silver-Coated Glass Microspheres

M. Koenig; U.S. Patent 4,098,652; July 4, 1978; assigned to M. Argueso & Co., Inc. describes a method for electroforming and electrodischarge machining (EDM) using an electrically conductive thermoplastic wax composition which can act as an electrode. The electrically conductive thermoplastic wax composition is both economical and easy to use and, most importantly, can be reused in electroforming and EDM where it does not form a part of the final article.

This is accomplished by selecting a thermoplastic wax material and incorporating therein spherical particles the surfaces of which have been treated or coated to make them electrically conductive. The treated coated spheres are added in an amount sufficient to make the thermoplastic wax material electrically conductive but insufficient to adversely affect the ability of the thermoplastic wax material to properly flow when in the fluid state to achieve the desired configuration.

Advantageously, the thermoplastic wax material may be similar to those suitable for use in investment casting procedures, so as to retain a molded shape or form at ambient temperatures. The glass spheres are solid glass microspheres all smaller than size 325 mesh, i.e., 44 microns in diameter or less, and coated with at least 4% silver by weight. The electrically conductive wax composition advantageously contains 60 to 75%, by weight, of the silver-coated glass microspheres.

The spherical particles contribute to the flow properties of the composition while at the same time imparting isotropic properties enabling effective shaping of designs and patterns on which it is desired to deposit the metal. Due to their spherical shape, the microspheres provide reliable contact between one another when packed rather densely together, so as to provide multiple electrically conductive paths in the thermoplastic wax material. The packing characteristics of spheres are such that voids will always exist between spheres of a generally similar size, so that good contact with low bulk density is achieved resulting in a lightweight conductive composition. Moreover, the density of glass spheres, even when coated with silver, is less than that of other conductive particulates such as metal powders.

When it is desired to separate the electrically conductive thermoplastic wax composition from the electroformed article which has been deposited thereon, the composition may be readily removed by heating above the melting point of the wax and allowing it to flow out of the resultant article. In all cases, a suitable solvent for the wax is used for removal of any residuals following melt-out.

To electroform, according to this process, the electrically conductive thermoplastic wax composition is heated to a fluid state, usually at a temperature above that at which the wax material without the presence of the electrically conductive spherical particles would be molded, and poured or injection molded to produce the desired molded wax pattern for electroforming metal deposition. The electrically conductive thermoplastic wax pattern is then used as the cathode in an electroforming circuit and a metal article deposited thereon. The conductive wax composition is removed from the hollow electroformed article and recovered.

To EDM according to this process the electrically conductive thermoplastic wax composition serves to provide a low impedance electrical connection to a work piece of intricate shape which forms one of the electrodes. This conductive wax composition is flowed into position and sets around the work piece which is thereby held at the desired attitude on a conductive support to which the work piece is electrically joined by the solidified conductive wax. Following the desired electric discharge machining of the work piece, the major portion of the solidified wax is recovered by melting it away from the work piece. Then, a suitable solvent is used to remove the residual conductive wax composition from the work piece.

Example 1: Various amounts of silver-coated glass microspheres were incorporated into a thermoplastic wax material, the samples molded into cylinders, the resistance measured and the conductivity observed. The specific composition of the thermoplastic wax material used in this example was as follows:

Material	Weight Percent
Chlorinated terphenyl resin*	75.23
T-57-N	8.20
Carnauba wax	12.15
Elvax 250	4.42

*Containing 60% chlorine by weight

T-57-N (Ashland Chemical Company) is a hydrosol glyceride. Elvax 250 (E.I. DuPont de Nemours & Co.) is an ethylene vinyl acetate resin. Carnauba is a well known vegetable wax. The above wax composition has a ball and ring softening point of approximately 170° to 180°F.

Using the thermoplastic wax material set forth above, samples were prepared containing various amounts of silver-coated solid glass microspheres smaller than 325 mesh and containing a coating of 4% silver, by weight. These glass spheres known as S-3000-S (Potters Industries, Inc.) are commercially available. The samples were molded into cylinders 2 inches long and 0.6 inch in diameter and the resistance of each cylinder measured using a Simpson Model 260 ohmmeter.

In addition, in order to determine whether the composition of thermoplastic wax material and silver-coated glass spheres was electrically conductive, a simple measurement using the cylinder as part of an electrical circuit containing a 100 watt light bulb was made. If the light bulb lit, the composition was determined. to be electrically conductive at an acceptable level.

The results are set forth in the table below showing the sample compositions and the resistance measurements and electrical conductivity observed.

Sample No.	Wax, weight %	Glass Spheres, weight %	Resistance, ohms	Electrically Conductive
1	50	50	*	No
2	45	55	105,000	No
5	42.5	57.5	200	Yes
3	40	60	8.75	Yes
4	35	65	0.55	Yes

*Too high to measure

The results show that a thermoplastic wax composition can be made electrically conductive through the addition of silver-coated glass spheres thereto and that there is a certain minimum amount of glass spheres which must be added before satisfactory conductivity is achieved.

Example 2: (a) An electrically conductive wax having the composition set forth below showed a measured resistance of less than 0.1 ohm. Although the electrically conductive wax was highly viscous, it worked well in actual field experimental use.

Material	Weight Percent
Chlorinated terphenyl resin*	23.61
T-57-N	2.58
Carnauba wax	3.81
Glass spheres, S-3000-S	70.00

*Containing 60% chlorine by weight

(b) A composition of electrically conductive thermoplastic wax was prepared containing a lesser amount of coated glass spheres. The resistance was measured as 1.5 ohms and although the composition was still highly viscous in the pourable state, it worked successfully in actual field experimental use in electrodeposition. The composition used is as follows:

Material	Weight Percent
Chlorinated terphenyl resin*	27.55
T-57-N	3.00
Carnauba wax	4.45
Glass spheres, S-3000-S	65.00

*Containing 60% chlorine by weight

Solid Spherical Particles of Coated Boron Carbide

The process of *H. Bildstein, K. Knotik and P. Leichter; U.S. Patent 3,939,233; February 17, 1976; assigned to HOBEG Hochtemperaturreaktor-Brennelement GmbH, Germany* relates to the production of spherical particles, using as starting material particles and organic substances which form a liquid, aqueous mix, spraying this mix or allowing it to drain off to form drops which are solidified during their downward passage through a column. The starting materials are ground to a fine powder and this powder is then introduced into an aqueous solution containing condensable or curable organic substances; a suspension is formed by stirring. To the resulting suspension, catalysts and crosslinking agents can be added. By the method it is possible to produce particles of a neutron-absorbing material or a reaction-moderating material.

For producing the carbon matrix of the particles, the known condensation reaction of phenols and aldehydes can be utilized. The utilization of resorcinol and/or urea has been proved to be advantageous. For the condensation agent formaldehyde solution or glyoxalic solution is used. For a complete condensation of 1 mol resorcinol about 1.2 to 1.4 mols formaldehyde are needed.

For adjusting the reaction time of the curing process necessary for the method, catalysts have to be added to the mixture to regulate the initiation of the polycondensation which follows an ionic reaction mechanism. Carboxylic acids and sulfonic acids especially toluene sulfonic acids, cyclohexane sulfamic acid, mellitic acid, and pyromellitic acid have been found suitable; by the addition of the two last-mentioned acids an advantageous three-dimensional linking of the resin is effected.

On account of the special utilization of the particles the desired fillers, like graphite, soot, boron, boron oxide, boron carbide, silicon, silicon carbide are added to the mixture in the form of highly ground powders and are mixed to a suspension by thorough stirring. Preferably the aldehyde is mixed with the suspension mixture immediately before the droplets are formed in a jet.

For ensuring complete condensation of the droplets the oil is heated to about 80° to 100°C. At this temperature it is possible to convert the droplets of the mixture to firm particles during their sinking in a column of a height of about 2 to 3 meters filled with oil. By fixing the diameter of the jet, the grain size of the powder and by adjusting the pressure, temperature, viscosity and surface tension in the mixture, particles having a determined size and a good uniformity can be produced. After having been cured, the particles are washed free from oil, dried and heated to 600°C to carbonize the resin.

In a further step the carbon matrix is graphitized at a temperature from 1800° to 2600°C; where boron or silicon is present the same is converted to the carbide. The resulting graphitized particles are flawless and extremely fine pored. Particles containing boron carbide, according to this process, are in the form of coated particles, i.e., particles which have been covered by a gas-impermeable layer of pyrocarbon or pyrocarbon and silicon carbide, which is especially suitable for the production of absorber elements for gas-cooled high temperature reactors.

For the production of boron-carbide-containing carbon particles, the suspension mix contains the following composition: 1,000 grams water, 375 grams resorcinol, 5 grams mellitic acid, 40 grams cyclohexane sulfamic acid and 45 grams boron (amorphous). For the curing agent 400 ml formaldehyde (40%) are added.

For carbon particles the following mix is given: 1,000 grams water, 410 grams resorcinol, 25 grams cane sugar, 5 grams pyromellitic acid, 35 grams toluene sulfonic acid, and 40 grams soot or graphite powder. 425 ml formaldehyde (40%) are added as curing agent. An apparatus for producing the particles is shown in Figure 8.2.

Figure 8.2: Apparatus for Production of Spherical Particles

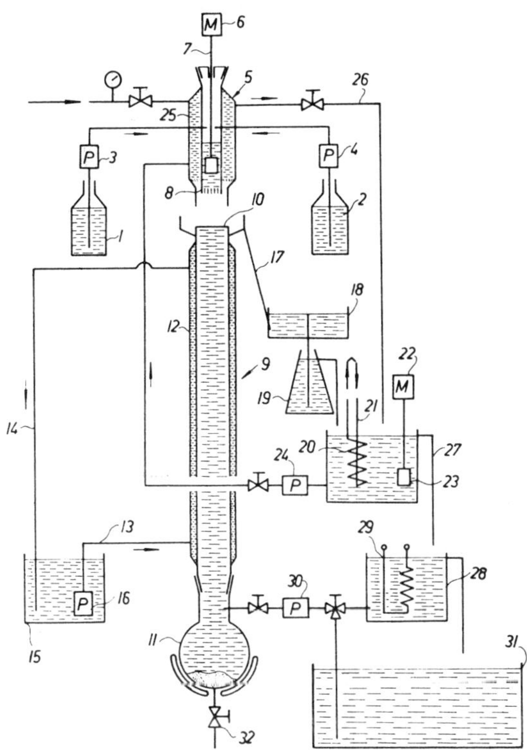

Source: U.S. Patent 3,939,233

A container **1** for the suspension mixture and a container **2** for curing agent are connected to a jet (mixing) vessel **5** by way of a proportioning pump **3** or **4**. The contents of the vessel **5** are thoroughly stirred by an agitator **7** driven by a motor **6**. The mixture in vessel **5** is forced through the jet openings **8** into a receiving vessel **9**. Droplets are thus formed which sink in a tube **10** being filled with paraffin oil, solidify and are collected in a vessel **11** attached to the end of the tube.

Besides oil also other liquids can be used such as organic solvents. The liquids can also contain dissolved amines or dissolved NH_3. In the drawing the receiving tube column **10** is surrounded by a jacket **12** through which a heating medium is passed and which is provided with conduits **13, 14**. The conduits **13, 14** discharge into a collecting tank **15**, the circulation being ensured by a pump **16** with a thermostat.

The diameter of the jet can for instance be between 0.2 and 0.7 mm. A height of drop of about 800 mm has proved sufficient for the particles ejected. The oil level is kept constant by the continuous supply of oil and an overflow tube

17. The overflow **17** is connected to a separator **18** which passes the oil to a second separator **19.** From there the oil is passed to a container **20** where a cooling device **21** and an agitator **23** are provided. The agitator is driven by a motor **22.** The cooled oil is moved by a pump **24** into the cooling jacket **25** of the jet (mixing) vessel **5**, from which it is returned into the container **20** by way of a conduit **26.** The container **20** is connected to a further container **28** by way of an overflow **27**; the container **28** contains a heating device **29.** A pump **30** brings the heated oil into the receiving tube **10.** A storage tank **31** serves for equalizing the oil level in the individual containers.

The collecting vessel **11** for the particles produced has an outlet **32** through which the particles can be removed from time to time. After they have been removed from the collecting vessel the cured particles are washed free from oil, are dried at 100°C and are screened. The screened particles are put into a graphite crucible and heated in an inert atmosphere (N_2-gas) to 600°C, during which step the resin and the carbon-containing additives are carbonized. Then the particles in the graphite crucible are sintered in an inductively heated high temperature furnace at 2000°C converting any boron and silicon respectively to boron or silicon carbide.

In the production of graphite-carbon-particles the charges are graphitized at 2500° to 2800°C. The size of the particles is determined by a number of factors, like pressure, shape of the jet, distance of the jet from the surface of the receiving liquid, temperature, density, viscosity and surface tension of the used mixture, ability of wetting and grain size of the used powder, temperature, density, viscosity and surface tension of the receiving liquid.

Temperature, density and viscosity can be kept constant without difficulties. The shape of the jet and the distance from the surface of the liquid are not altered and are therefore also constant. However, the surface tension is subjected to considerable fluctuation which can be removed if a tenside is added in a concentration which is not too low. Thereby the surface tension is kept at very low value which remains constant to a large extent on account of the surplus of the tenside. The concentration of the tenside should be, according to the effectivity, 0.5 to 2 g/l.

Solid Evacuated Microspheres of Hydrogen for Use as a Laser Fusion Target

An energy source under active investigation is laser fusion. In laser fusion a pellet of deuterium-tritium is imploded by intense beams of laser light. If the pellets can be imploded to 10,000 times their normal densities, efficient generation of fusion energy can be obtained. If the pellets are hollow rather than solid, the implosion should require significantly less peak laser power. It is therefore desirable to be able to produce small, evacuated, solid spheres of liquid hydrogen for use as laser fusion targets.

R.J. Turnbull, C.A. Foster and C.D. Hendricks; U.S. Patent 3,985,841; Oct. 12, 1976; assigned to the U.S. Energy Research and Development Administration provide a method for producing solid, evacuated microspheres comprised of hydrogen. The spheres are produced by forming a jet of liquid hydrogen and exciting mechanical waves on the jet of appropriate frequency so that the jet breaks up into drops with a bubble formed in each drop by cavitation. The drops are exposed to a pressure less than the vapor pressure of the liquid hydrogen so that the bubble which is formed within each drop expands. The drops which contain bubbles are exposed to an environment having a pressure just below the triple point of liquid hydrogen and they thereby freeze giving solid, evacuated spheres of hydrogen. The process is described with reference to Figure 8.3.

Figure 8.3: Production of Solid Evacuated Microspheres of Hydrogen

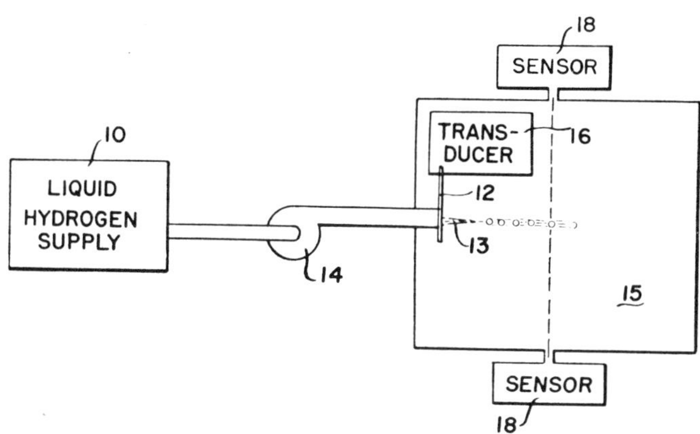

Source: U.S. Patent 3,985,841

Liquid hydrogen is provided by a liquid hydrogen supply **10** and should be of very high purity to avoid fouling the equipment. The liquefication may be done, for example, by passing gaseous hydrogen through a series of heat exchangers using liquid helium as the coolant. Liquid hydrogen then flows through a nozzle or orifice to form jet **13**. The orifice may simply be a glass capillary, a plate with a hole drilled into it or a hypodermic syringe. Means such as a gas pressure system provides sufficient pressure to form the jet. A pump **14** could also be used. The pressure applied to the liquid hydrogen should be sufficient to form and maintain the integrity of a cylindrical jet extending from the plane of plate **12**. The size of the orifice and the velocity of the jet are the variables for determining the quality of the jet formed. Generally, for a 50 micrometer diameter nozzle differential pressures from 1 to 3 psi absolute produced a satisfactory jet.

The jet **13** is formed within a chamber **15** wherein the pressure is controlled. Since the temperature of the gas in chamber **15** should be in the cryogenic region, chamber **15** is limited to containing either helium gas or hydrogen gas or a combination of the two since only these two gases are capable of being gaseous at such low temperatures.

A liquid jet, such as the hydrogen jet described, is unstable and will break up into drops. To control this breakup, so that drops of a desired uniform size and distribution are formed, it is necessary to mechanically excite waves upon the jet. This may be done in a variety of ways. In the figure, a transducer **16** is coupled to plate **12** and causes the orifice to vibrate at the desired frequency. Another means for exciting the jet could be to position a diaphragm upstream from the orifice and vibrate the diaphragm. This produces pressure waves in the fluid entering the orifice. The excitation of the jet produces a wave on the jet which grows in amplitude as driven by the surface tension of the jet. Considering the jet as a column or cylinder held together by the surface tension of the fluid, the wave imposed on the jet induces the surface tension to break the cylinder into small segments. The optimum frequency of excitation depends on the density of the fluid, the radius of the jet and the surface tension of the liquid. The optimum frequency depends inversely on the density and radius and directly upon the surface tension. The jet can be induced to break up over a wide range of frequencies.

The amplitude of the wave is also a variable. Too low an amplitude will not produce the desired breakup and cavitation while too high an amplitude will cause the drops to be disintegrated. The desired breakup of the jet should be done so that drops of uniform size and distribution are developed. Detection of drop character can be by eyeballing or microphotographic techniques. In addition, a photocell electric sensor **18** could be used to detect drop position or the drops could be charged and then the sensing of their presence could be done electronically.

If the pressure on a liquid jet is less than the vapor pressure of the liquid jet at the temperature of the jet, there is a critical radius for any bubbles within the liquid, r_c, at which bubbles with a radius larger than r_c grow in size due to the evaporation of the liquid into the bubble. The critical radius is given by the expression $r_c = 2\sigma/(p_v - p)$ where σ is the surface tension, p_v is the vapor pressure of the liquid at that temperature and p is the hydrostatic pressure imposed on the liquid.

The excitation of the jet produces waves on the jet and regions of low instantaneous pressure in the jet. In these regions of low pressure, cavitation nuclei form and begin to grow and, if they reach the critical radius, the bubbles continue to grow. For example, if the external pressure on the jet in the atmosphere in which the jet is formed is about 70 torrs and the frequency of excitation is 63,000 Hz so that uniformly sized and distributed drops are formed, it was observed that with a temperature of the liquid hydrogen at 14.7°K no bubbles formed. However, at 15.3°K the vapor pressure of the liquid is 110 torrs resulting in a bubble radius of 1.1 micrometer and the desired bubbles formed.

A temperature of 16.3°K produced bubbles so large that they broke through the liquid shell shattering the hollow drop. The desired condition of the liquid of the jet is that it is slightly superheated. Thus, the rate of expansion of the bubble needs to be controlled because if the expansion occurs too quickly, the drops will coalesce again. By controlling the temperature of the liquid hydrogen the rate of expansion is controlled. But utilizing the proper frequency of excitation and the proper temperature the proper breakup of the drops and the desired rate of expansion is ensured.

Formation of the solid sphere by freezing of the liquid drops with the desired bubble can be done in two ways. The freezing may take place in chamber **15** in which the drops are formed by having the desired pressure of the environment less than the triple point pressure of hydrogen. At such a pressure the drops freeze with the gaseous hydrogen of the bubble condensing on the sphere wall thereby producing solid evacuated microspheres, i.e., spheres having a vacuum within the outer solid shell. Alternately evaporation of the drops in chamber **15** can be prevented by having the pressure therein at the triple point. The drops can then be extracted through a small tube into a second chamber. In the second chamber the pressure may be reduced below the triple point giving greater pressure control. This is because the breakup of the jet which is determined by the pressure in the first chamber is not a limiting factor in the second chamber. Thus, a greater range of pressures may be utilized with a second chamber.

Using the method herein described with a 50 μ orifice diameter, microspheres 50 to 200 microns diameter with wall thickness as low as about 10 microns were produced. Of course depending upon orifice diameter, among other things, other sizes of microspheres are realizable. These spheres were of high purity hydrogen of at least 99.9% pure. Of course, isotopes of hydrogen and mixtures thereof are readily usable in this process. The changes in the operating conditions are according to the guidelines established. For example, the triple point of deuterium is about 18°K and 128.6 torrs, and that of tritium 28°K and 162 torrs so that these would be the benchmark temperatures and pressures for controlling bubble expansion.

Likewise, the pressure in which the jet forms to induce expansion of bubbles will be determined according to the vapor pressure of the liquid. Mixtures of the isotopes require determination of their triple point and their vapor pressures by empirical means.

OTHER

Microencapsulated Liquid Lubricants for Powder Metallurgy

Powdered metals, for example, powdered iron, are used to make small, fairly intricate parts, for example, gears. The fabrication of such metallic parts by powdered metal technology involves the following steps:

(a) the powdered metal is blended with a lubricant and other additives to form a mixture;

(b) the mixture is poured into a mold;

(c) the mixture is compacted in the mold to form a part using a high pressure, usually of the order of 30 tons per square inch;

(d) after compaction the part is ejected from the mold;

(e) the ejected part is subjected to a high temperature to decompose and remove the lubricant;

(f) the part is heated to a higher temperature to cause all the particles of metal in the part to sinter together; and

(g) the part is cooled, after which it is ready for use.

Commonly used lubricants include zinc stearate and lithium stearate. The lubricant is added to the powdered metal for several reasons. It increases the bulk density of the uncompacted powdered metal. This means that the molds can be shallower, for a given thickness of the final part. The bulk density is generally referred to as the apparent density.

The lubricant allows the compacting pressure to be reduced to attain a specified density before sintering. This is very important because it means that for a given pressure a larger part can be made. Because of the very large pressures required to compact powdered metal, only relatively small parts are made. The density of the compacted part is called the "green density."

The ejection force to remove the compacted part from the mold is much lower when a lubricant is present and this lower force results in less mold wear. Unfortunately, the lubricant also has a few adverse effects. It often reduces the flow rate of the powdered metal and therefore the rate at which a mold can be filled; it reduces the strength of the compacted part, referred to as the "green strength;" further, it can cause an unattractive surface finish on the sintered part. Zinc stearate is commonly used as a lubricant and slowly deposits a thin coating of zinc and zinc oxide on the walls of the oven used to burn off the lubricant or on the walls of the sintering oven.

This last disadvantage is often serious, and because of it a wax is sometimes used instead of zinc stearate. The most commonly used wax is ethylenebis-stearamide; however, it is not as good a lubricant as zinc stearate, especially with regard to compressibility, i.e., it gives a lower green density for a given compacting pressure. It can only provide the same compressibility as zinc stearate if it is ground to a very fine powder using a special grinding mill which is expensive and consumes a great deal of energy.

J. Blachford; U.S. Patent 4,106,932; August 15, 1978; assigned to H.L. Blachford Limited, Canada found that small capsules called microcapsules consisting of a liquid lubricant surrounded by a solid shell material, having certain properties, provide an excellent lubricant for powdered metals. The addition of a liquid lubricant to powdered metal results in high compressibility and low ejection pressure; however, it also causes very poor flow and very low apparent density which are unacceptable.

When the liquid lubricant is encapsulated, however, it does not have an opportunity to reduce the flow rate or the apparent density of the powdered metal; however, when the mixture of powdered metal and encapsulated lubricant is subjected to high pressure during the compaction stage, the shell of the capsule is ruptured or broken and the liquid lubricant is released to coat the particles of powdered metal and the die wall, and thereby results in high compressibility and low ejection pressure.

The process provides discrete pressure-rupturable microcapsules for lubrication in powder metallurgy comprising a core and a solid shell surrounding the core. The core comprises an organic liquid lubricant able to wet powdered metals, and the shell comprises a thin non-atmospherically-degradable polymeric material. The shell is impermeable to the lubricant and has a smooth, outer surface resistant to abrasion by sinterable powdered metal, to the extent that the microcapsules can be thoroughly mixed with sinterable powdered metal without release of lubricant. The shell is rupturable when the microcapsules are in admixture with sinterable powdered metal and are subjected to powder metallurgy compacting pressures. The lubricant and the shell are heat-decomposable to gaseous products which are noncorrosive to sinterable metal with a low residue of carbon at elevated temperatures below the sintering temperature of a powdered metal to be sintered.

The shell of the microcapsules can be coated with a thin layer of a solid which is a good lubricant for powdered metals, for example, stearic acid or carnauba wax. This coating can result in an improvement in the apparent density and flow rate, without harming the other properties. Preferably, the coating constitutes between 5 and 15% of the total weight of the microcapsules. If it is much less, the coating will not completely cover the shell; if it is much more, the beneficial effects of the encapsulated liquid lubricant will be reduced.

The microencapsulated lubricant can also be mixed with an unencapsulated solid particulate lubricant because synergism occurs with respect to certain properties; for example, the compressibility may reach a maximum at a particular concentration of microcapsules, and the ejection force may reach a minimum at another, usually different, concentration of microcapsules; the values of these concentrations depend upon the particle size and the composition of the microcapsules and of the unencapsulated solid particulate lubricant. The compositions giving optimum properties can vary over a wide range, depending on the property considered and the powder used, but usually the microcapsule content is from 1 to 99, preferably 5 to 95%.

Suitable solid particulate lubricants include waxes (for example, ethylenebis-stearamide wax, carnauba wax, Fischer-Tropsch wax), fatty acids, zinc stearate and lithium stearate.

Microcapsule Production: There are several methods of microencapsulating a liquid and most of these can be applied to the microencapsulation of liquid lubricants. The microcapsules may be manufactured by a method comprising the following steps:

(1) If necessary, mix an emulsifying agent with either the liquid lubricant, the water phase, or both.

(2) Mix a lubricant-soluble monomer with the liquid lubricant.

(3) Add the resulting mixture to the water phase.

(4) Mix at room temperature using vigorous agitation to form an emulsion of the desired droplet size, 5-100 μ diameter.

(5) To the emulsion add, with mixing, a water-soluble monomer reactive with the lubricant-soluble monomer or a polymerization catalyst for the lubricant-soluble monomer.

(6) Mix, but not so vigorously that the capsules are destroyed, for several hours, with heating to about 80°C, if desired, to accelerate the reaction.

(7) Filter the mixture to separate the microcapsules from the water.

(8) Wash the microcapsules to remove emulsifying agent and any excess water-soluble monomer.

(9) Dry the microcapsules.

The liquid lubricant should, of course, be inert to and not interfere with the polymerization. In this respect fatty acids should be avoided as the liquid lubricant when an isocyanate/amine reaction is employed because the fatty acids and amines tend to react together preventing or hindering the formation of microcapsules, and the fatty acid can also react with the isocyanate.

To coat the microcapsules with a thin layer of a solid lubricant, the mass of dried microcapsules is heated to a temperature a little above the melting point of the solid lubricant; the solid lubricant is then added, preferably as a fine powder, and the mixture is mixed gently for about an hour while the temperature is held constant.

Finally, with continuous mixing, the temperature is allowed to slowly decrease to that of the room. It is generally found that several aggregates of microcapsules have formed during this process because of the bonding nature of the solid lubricant. These can easily and completely be broken by grinding lightly in a hammer mill.

In the preferred method a di- or polyfunctional isocyanate is dissolved in the liquid lubricant, the resulting solution is emulsified in water containing an appropriate emulsifying agent, and an aqueous solution of a di- or polyfunctional amine is added. Among the isocyanates that can be used there may be mentioned: toluene diisocyanate, dianisidine diisocyanate, xylylene diisocyanate, o-, m- and p-phenylene diisocyanate, etc.

Examples of amines that can be used in the method are the following: ethylenediamine, 1,3-diaminocyclohexane, diethylenetriamine, etc. Examples of liquid lubricants which can be used in the preferred encapuslation method are as follows: rapeseed oil, soybean oil, epoxidized soybean oil, etc.

Example 1: Rapeseed Oil Encapsulated in Reaction Product from Ethylenediamine and Toluene Diisocyanate – 30 grams toluene diisocyanate (known as Nacconate 80) was dissolved in 120 grams of refined rapeseed oil. The solution was added with stirring to a solution of 3 grams of polyoxyethylene thioether (known as Siponic 218) in 700 grams of water. When the emulsification was complete, the stirring rate was reduced and 30 grams of ethylenediamine dissolved in 70 grams of water was added. The temperature was then increased to 80°C and maintained constant while the mixture was stirred for 4 hours.

The resulting dispersion of microcapsules in water was filtered and the microcapsules dried at 60°C. Aggregates of microcapsules were broken by light grinding through a hammer mill. The microcapsules were white, spherical, free-flowing, had an average particle size of about 50 microns and contained about 66% by weight of rapeseed oil.

Example 2: Methyl Oleate Encapsulated in Reaction Product from Ethylenediamine and Toluene Diisocyanate – 30 grams of toluene diisocyanate was dissolved in 120 grams of methyl oleate. This solution was added with stirring to a solution of 3 grams of Siponic 218 in 700 grams of water. When the emulsification was complete the stirring rate was reduced and 30 grams of ethylenediamine dissolved in 70 grams of water added. The temperature was increased to 80°C and maintained constant while the mixture was stirred for 4 hours.

The microcapsules were separated from the water by filtration and then dried at 60°C. Aggregates of dried microcapsules were broken by light grinding with a hammer mill. The microcapsules were white, spherical, free-flowing, had an average particle size of about 50 microns, and contained about 66% by weight methyl oleate.

Example 3: Testing of Microcapsules – The microcapsules prepared in Examples 1 and 2 were tested as lubricants for two different powdered metals using the following formulations:

Ingredients	. . . Formulation (% by wt). . . A	B
Iron powder		
(Atomet 29, QMP)	95.10	-
(MP32, Domtar)	-	96.28
Graphite		
(1845, Southwestern)	0.94	0.99
Copper		
(MD151, Alcan)	2.96	1.98
Lubricant	1.00	0.75

Standard test methods were used to determine the effects of the lubricant, namely apparent density by ASTM B212-48, compressibility by ASTM B331-64, green strength by ASTM B312-64, transverse rupture strength by ASTM B528-70 and tensile strength by ASTM E8.

A compacting pressure of 27.5 tons per square inch was used to prepare specimens of Formulation A for tensile strength determinations and of 30 tons per square inch for transverse rupture. A compacting pressure of 25 tons per square inch was used to prepare specimens of Formulation B for tensile and transverse rupture strength determinations.

Following compaction the samples were subjected to 1000°F in a pure hydrogen atmosphere for 20 minutes to burn off the lubricant, and subsequently to 2050°F for 30 minutes to sinter the metal.

Tables 1 and 2 present the results, along with the corresponding results for two commercially used lubricants, zinc stearate and ethylenebisstearamide wax. It can be seen that compared to the stearate and the wax the use of microcapsules leads to much lower ejection force, to lower apparent density and to greater shrinkage. With regard to the other parameters the results are comparable. A high shrinkage is frequently desirable, and although the tensile strength obtained using encapsulated rapeseed oil is low, it is still acceptable.

Table 1: Comparison Between Effects of Standard and Microcapsule Lubricants for Formulation A

	Zinc Stearate	Ethylene-Bisstearamide Wax	. . Microcapsules from. . . Example 1	Example 2
Apparent density, g/cc	3.08	2.66	2.30	2.37
Ejection force, tons/in^2	4.2	4.9	4.2	4.0
Green density, g/cc	6.57	6.53	6.49	6.49
Shrinkage, in/in x 10^{-4}				
Length	7	13	24	39
Width	6	10	24	36
Thickness	29	26	55	93
Tensile strength, psi	54,140	61,050	57,000	56,390
Transverse rupture strength, psi	111,130	111,180	111,080	121,230

Table 2: Comparison Between Effects of Standard and Microcapsule Lubricants for Formulation B

	Zinc Stearate	Ethylene-Bisstearamide Wax	. . Microcapsules from. . . Example 1	Example 2
Apparent density, g/cc	2.73	2.57	2.15	2.25
Ejection force, tons/in^2	4.3	4.8	3.2	3.6
Green density, g/cc	6.35	6.30	6.30	6.28
Shrinkage, in/in x 10^{-4}				
Length	20	6	6	16
Width	12	6	4	14
Thickness	23	13	43	60
Tensile strength, psi	37,890	37,260	28,640	37,730
Transverse rupture strength, psi	77,410	80,360	74,930	79,290

Example 4: Soybean Oil Encapsulated in Reaction Product from Ethylenediamine and Toluene Diisocyanate – 30 grams of toluene diisocyanate was dissolved in 120 grams of soybean oil. The solution was added with stirring to a solution of 3 grams of Siponic 218 in 700 grams of water. The resulting coarse emulsion was then mixed very vigorously in a high intensity colloid mill to produce an emulsion containing very fine droplets of oil. The stirring rate was then reduced and 30 grams of ethylenediamine in 70 grams of water was added. The temperature was then increased to 80°C and maintained constant while the mixture was stirred for 4 hours.

The microcapsules were separated from the water by filtration and dried at 60°C. Aggregates of dried microcapsules were broken by gentle grinding. The microcapsules were white, spherical, free-flowing, had an average diameter of 5 microns and contained about 66% by weight oil.

Example 5: Coating of Microcapsules from Example 4 with Thin Layers of Lubricants – A 166 gram sample of fine microcapsules from Example 4 was heated to 150°F and to half of this was added, with mixing, 17 grams of double pressed stearic acid and to the other half was added, with mixing, 17 grams of a Fischer-Tropsch wax (Paraflint). The samples were held at 150°F and mixed for 30 minutes. The heat source was then removed and the samples allowed to cool to room temperature, at which point the mixing was stopped. The aggregates that had formed as a result of this treatment were broken by light grinding. The coated microcapsules were tested as lubricants for iron powder (Atomet 29) using a lubricant concentration of 0.75% by weight.

Table 3: Effect of Thin Coating on Lubricant Properties

	Zinc Stearate	Ethylene-Bisstearamide Wax	Uncoated Capsules	Coated Capsules Stearic Acid	Wax
Flow rate, sec/50 g	34.5	41.0	no flow	no flow	no flow
Apparent density, g/cc	3.24	2.94	2.58	2.95	2.66
Green density, g/cc	6.60	6.55	6.55	6.60	6.52
Ejection force, tons/in^2	5.4	6.4	5.6	4.9	5.7
Green strength, psi	1,664	2,218	1,437	1,175	1,423

The results show that the stearic-acid-coated microcapsules give higher apparent densities and green densities than do the uncoated.

Bearing Material Containing Encapsulated Lubricant

The process of *A.J. Capelli; U.S. Patent 4,056,478; November 1, 1977; assigned to Sargent Industries, Inc.* makes it possible to use nonsolid lubricants in bearing material. This is accomplished by microencapsulation of the nonsolid lubricant in the body of the bearing material. As used herein nonsolid lubricant includes liquid lubricants such as oil and readily extrudable paste-like lubricants such as grease and excludes solid and powdered lubricants such as polytetrafluoroethylene (Teflon) powder. An important advantage of using nonsolid lubricants is that the number of applications for bearing materials is substantially increased. The bearing material of this process can be used as a bearing liner, a bearing, or a portion of a bearing such as a race for a spherical bearing. The process is described with reference to Figure 8.4.

Figure 8.4: Bearing Material Containing Encapsulated Lubricant

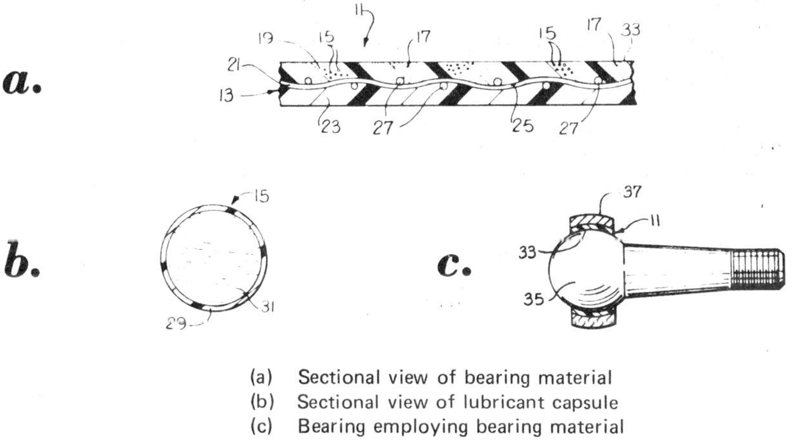

(a) Sectional view of bearing material
(b) Sectional view of lubricant capsule
(c) Bearing employing bearing material

Source: U.S. Patent 4,056,478

Figure 8.4a shows a bearing material **11** which includes a body **13**, lubricant capsules **15**, and lubricant particles **17**. Except for the presence of the lubricant capsules **15**, the bearing material **11** may be identical to the bearing material disclosed in U.S. Patent 3,594,049.

The body **13** includes a matrix **19** constructed of a binder or adhesive, a fabric backing member **21**, and an adhesive layer **23** for attaching the bearing material **11** to an external member. The matrix **19** must be constructed of a material which is capable of binding or holding the lubricant capsules **15** and the lubricant particles **17**. For example, a phenolic base adhesive such as Rabond R-84015 (Raybestos-Manhattan) or Resiweld R-7119 (H.B. Fuller Co.) may be employed. Both of these adhesives are thermosetting two-stage adhesives which give a strong chemical bond. Both of these adhesives can be hardened without curing by heating to a temperature under 212°F and can be cured in two stages by heating to temperatures of 330° and 375°F respectively. Of course, the material selected must cure at a low enough temperature to prevent destruction of the lubricant capsule **15**. In addition, the binder must cure at less than 300 psi to avoid breaking of the capsules **15**.

The matrix **19** and the adhesive layer **23** are bonded to the opposite faces of the backing member **21**. The adhesive layer **23** may be constructed from the same material as the matrix **19**. The backing member **21** can advantageously be in the form of a woven sheet and includes a plurality of warp strands **25** (only one being shown) and a plurality of filler strands **27**. The strands **25** and **27** can be woven together in any suitable manner to provide a strong backing member. Each of the strands **25** and **27** is made up of many small fibers (not shown). The backing member **21** is preferably constructed of a synthetic material such as Dacron, nylon or rayon. As illustrated, the backing member **21** is 6.5 oz plain weave, 100% Dacron fiber designated by Style No. 5133 and obtainable from the Texlon Corporation. This fabric provides pores of a proper size for purposes which are described in U.S. Patent 3,594,049.

The woven backing member **21** has tensile strength in substantially all directions lying in the plane of the backing member. The matrix **19** preferably has a thickness of 0.0024 to 0.0035 inch with 0.003 inch being considered optimum and with these dimensions being from the uppermost part of the backing member **21** to a wear surface **33**.

The lubricant capsules **15** and particles **17** are uniformly distributed throughout the matrix **19**. Each of the lubricant capsules **15** includes a frangible shell or capsule **29** and a nonsolid lubricant **31**. The shell **29** is generally spherical, very tiny, and frangible (see Figure 8.4b).

The shell **29** must be constructed of a material which is suitable for microencapsulation and which does not adversely affect the properties of the lubricant **31**. For example, polyvinyl alcohol may be used as the encapsulating material. The lubricant **31** may be encapsulated in accordance with known microencapsulation processes such as the process described in NCR technical publication "Microencapsulation—The Process and Its Capabilities."

The characteristics of the lubricant **31** within the shell **29** will be selected in accordance with the contemplated use of the bearing material **11**. The nonsolid lubricant **31** may have particular environmental capabilities such as desirable high and low temperature characteristics or it may be a general purpose lubricant. A liquid lubricant known as Dow-Corning 200 is a suitable general purpose lubricant. Examples of nonsolid, low temperature lubricants which can be encapsulated and used at temperatures down to about -60°F are identified by the following military specifications MIL-L-7870A, MIL-L-10295B, MIL-L-10324A and MIL-L-14107B.

Examples of nonsolid, high temperature lubricants which can be encapsulated and used at temperatures up to about 500°F are identified by the following military specifications MIL-A907D, MIL-G-81322A, MIL-G-27617A, MIL-G-3545C (MR) and MIL-L-25681C.

The lubricant particles **17** are dry. Examples of suitable dry lubricant materials are polytetrafluoroethylene, fluoroethylene propylene, polyethylene, graphite, molybdenum, nylon and Dacron. Nylon and Dacron are generally considered to be abrasive when used with a steel bearing but they may be used, for example, with ceramic bearings which are quite abrasion-resistant. For many applications, a fluorocarbon, such as polytetrafluoroethylene is preferred. The dry lubricant may also include minor proportions of a metal powder additive such as bronze, Babbitt or lead. In this embodiment, the dry lubricant is composed of five micron polytetrafluoroethylene pure powder.

The particles **17** may be omitted from the bearing material **11** depending upon the results desired. Stated differently, if the dry lubricant particles **17** provide a desired lubricating characteristic, they may be used; however, if they do not provide a characteristic which is necessary or desirable for a particular application, only the lubricant capsules **15** may be employed in the bearing material **11**.

The bearing material **11** can be used as a bearing liner as shown in Figure 8.4c. The wear surface **33** slidably engages the surface of a spherical ball **35**. The bearing material **11** is adhered by the adhesive layer **33** to a race **37**. The bearing liner **11** allows low-friction, sliding, universal movement between the ball **35** and the race **37**.

Forcible contact between the wear surface **33** and the ball **35** causes the shells **29** closely adjacent the wear surface to break, thereby freeing the lubricant **31**. The lubricant **31** so freed acts to lubricate the wear surface **33**. The shells **29** which are more remote from the wear surface **33** are not broken by the contact between the wear surface and the ball **35**. However, as the bearing material **11** wears, its thickness is reduced. This brings unbroken shells **29** closer to the wear surface **33** with the result that these additional shells are broken thereby freeing additional lubricant **31**. Thus, the capsules **15** are progressively broken as the bearing liner **11** wears to assure that the surface **33** will remain lubricated.

The lubricant **31** and the lubricant particles **17** can cooperate to provide a wide range of environmental conditions under which the bearing material **11** can be used. For example, a first group of the shells **29** may have a low temperature nonsolid lubricant and a second group of the shells may have a high temperature nonsolid lubricant. The dry lubricant particles may be suitable for a middle temperature range such as about -20° to 350°F. This means that all three kinds of lubricant will be present at any one time at the wear surface **33**. However, at very low temperatures the dry particles **17** become very rigid and are themselves lubricated by the low temperature lubricant. Similarly, the high temperature liquid lubricant freezes at low temperatures and is also lubricated by the low temperature lubricant.

At high temperatures, the low temperature lubricant boils off at the wear surface **33** and the lubricant particles **17** deteriorate. Accordingly, only the high temperature lubricant is effective to lubricate the wear surface **33** under these conditions.

Similarly, in the middle temperature range, the low temperature lubricant boils off and the high temperature lubricant is frozen or too viscous to be effective. Accordingly, the lubricant particles **17** lubricate the wear surface **33** under these conditions. Other combinations of lubricants can be employed to further expand the range of environmental applications for the bearing material **11**.

Encapsulated Thermonuclear Fuel Particle

Work in connection with energy studies and development has indicated the desirability of an improved fuel particle embodying deuterium or tritium, or combinations thereof, which would afford the opportunity of custom-loading same. Such would provide for quantized "mini-explosions". One area in which such is desired is that wherein the particle is subjected to laser beams. Particulate fuel material for the above would provide a fuel for use in fusion reactor development, and additionally for plasma, material and gas studies.

W.H. Smith, W.L. Taylor and H.L. Turner; U.S. Patent 3,953,617; April 27, 1976; assigned to the U.S. Energy Research and Development Administration describe a method for making an encapsulated fuel, and the product formed thereby having an exterior shell of a relatively high atomic number material (relative to the fuel atomic mass), an inner concentric shell of fuel at the inside surface of the high atomic number shell, and the interior volume being at least partially evacuated. Figure 8.5 illustrates an enlarged view of a loaded microsphere **10** or otherwise generally spheroidal fuel particle.

Figure 8.5: Encapsulated Thermonuclear Fuel Particle

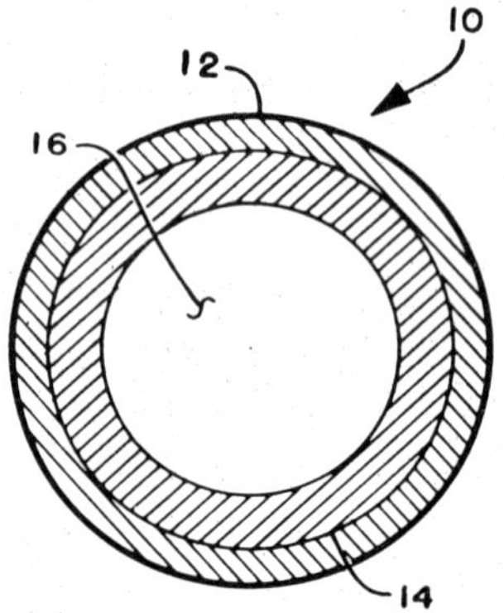

Source: U.S. Patent 3,953,617

The fuel microsphere includes an exterior shell **12** of a suitable high atomic number material or metal. Those materials or metals which may be used may be such as nickel, gold, uranium, etc., and may have an atomic number above mass 50. Preferred materials have the higher atomic numbers. The thickness of the shell **12** wall of the metal microsphere may range from about 1 to 30 microns. The diameter of the microsphere in the finished product may be from about 100 to several thousand microns, depending upon intended usages to be made thereof. Although microspheres are herein referred to, it should be understood that the particles may not necessarily be perfectly spherical but may be generally spheroidal, oblate, etc.

The fuel **14** within the metal shell or exterior **12** preferably in the form of a deposit or coating may be of a wall thickness which is any fraction of the sphere radius depending upon the amount of fuel or effects sought from the microsphere. The maximum thickness may be limited by the loading process.

Typical materials which may be used as a fuel are such as deuterium-tritium (DT), deuterium (D_2), and tritium (T_2). Mixtures of the above may be used in order to achieve or provide desired properties or reactions and the same may not necessarily be entirely condensed as a coating to provide the desired results. The volume **16** within the hollow thermonuclear fuel may be partially evacuated as a result of deposition of the fuel upon the metal shell, i.e., a partial vacuum forms as gas provided within the material or metal shell **12** solidifies due to reduction in temperature. Evacuation of this volume may also be accomplished by the process used in preparing the microspheres or particles. Evacuation may be such as to be considerably less than 1 torr but in any event should be such that substantially all of the fuel is deposited on the inner wall of the metal shell **12**.

The method of making the described microspheres, or encapsulated, generally spheroidal, particulate fuels, may be by such as:

(a) grinding and sieving of the selected material to obtain the required uniform size particles, to be preferably from about 75 to 500 microns, and passing the particles through a plasma or high temperature zone of an induction-coupled plasma torch to form hollow, generally spheroidal fuel shells having diameter sizes ranging from about 100 to several thousand microns and preferably from 100 microns to 700 microns; and

(b) physical entrapment or dissolution of a hydrogen isotope or other suitable gas by allowing the gas to diffuse into the material particles.

The preferred method of making the encapsulated fuel particle may begin with the hollow spheres of the material to be used. These hollow spheres or spheroids of suitable size and material, as described hereinabove, may be contacted with gaseous fuel which is to be used, at a temperature of about 370° to about 770°K and preferably from about 470° to 600°K for a period of from about 1 to 48 hours. The length of time in which contact between the gaseous and the solid hollow sphere is maintained will be determined by the extent of diffusion desired into the spheres. The microspheres would have been cleaned and sieved to appropriate diameters prior to diffusion processes.

In addition to maintaining the contact at a suitable temperature as recited, the gaseous fuels may be at or under a pressure of up to several thousand pounds per square inch in order to load the desired quantity of fuel into the hollow metal sphere. During the loading process, the pressure differential between the fuel on the outside and within the hollow sphere may be maintained within the range of two to several hundred pounds per square inch, limited by the ultimate tensile strength of the metal spheroids, in order to cause the fuel to diffuse inward at an acceptable rate.

Once the desired quantity of fuel has permeated through the hollow metal shell wall, the pressure and temperature may be reduced by suitable means such as by quenching in a suitable cryogenic fluid such as liquid nitrogen. If desired the gas may be solidified and deposited on the wall of the metal sphere by further cooling in liquid helium.

In order to store the bulk of the fuel as a solid the temperature to which the material is cooled will be dependent upon the type of gas utilized. For example, if deuterium is used, cooling should be effected to at least less than about 18.7°K and preferably less than about 18°K. If deuterium-tritium is used, then cooling should be effected or maintained at least less than about 19.7°K and preferably less than about 19°K.

This temperature should be maintained until the fuel is used. Effective storage of the fuel as a dense gas can be accomplished at temperatures from about 77° to about 4°K.

The amount of fuel within a given size sphere may be varied as desired for achieving different energy outputs, but the amount of fuel which may be loaded also depends upon the molar volume (or density) of the fuel in its final form under the specified cryogenic storage conditions prior to use. Typical values for solid hydrogen, deuterium, deuterium-tritide, and tritium are as follows:

	Molar Volume (cm^3/mol)	Density (g/cm^3)
H_2	22.65	0.0888
D_2	19.65	0.204
DT	18.02	0.278
T_2	16.48	0.365

The above values are at a storage condition of about 4.2°K. As an illustration, a 10 to 30% volume packing fraction may be assumed. The volume packing fraction (expressed as %) is equal to the volume occupied by fuel divided by internal volume of sphere times 100. For example, a hollow sphere of fuel such as DT whose thickness is approximately about 5 to 10% of the inner radius of the metal shell may be formed by depositing or freezing out the fuel as a coating, onto the interior of the shell. Specifically, hollow spheres approximately 350 microns in diameter containing DT fuel with a 15% packing fraction when "burned" (ignited to effect a fusion reaction) at a rate of 50 per second will release energy at a gross power level of approximately one megawatt.

Encapsulated Liquid Explosive Compositions

K. Inoue, H. Sato and F. Matsui; U.S. Patent 3,977,922; August 31, 1976; assigned to Nippon Oils and Fats Company Limited, Japan have found that when an explosive liquid compound or a gelatinized product thereof is microcapsulated with a high molecular weight compound, the explosive liquid compound is fixed and an explosive composition, which has a low sensitivity and a high chemical stability and can be easily handled, can be obtained.

As the explosive liquid compounds to be used for the production of microcapsules mention may be made of glycerin trinitrate, glycerin dinitrate, ethylene glycol dinitrate, diethylene glycol dinitrate, triethylene glycol dinitrate, trimethylene glycol dinitrate, diglycerin tetranitrate, monochlorohydrin dinitrate, acetylglycerin dinitrate, 1,2,3-butane-triol trinitrate, 2-nitro-2-oxymethyl-1,3-propanediol trinitrate, 2-methyl-2-oxymethyl-1,3-propanediol trinitrate, trinitrobenzene, tetranitromethane and the like, and mixtures thereof.

Further, gelatinized products of the abovedescribed explosive liquid compounds with gelatinizing agents, such as nitrocellulose and the like, for example, gelatinized products obtained by absorbing glycerin trinitrate, glycerin dinitrate, ethylene glycol dinitrate and the like in nitrocellulose can be used for the production of microcapsules.

As the high molecular weight compounds to be used for the production of microcapsules, mention may be made of thermosetting resins, such as polyurethane, polyurea, epoxy resin and the like, and thermoplastic resins, such as polystyrene, polyvinyl alcohol and the like.

The microcapsules are produced in the following manner. An explosive liquid compound is dispersed in water together with methylcellulose, a surfactant and the like, monomer of a high molecular weight compound, which forms the capsule wall, is added to the dispersed system, and, if necessary, a polymerization initiator or a reactive monomer is added thereto, and the resulting mixture is subjected to a polymerization reaction.

According to the abovedescribed method, it is possible to produce microcapsules containing an explosive liquid compound in an amount as large as about 80 to 95% by weight.

The microcapsules produced by the abovedescribed method have the following excellent properties: (1) the power is high; (2) the sensitivity is low; and (3) the vapor pressure is low. Moreover, since the microcapsules are solid, they can be easily handled in transportation and weighing. The microcapsules are particularly useful as a propellant for small arms or artilleries, a propellant for rockets and a high explosive for special use.

Microencapsulated Vulcanizing Agent

Alkylated phenol sulfides are well known, versatile, rubber processing chemicals which can be used as vulcanizing agents for both natural and synthetic rubbers and for blends thereof. Such sulfides act as resinous type plasticizers during processing and tend to equalize the rate of cure of blends of natural and synthetic rubber. When used as vulcanizing agents with or without sulfur, they show an activity proportional to their sulfur content. The alkylated phenol sulfides, have, however, one serious disadvantage; they are tacky, relatively low-melting solids and are therefore difficult to handle.

I.C. Popoff and C.B. DeSavigny; U.S. Patent 4,102,800; July 25, 1978; assigned to Pennwalt Corporation describe an improved vulcanizing agent composition which is comprised of microcapsules in which the capsule wall is composed of crosslinked polyamide, polyurea, or polyamide-polyurea resin, and, contained within these capsules, alkylated phenol sulfide. This encapsulated form of alkylated phenol sulfide is a free-flowing, dust-free, easily dispersible product which can be incorporated into the elastomer much easier and faster than the conventional unencapsulated sulfide, without tearing the rolling bank. Because the encapsulated product readily disperses in the rubber, excessive milling and resultant breakdown of the elastomer polymer chain are avoided. The excellent dispersibility of the composition can be observed visually during the rubber milling process, and this advantage results in a narrow range of tensile breaks of samples of the elastomer vulcanized therewith. The encapsulated vulcanizing agent is a more active and faster vulcanizing agent than unencapsulated sulfide, producing vulcanizates with better physical properties.

The method and technique of preparing crosslinked-wall microcapsules are disclosed in U.S. Patent 3,577,515 and the corresponding British Patent 1,091,141. The particle sizes of the microcapsules will generally range from about 50 to 1500 microns with a preferred average particle size of about 300 to 800 microns. The wall thickness of the capsule will range from about 0.5 to 20 microns, with from about 1 to 5 microns thickness preferred.

Example: (a) Preparation — A solution of 100 grams p-tert-amylphenol sulfide (a tacky brown solid melting in the range of 50° to 60°C and containing 22.5% sulfur), 7.2 grams of sebacoyl chloride, and 2.7 grams Papi polyisocyanate reactant in 100 grams methylene chloride is added with vigorous stirring to 1,600 ml of water containing in solution 0.5% of polyvinyl alcohol dispersing agent (Elvanol 50-42 G, a 4% aqueous solution with a viscosity of 35 to 45 cp at 20°C, determined by the Hoeppler falling ball method) in a 3-liter baffled resin flask. To the resulting emulsion is added a solution of 3.6 grams ethylenediamine, 4.2 grams of diethylenetriamine, and 6.4 grams of sodium carbonate in 100 ml of water. After an additional 30 minutes stirring, the reaction mixture is cooled down to 10°C and acidified with sulfuric acid to about pH 6.

The encapsulated alkylated phenol disulfide is recovered by filtration. It is a free-flowing, non-dusty product free of tack and contains about 60% alkylated phenol sulfide, 18 to 20% capsule wall consisting of a nylon-type crosslinked polyamide-polyurea, and about 20% solvent. The size of the microcapsules ranges from about 100 to 1,000 microns, average about 300 to 500 microns. When the solvent is removed by evaporation, a capsule containing about 75% alkylated phenol sulfide and about 25% capsule wall is obtained.

(b) Evaluation — Representative rubber vulcanizates are prepared to confirm that the microencapsulated alkylated phenol sulfides of this process give better results as vulcanizing agents than unencapsulated material. The following elastomer vulcanizate formulation is used in the comparisons:

	Parts by Weight
Raw elastomer (SBR 1500)	100
Carbon black (FEF)	52
Highly aromatic rubber processing oil	10
Zinc oxide	5
Stearic acid	2
Accelerator (Ethylac)	1
Vulcanizing agent	7*

*Based on weight of active agent therein

The compounded rubber is cured at 320°F with samples taken after 10, 20, and 40 minutes cure time for determination of physical properties, as set forth below in the table which shows that the encapsulated sulfide is even faster curing than before encapsulation. The ease of handling the encapsulated sulfide, is however, the most important advantage over the unencapsulated material; this advantage is particularly noticeable and results in safer and more economical use when practiced on the commercial scale of rubber processing.

Physical Properties of Vulcanizates Made with the Vulcanizing Agents

	Microencapsulated*	Unencapsulated**
	.... Alkylated Phenol Sulfide	
Modulus, 300%, psi		
10 min cure	675	475
20 min cure	850	750
40 min cure	1,100	875
Tensile, psi		
10 min cure	2,025	1,700
20 min cure	2,475	2,325
40 min cure	2,850	2,800
Hardness, Shore A		
10 min cure	56	50
20 min cure	57	53
40 min cure	60	54

*Containing 60% sulfide; 11.6 g used.
**7 g used.

Encapsulated Flame Retardant

The process of *D.N. Vincent and R. Golden; U.S. Patent 4,138,356; Feb. 6, 1979; assigned to Champion International Corporation* relates to extremely small, compatible, encapsulated flame retardant particles and polymeric systems including the microcapsules.

When comparatively large diameter microcapsules are introduced into the polyurethane foamable mixture, the resulting foam contains numerous stress points in the foam at the points where the microcapsules have been introduced into the cell walls. By employing microcapsules having an average particle diameter less than 5 microns, only a relatively small fraction of the total thickness of the cell wall or rib of the foamed structure contains the microcapsules. Thus, the stress points are obviated providing a finished article having antiflammability properties without a reduction or weakening of the physical properties of the foamed material.

The small particle diameter, flame retardant microcapsules can be employed in the production of polymeric fibers, the microcapsules being sufficiently small to avoid clogging the extrusion equipment for producing such fibers, e.g., the spinneret. Additionally, the microcapsules do not materially alter the physical properties of the resulting fibers while rendering them flame resistant. The small diameter flame retardant microcapsules can be incorporated in paints, such as latex base paints, the microcapsules providing opacity or hiding power to the paints as well as providing flame resistant properties thereto.

Any suitable fire retardant may be employed in the microcapsules whether in liquid or solid form. Thus, the liquid fire retardant material or solution of such fire retardant material may be any one or a mixture of several classes of fire retardant chemical compounds such as phosphate esters, halogenated phosphate esters, phosphonate esters, halogenated phosphonate esters, phosphites, halogenated paraffins, halogenated olefins, halogenated aromatics and other halogenated organic compounds generally recognized as having fire retardant properties.

The microcapsular walls of the microcapsules to be employed in polyurethane foams are formed from polyhydroxy polymers, such as methylcellulose, poly(vinyl alcohol), and starch. Polyurethanes are commonly made by a reaction between a polyisocyanate and hydroxyl-group-containing polyethers and/or polyesters. Accordingly, by employing polyhydroxy-bearing polymers in the formation of the microcapsular walls, there are hydroxyl groups available to chemically react with the polyisocyanates of the polyurethane foam-forming mixture to result in a chemical bonding between the microcapsular walls and the polyurethane structure.

An especially preferred process for forming microcapsules involves admixing: (a) a water-immiscible oily material containing an oil-soluble, nonpolymeric, crosslinking agent selected from the group consisting of a polyfunctional isocyanate and an orthoester of a Group IV element, and a water-immiscible, oily flame retardant material; and (b) an aqueous solution of an hydroxyl-group-containing polymeric, emulsifying agent.

The materials are admixed to form an oil-in-water emulsion wherein the oily, flame retardant material is dispersed in the form of microscopic emulsion droplets in an aqueous, continuous phase, and the crosslinking agent reacts with the polymeric emulsifying agent to provide each of the flame-retardant-containing emulsion droplets with a solid, crosslinked capsule wall. A curing step is employed wherein the crosslinking agent and the polymeric emulsifying agent are subjected to temperatures in the range of ambient temperature to 100°C for periods of time between 1 and 24 hours; preferably reaction is in the range of 40° to 80°C for a period of 1 to 3 hours.

The ratio of the emulsifying agent to crosslinking agent is at least one part by weight of emulsifying agent per part of crosslinking agent, preferably between about 4 and 20 parts by weight of emulsifying agent per part of crosslinking agent.

Suitable oil-soluble polyfunctional isocyanates include, 4,4'-diphenylmethane diisocyanate, toluene diisocyanate, hexamethylene diisocyanate, triphenylmethane triisocyanate, mixtures of such isocyanates, polyphenylene polyisocyanate (Papi), and adducts of such isocyanates with polyhydric alcohols, such as trimethylolpropane.

Example 1: (a) Preparation – 32 grams of a 3:1 molar adduct of toluene diisocyanate and trimethylolpropane are dissolved in 64 grams of a low viscosity chlorinated aliphatic hydrocarbon (known as Exchlor 4, containing 45% chlorine) and then admixed thoroughly with 800 grams of tris(2,3-dibromopropyl)phosphate (known as Fyrol HB-32). The resulting oily solution is emulsified in 3,434 grams of a 7% by weight, high molecular weight, 87% hydrolyzed, poly(vinyl alcohol) solution (known as Elvanol 50-42 G) containing 240 grams on a dry basis, in a large Waring-type blender until the emulsion droplets have an average particle size of 3 microns. The emulsion is then cured for 2 hours at 60°C to harden the capsule walls. The cooled product is diluted at a ratio of 1:3 with water and allowed to stand for 3 days.

The supernatant liquid is poured from the sediment, and the sediment is redispersed in 3 liters of fresh water and permitted to settle once again. The sediment is then spray-dried at 52% by weight solids at a temperature of 65° to 93°C to give a dry, free-flowing powder containing 85% by weight volatile oils. The dry powder comprises microcapsules having an average particle diameter of 3 microns and containing the flame retardant bis(2,3-dibromopropyl)phosphate.

(b) Incorporation into Paint — 16 grams of the microcapsules as produced in (a) are combined with 300 grams of a latex flat paint. The mixture is stirred at high shear to provide a flame retardant, water-based paint. When applied to a substrate, the paint provides an opaque, flame-resistant coating.

Example 2: (a) Preparation — Microcapsules having an average particle diameter below one micron are provided by dissolving 4 grams of the adduct of toluene diisocyanate and trimethylolpropane employed in the previous example in 45 grams of a chlorinated aliphatic hydrocarbon. The resulting solution is emulsified in 150 ml of a 7% by weight, high molecular weight, 87% hydrolyzed poly(vinyl alcohol) solution containing 0.25 gram of the surfactant, sodium lauryl sulfate (30% by weight). The resulting emulsion has a uniform particle diameter of one micron and less. The emulsion is cured for 3 hours at 60° to 70°C.

(b) Incorporation into Regenerated Cellulose Fibers — 10 grams of filter paper are treated with caustic, then with carbon disulfide, and finally dissolved in dilute caustic in order to form an aqueous solution of sodium cellulose xanthate. After suitable aging or ripening of the viscose solution, 1.5 grams of microcapsules made in the manner of (a), but containing tris(2,3-dibromopropyl)phosphate and spray-dried are dispersed in the sodium cellulose xanthate solution. The resulting mixture is filtered and then passed through a spinneret and extruded into a spinning solution containing 8 to 10% sulfuric acid, about 15% sodium sulfate, 1% zinc sulfate and about 6% glucose.

The resulting solution from the spinneret is coagulated in the bath as a filament of regenerative cellulose containing the flame retardant microcapsules. The rayon fibers are then collected and upon testing have greatly reduced flammability, while their other physical characteristics remain similar to untreated rayon.

Example 3: Production of a Urethane Foam Containing Fire Retardant Microcapules — Rigid, Freon-blown urethane foam is prepared by admixing 11.7 grams of a polyol resin component, i.e., a polypropylene glycol and 18.3 grams of polyisocyanate. This results in a rapid initiation of an exothermic reaction and production of a rigid foam.

A second batch is prepared with the same proportions, but additionally, 3 grams of the spray-dried capsules of Example 2(b) containing 85% active flame retardant are thoroughly dispersed in the resin component before admixing the resin and the isocyanate.

The resulting foam shows no impairment of physical properties due to the presence of the microcapsules. On the other hand, the untreated foam burns vigorously when ignited, while the foam containing the flame retardant microcapsules is self-extinguishing.

Chemiluminescent Warning Capsules

A method for detecting hostile troop movements in particular areas involves distributing encapsulated air-reactive chemiluminescent material in the area where detection is desirable so that when troops or the like moving across the area crush the capsules a chemiluminescent reaction will be produced.

U.S. Patent 3,850,836 discloses chemiluminescent systems made up of: (1) an organic compound selected from the group consisting of anthrahydroquinone, 2-ethylanthrahydroquinone, 2-tertiary-butylanthrahydroquinone and benzoin, (2) an oxalate ester, and (3) a fluorescer. When solutions containing these three ingredients are reacted with oxygen (from the air) in the presence of a catalyst such as sodium salicylate or tetrabutylammonium salicylate high intensity light is produced rapidly. These systems have light capacities in the range of from 30 to 50 lumen-hours/liter.

However, the use of a salicylate catalyst presents a problem in that its incorporation directly into the system tends to cause the system to decompose. It would be advantageous to omit the catalyst. However, a catalyst is necessary for rapid production of high intensity light in situations where the encapsulated material is to be used as an infiltration detection device.

According to *C.A. Heller, H.P. Richter and R.J. Marcus; U.S. Patent 4,089,797; May 16, 1978; assigned to the U.S. Secretary of the Navy* a special capsule is provided for chemiluminescent systems made up of the aforementioned materials. The capsule has a catalyst incorporated on the outer surface of its wall. Thus, the catalyst and the rest of the chemiluminescent system do not come into contact until the capsule is crushed (by infiltrating troops or the like). In this way, storage problems which are present if the catalyst is incorporated directly into the chemiluminescent solution are avoided. Glass fibers, glass beads, cracked glass or powdered glass are suitable as catalysts. Also paper fibers which have been infiltrated with one of the salicylates may be incorporated on the outer surface of the wall so that a salicylate may be used as the catalyst. The capsule is described with reference to Figure 8.6.

Figure 8.6: Chemiluminescent Warning Capsule

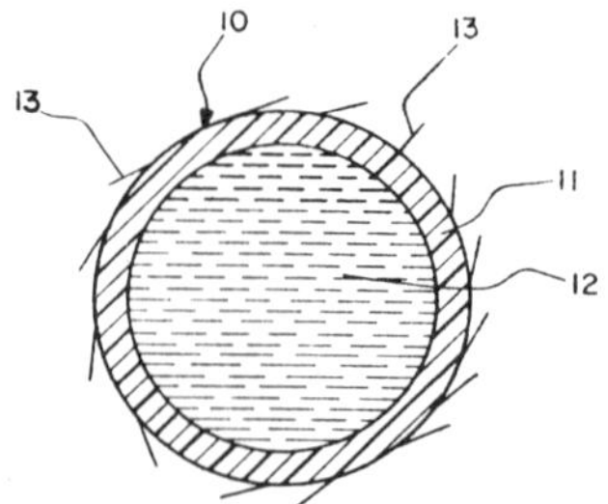

Source: U.S. Patent 4,089,797

The figure depicts, in cross section, a warning device **10** made up of a capsule **11**, a chemiluminescent system **12** within the capsule and catalytic material **13** affixed to the outside of the capsule. The capsule **11** is roughly spherical in shape (though it could have another geometrical shape if so desired) and is made of an easily crushed material which will not react with the chemiluminescent system contained within it. A mixture of paraffin wax and ethylene-vinyl acetate copolymer (75 to 95 wt % wax and 5 to 25 wt % copolymer) has been found to be suitable as a capsule material both from the standpoint of easy crushability and from the standpoint of nonreactiveness. Encapsulation of the air-reactive chemiluminescent material may be accomplished by any of the methods set forth in U.S. Patent 3,973,466.

The air-reactive chemiluminescent system **12** is made up of: (1) an organic compound selected from the group consisting of anthrahydroquinone, 2-ethylanthrahydroquinone, 2-tertiary-butylanthrahydroquinone, and 2-hydroxy-2-phenylacetophenone (benzoin), (2) an oxalate ester, and (3) a fluorescer as described in U.S. Patent 3,850,836.

Suitable oxalate esters include bis(2,3,5-trichloro-6-carbobutoxyphenyl)oxalate and bis(2,4,5-trichloro-6-carbopentoxyphenyl)oxalate. Suitable fluorescers include 9,10-bis(phenylethynyl)anthracene and rubrene. Dibutyl phthalate is a suitable solvent for the system.

Solutions of the quinone or benzoin, the oxalate ester, and the fluorescer in concentrations as utilized in U.S. Patent 3,850,836 are contemplated for this process, as well as solutions having different molar quantities of the various components. The solutions are made by dissolving the quinone or benzoin, and the oxalate ester, in a solution of the fluorescer in dibutyl phthalate.

The catalytic material **13** may be either glass alone or paper fibers which have been impregnated with a salicylate such as sodium salicylate or tetrabutylammonium salicylate. Glass may be attached in any form having a large active surface. Soda-lime, borosilicate ore and other glasses may be used.

Paper fibers may be readily impregnated with a salicylate by contacting a solution of the salicylate with the fibers and then allowing the fibers to dry. The catalyst (either glass or salicylate impregnated paper fiber) may be attached to the outer surface of a capsule in any convenient manner. For example, fibers, beads or powdered catalytic material may be attached by means of an adhesive. As another example, heated glass fibers or beads may be mixed with already formed capsules whereupon hot material coming into contact with the capsule surfaces will partially melt the surfaces and the catalytic material will be entrapped on or near the surface as the surface material flows around the catalytic material.

U.S. Patent 3,973,466 describes a method for forming capsules wherein a liquid rod of filler material is encased within a sheath of shell solution. When the rod leaves a nozzle it breaks into capsules under the force of gravity, after which the capsules are caught in a hardening bath. Catalytic material may be affixed to the surface of capsules formed in this manner by contacting the still soft capsules with the catalytic material subsequent to the time when the capsules leave the nozzle and prior to the time when the capsules enter the hardening bath.

In operation, when a device is crushed the formulation within the capsule is brought into substantially simultaneous contact with air and the catalytic material affixed to the outside of the capsule. When this occurs, high intensity light is produced rapidly. The amount of the light produced is in the range of from 30 to 50 lumen-hours/liter and the light can be readily observed by troops in almost any situation.

The mixture of paraffin wax and ethylene-vinyl acetate copolymer set forth above is a particularly desirable encapsulating agent for several reasons. First, it is not reactive with the air-reactive chemiluminescent formulation. Further, it withstands the conditions it will have to withstand if it is to be used in a warning situation well. That is, it withstands temperatures in the range of from about 0° to 40°C without deterioration and it is not soluble in water (in case of rain).

Polytetrafluoroethylene and certain polyethylenes could conceivably be used in lieu of the mixture set forth. They are also nonreactive with the chemiluminescent formulation. However, the capsules would have to be very thin-walled to provide the crushability desired.

If it is desired to insure long life once capsules have been scattered on the ground or the like to provide a warning system, it may be desirable to incorporate a brown organic dye or the like into the capsule wall. This will have the effect of filtering out sunlight during the day. Long exposure to intense sunlight tends to decompose the chemiluminescent formulations used.

Encapsulated Electron-Absorbing Substances in Tagging Technique for Identifying Oil Spills

The process of *F.H. Shair, P.G. Simmonds, R.B. Leighton and P.J. Drivas; U.S. Patent 3,964,294; June 22, 1976; assigned to California Institute of Technology* relates to coded tagging of substances for identifying the source of oil spills and slicks.

Containerized products (such as an oil tanker cargo) are tagged and coded by dispersing coded, volatile electron-absorbing substances microencapsulated in microspheroids throughout the oil tanker cargo to be regulated. A sample of the coded cargo such as an oil spill is collected and the source of the cargo and the identity of the polluter is determined by electron capture gas chromatographic detection of the coded, electron-absorbing substances.

The encapsulation of the electron-absorbing tag protects the tag from evaporation, oxidation, microbial attack, etc. By removing many restrictions heretofore deemed necessary for electron-absorbing coded compounds such as the halogenated aromatic tagging system, only very small amounts, on the order of a pound of coded microcapsules would be needed to label a 500,000 ton tanker. The average cost of such a tag including microcapsulation would be below $15 per pound. The cost of the laboratory equipment is not high. The use of microencapsulated tags permits the use of more volatile compounds which significantly aids the analysis. There are many such compounds suitable for use such as halogenated, aliphatic compounds. With only 10 compounds, there can be 10^6 different and distinct tags available for microcapsules containing up to six different compounds in varied and carefully controlled relative amounts. Further variation in distinction can be provided by the use of 10 separate particle sizes which would further permit up to 10^7 different and distinct tags.

Since detection of the tag can be performed after it has been physically removed from the oil slick sample, no interference of the oil slick is possible. Thus, the final chromatogram will show those, and only those peaks associated with the tag. The forensic record would be conclusive and limited to the reliable information actually needed for the identification of the source, for example, six peaks, particle size and potentially the character of the encapsulating material. This type of data can be readily comprehended by laymen. At least three levels of redundancy can be built into the tagging system through the use of particle size, density, encapsulating coating and electron-absorbing compounds.

Positive identification of the tag can be obtained and recorded in less than one hour after the sample has been collected. The detection technique is so sensitive that only one particle is actually needed to provide the identification. Thus, even if 90% of the particles were lost in some manner, the volume of oil slick sample needed to provide identification would still be less than 10 cm^3. By using volatile compounds for the tag and an encapsulating material that would slowly decompose over an extended period, for example, a few years, buildup on the ocean surface could be completely avoided.

The electron-capture (EC) detector is a substance-specific device. It is extremely sensitive to any molecular species which reacts with free electrons to form stable negative ions. The tag molecules are certain types containing electron-absorbing atoms or groups, such as halogens, carbonyl, nitro groups, or certain condensed ring atomatics. The EC detector has very low sensitivity for hydrocarbons other than fused ring aromatics and very importantly the detector is extremely sensitive to halogen atoms. It can reliably detect halogenated hydrocarbons in quantities as low as 10^{-10} to 10^{-12} gram and under optimized conditions 10^{-14} gram has been detected.

Compounds which strongly capture the electrons have one or more of the following electrophore structures or substituents in their molecules: (1) –COCO–, (2)–COCH=CHCO–, (3) the quinone structure, (4) $-NO_2$ and (5) –X where X is halogen. With substitution, the halogen affinities fall in the order $I > Br > Cl > F$. Multiple substitution by halogen or nitro groups more than linearly enhances the affinity for electrons. It appears that –CO in the electrophores listed above can be replaced by a phenyl group without great loss of affinity. Similarly, nitrogen can be substituted for carbon.

SF_6 and its telomers are a series of compounds very suitable for use as active tags in the system. The homologous telomers of the formula $SF_5(CF_2)_nZ$ where n is an integer from 0 to 25 and Z is F, Br or I give very high responses. With only 10 of these compounds there can be 10^6 distinctly distinguishable tagging permutations for microcapsules containing up to 6 compounds in controlled quantities. These compounds further satisfy the design criteria since they are not normally present in crude oil. Moreover, they exhibit a substantial vapor pressure at room temperature.

The coded compounds are encapsulated in microcapsules by state of the art techniques. The microcapsules are preferably smooth spheroids of well classified particle sizes so as to be able to further identify the particles by microscopic inspection or particle size analysis. Suitably the capsules are formed from an organic synthetic polymer having low solubility in the liquid tagged material and having low permeability to the volatile code material. A suitable encapsulating material for the halogenated aliphatic telomers is a urea-formaldehyde copolymer. If the permeability is suitably adjusted the volatile tag compounds can escape to the atmosphere over a period of several months and thus avoid buildup of the halogenated code compounds on the surface of the ocean. The wall thickness may vary over wide ranges but is suitably about 0.5 to 2 μ so as to be sufficient to encapsulate the code material yet allow crushing by ordinary force to release the volatile coding material for analysis. The microcapsule particles should range in size from about 5 to 500 microns in diameter.

An index of codes is prepared and each code is assigned an identification number. When the code is added to the cargo, the identity of the transporting vessel, shipper, ports of call and route are recorded. When an oil spill is sampled and analyzed, the index will be able to absolutely identify the source of pollution. It would be preferable to maintain the regulation of the index and addition of the code by government authority, whether of national or international jurisdiction to avoid duplication of codes and to assure that each and every cargo is appropriately labeled. It is also possible that some companies or an industry would adapt and implement the system on a voluntary basis to be able to avoid false accusation of pollution.

Apart from the type of material used for tagging, codes and tagging profiles will be involved in the system. Oil shipped into one port will be mixed upon unloading with oil from other tankers and hence the stored oil with its mixture of tagging codes will have its own unique tagging profile at a given time. Oil subsequently loaded onto a tanker will be retagged by the unique code assigned to the tanker. Thus, the retagged oil has a new tagging profile whose dominant code will be that of the tanker that last tagged the oil. As a result, any oil or oil slick from a tanker will have an underlying tag noise with a superimposed tanker code. To identify the source-last jurisdiction-of the oil not only must the individual tags be identified but also the relative abundance of each tag.

Encapsulating Individual Fibrils of Chrysotile Asbestos

M. Xanthos and R.T. Woodhams; U.S. Patent 3,965,284; June 22, 1976; assigned to Canadian Patents and Development Limited, Canada found that chrysotile asbestos is chemically opened into the individual fibrils by soluble vinylic polymer polyelectrolytes containing carboxylic acid groups in aqueous media.

Polyacrylic acids, polymethacrylic acid, maleic anhydride polymer and water-soluble copolymers thereof are preferred polyelectrolytes and form stable colloidal dispersions. The polyelectrolytes are neutralized to alkaline pH with inorganic or organic bases, but preferably with basic vinylic monomers when complete encapsulation is desired. The polyelectrolyte-coated fibrils in aqueous dispersion are encapsulated by copolymerization with (a) a basic vinylic comonomer (used for pH control) such as dimethylaminoethyl methacrylate, tert-butylaminoethyl methacrylate or a vinylpyridine; and (b) a nonbasic vinylic comonomer such as styrene, divinylbenzene, vinyl chloride or fluoride, vinyl acetate, methyl methacrylate, ethyl acrylate, acrylonitrile and methacrylonitrile.

Example: (a) 3 grams chrysotile asbestos, grade Plastibest No. 20 were added to 300 cc of a 0.3% aqueous polyacrylic acid solution (known as Acrysol A-3) and the mixture was agitated for 3 minutes at low speed in a Waring Blendor. 1.96 grams dimethylaminoethyl methacrylate were then added dropwise to pH 8 and stirring was continued at high speed for a total period of 10 minutes. A stable dispersion of colloidal chrysotile (average diameter 500 A) was produced. 5.88 grams styrene containing 0.5% azobisisobutyronitrile (AIBN) were then added. After 16 hours at 60°C, completely coated asbestos fibers precipitated. The material was then filtered, dried and molded to give excellent translucent specimens. The asbestos content of the encapsulated material, determined by ashing, was found to be 27.8% by weight, in good agreement with the feed composition.

(b) The same procedure was repeated as in (a), but in this case methyl methacrylate was used instead of styrene. A very desirable product was obtained.

Photomicrographs of (a) at magnification of 6,340 show individual fibrils opened and dispersed with polyacrylic acid and completely coated with copolymer formed in situ from styrene/dimethylaminoethyl methacrylate (3/1) using AIBN initiator.

Photomicrographs of (b) at magnification of 7,940 show that the fibrils were opened and dispersed with polyacrylic acid, and coated with copolymer formed from methyl methacrylate/dimethylaminoethyl methacrylate (3/1) and AIBN initiator. In both (a) and (b) the polymer is seen to completely encapsulate and adhere to the individual fibrils.

Encapsulated asbestos fibrils may be partially fused into sheets, tubes, or other shapes to be used as porous filter webs of extreme fineness such that only the finest particles may pass through the reticulated structure. The type of polymeric encapsulation may be selected to resist acids or bases, or other corrosive environments which would normally destroy the asbestos. Solvent-resistant sheaths may be provided using acrylonitrile copolymers as the encapsulating material. It is apparent that only a continuous coating would provide a coherent network, and that encapsulation must be essentially complete. The individual coated fibrils may be fused or joined together at their crossover points by the mild application of heat and pressure.

Ferrocene Encapsulated in a Urea-Formaldehyde Polymer Shell

S. Wojciak; U.S. Patent 4,093,556; June 6, 1978; assigned to Loctite Corporation describes a process for producing metallocenes encapsulated by a urea-formaldehyde polymer shell. The presence of a small amount of a cationic surfactant, preferably an alkyl hydroxy amine, is required during the condensation polymerization which forms the shell.

The metallocenes comprise a fairly common class of organo-metal compounds having the formula $(C_5H_5)_2M$, wherein M is a metal having a bonding capacity of at least 2. These compounds find use in a variety of ways, e.g., catalysis, synthetic intermediates, antiknock additives, etc. Of the metallocenes, perhaps the most useful and the preferred one is ferrocene, also known as dicyclopentadienyl iron. In addition to its other known uses, this material has been found useful as an accelerator for the cure of anaerobic adhesive and sealant compositions, such as those described in U.S. Patent 3,855,040. Encapsulation of such a ferrocene accelerator permits its use in mixture with microencapsulated anerobic materials to provide highly desirable, rapid curing anaerobic adhesive systems.

The process for microencapsulating a water-insoluble metallocene, a water-insoluble metallocene ion, or water-insoluble metallocene derivatives (e.g., polymers), or mixtures thereof, comprises:

(a) providing an aqueous solution of a water-soluble precondensate of urea and formaldehyde wherein the precondensate concentration is about 15 to 50% by weight;

(b) adding to this precondensate solution a particulate metallocene in such amount that the weight ratio of metallocene to precondensate is between 1:1 and 8:1;

(c) adding to the precondensate solution or the mixture of precondensate solution with metallocene a cationic surfactant in such amount that the weight ratio of surfactant to metallocene is between 1:6,000 and 1:10;

(d) forming a slurry of the metallocene;

(e) adjusting the pH of the resultant dispersion to about 1 to 6.5 by addition of a water-soluble acid, thereby causing polymerization of the precondensate; and

(f) continuing the polymerization in the temperature range of about 15° to 80°C for at least 1 hour, i.e., until the metallocene particles are encapsulated with a shell of water-insoluble urea-formaldehyde polymer.

The ratio of urea to formaldehyde will be in the range of 0.9:1 to 1.8:1 by weight (preferably 1.1:1 to 1.5:1 by weight). It is preferred that the formaldehyde be used in the form of a 37% by weight aqueous solution known as formalin since this is readily commercially available.

Example: A mixture of 488.5 grams of a 37% by weight aqueous formaldehyde solution and 240 grams of urea was stirred and heated at 70°C for 1 hour. The pH was adjusted to 8 with triethanolamine. One liter of water was added and the precondensate solution thus formed was allowed to cool to room temperature.

To 150 ml of the above precondensate solution at room temperature were added, with good stirring, 50 grams of ferrocene. To this was added 1 ml of a 1% by weight solution of Priminox T-1M in styrene and the mixture was stirred well. The pH was adjusted to 2.5 with a 10% by weight aqueous solution of citric acid. The reaction was allowed to proceed at room temperature, with good stirring, for about 50 minutes, at which time the mixture was thinned by addition of 50 ml of water.

The reaction was continued for an additional 6 hours at room temperature, at which time 600 ml of water were added. The microencapsulated ferrocene thus formed was separated by filtration, was washed thoroughly with water, and the microcapsules were dried in an oven at low heat.

The microcapsules showed no sign of leakage during prolonged storage and were sufficiently durable to withstand normal handling but could be readily crushed upon application of localized pressure to release the ferrocene.

Light Reflective Dye-Containing Capsules for Photographic Film Unit

The process of *W.J. McCune, Jr.; U.S. Patent 4,137,194; January 30, 1979; assigned to Polaroid Corporation* relates to capsules adapted to retain solid and fluid materials and to the use of such capsules in photographic color processes for forming monochromatic and multichromatic images and to photographic products for carrying out the processes.

The process utilizes minute capsules for forming color images by transfer techniques wherein an imagewise distribution of one or more color-providing substances is formed in unexposed parts of a negative photosensitive element having one or more light-sensitive portions having silver halide therein and transferred to an image-receiving element, and wherein the imagewise distribution of each color-providing substance so transferred by imbibition and deposited upon the image-receiving element arranged in superposed relation to the negative photosensitive element colors the image-receiving element a predetermined color to provide therein a monochromatic or multichromatic image comprising one or more positive images of negative latent color images formed by the exposure of the photosensitive element.

The photosensitive element, usable in a color process comprises a support, one or more light-sensitive portions comprising a silver halide emulsion, capsules containing at least a predetermined color-providing substance, such as a dye which is capable of coupling with an oxidized silver halide developer or a dye which is itself a silver halide developer, associated with each light-sensitive portion, the color-providing substance employed adapted to be transferred at least in part to an image-receiving element for coloring the image-receiving element, the capsules having a light-reflecting coating for increasing the effective emulsion speed of the photosensitive element.

In the process there are provided capsules having the outer surfaces or walls thereof coated with a thin continuous film or layer of a metal such as, for example, aluminum or other material, for example, polymeric fluorocarbons which increase the impermeability of the capsule wall without at the same time (a) appreciably increasing the wall thickness or capsule size, (b) appreciably modifying the rupture or release characteristics of the capsule wall, and (c) undesirably modifying the wall-to-fill ratio. The thin continuous coating may be applied to any one of several methods such as, for example, spraying, electroplating, vapor deposition and the like.

The minute capsules of this process may be formed of film-forming polymeric material of a hydrophilic nature or character such as gelatin, or they may be formed of film-forming polymeric material of a hydrophobic nature such as polyvinyl chloride. Each capsule consists of a nucleus comprising, for example, a solid or substantially solid material, e.g., magnetic iron oxide or a fluid material, e.g., a color-providing substance in solution or dispersed in a suitable medium around which has been deposited a dense shell-like coating of film-forming polymeric material which may be pressure-rupturable.

The encapsulating material selected in any specific instance depends upon the encapsulating process employed and the particular material to be encased therewithin. The capsules may be formed by well-known methods.

The permeability of fluids through the capsule walls may be decreased by providing the outer wall or surface of the capsules with a thin continuous coating of suitable material, preferably a metal such as, for example, aluminum. One process for coating each capsule with a thin continuous film or layer of a metal or metal-bearing compound, e.g., metal oxide, or other material, e.g., Teflon, involves vacuum deposition. The step of vacuum depositing may involve either thermally evaporating or cathode sputtering at pressures below about 100 microns of mercury and usually within the range of from 0.1 to 100 microns of mercury and depositing the vaporized material as a thin continuous coating upon the outer wall of the capsules.

When the vacuum deposition is effected by thermal evaporation, pressures below 10 microns are usually employed. The temperature employed, in any case, is dependent upon the material being evaporated and pressure. When the vacuum deposition is effected by cathode sputtering, voltages of the order of 5 to 10 kilowatts and pressures of from 10 to 20 microns of mercury are common.

Among the large number of metals or metallic materials capable of being vacuum deposited upon the outermost surfaces of capsules are aluminum, silver, zinc, magnesium, cadmium, chromium, cobalt, copper, gold, nickel, iron, tin, platinum and palladium. Metal oxides such as aluminum oxide, tin oxide and other metal-containing compounds may also be employed as the capsule coating. Organic materials such as certain polymeric materials, e.g., Teflon, may also be vacuum deposited upon the capsules.

The thickness of the vacuum-deposited coating may be varied or controlled, suitable thicknesses generally being within the range of 0.1 to 1 micron. Thicker coatings, for example, between 1 and 10 microns may be deposited especially when maximum impermeability is desired. The capsule wall coating may comprise one or more materials. For instance, the coating may comprise a single metal or an alloy or it may comprise two or more distinct layers of different metals such as, for example, a first layer comprising copper and a second layer overcoated on the first layer comprising aluminum.

The process is described with reference to Figure 8.7. Figures 8.7a and 8.7b illustrate an apparatus for evaporating a material **20** onto capsules **22**. Material **20**, for example, is a metal in the form of a coating upon a wire gauze. Capsules **22** are contained within a cylindrical glass jar **24**, one end of which is closed at **26** and the other end of which is provided with an open mouth **28**. Gauze **20** is supported by a mounting arm **30** extending through mouth **28** and carried by a standard **32**. Jar **24** rests upon a pair of rollers **34** and **36**, the ends of which are journaled in bearing mounts **38** and **40**. A motor **42** is provided for rotating rollers **34** and **36** through gearing **37** in order to cause rotation of jar **24**, which is prevented from moving longitudinally by circular flanges **44** at the ends of the rollers. As shown, electrical leads **46** and **48** are connected to the opposite extremities of gauze **20** in order to transmit a suitable electric current through the gauze from a power supply (not shown). In operation, a sufficient current is transmitted by leads **46** and **48** through gauze **20** for generating sufficient heat to cause rapid evaporation of the coating of gauze **20**. At the same time, motor **42** causes causes rotation of rollers **34** and **36** so that capsules **22** are continuously agitated by movement of the inner surfaces of jar **24** as well as a plurality of ribs **50** projecting inwardly from the inner surfaces of the jar. The apparatus, including jar **24**, is mounted on a base plate **52** and enclosed by such means as a glass cylinder **54** and a cover plate **56**. O-ring gaskets **57** hermetically seal glass cylinder **54** between base plate **52** and cover plate **56**. A pump (not shown) continuously exhausts the region defined by base plate **52**, glass cylinder **54** and cover plate **56** through a conduit **60**. Capsules **22**, as a result, become coated with a thin continuous coating of the metal which initially was part of gauze **20**.

Figure 8.7: Photographic Film Unit

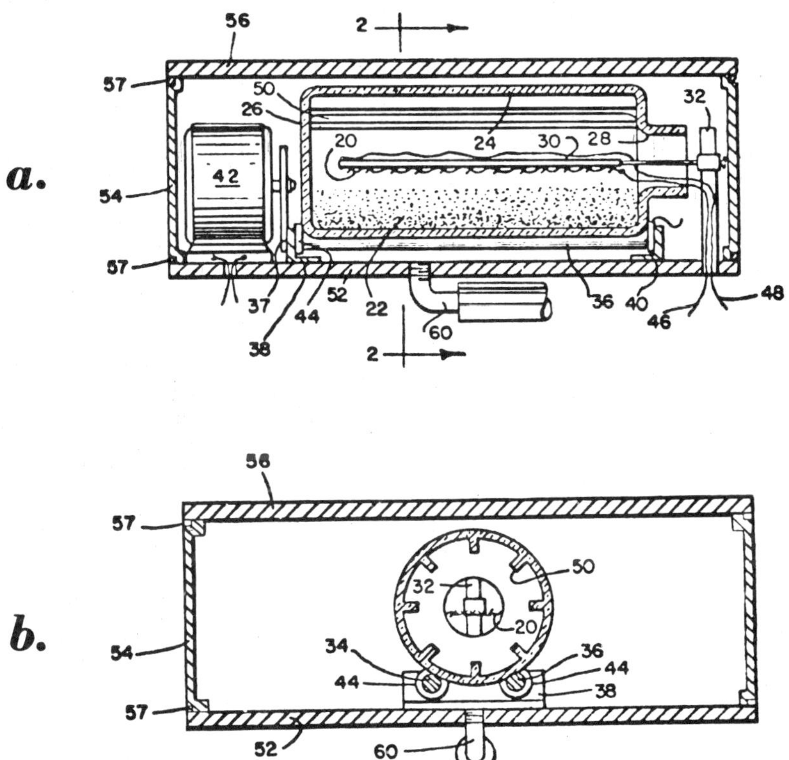

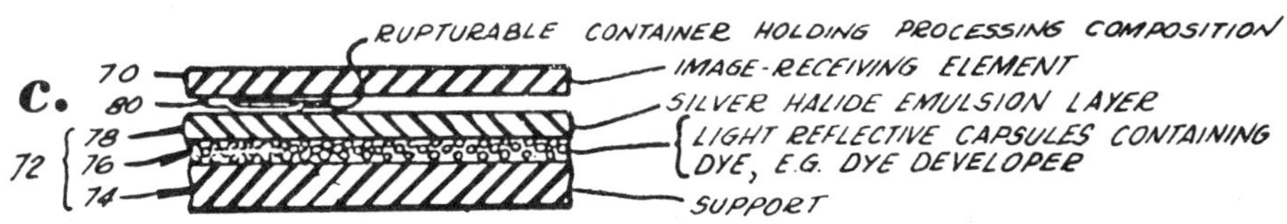

(continued)

Figure 8.7: (continued)

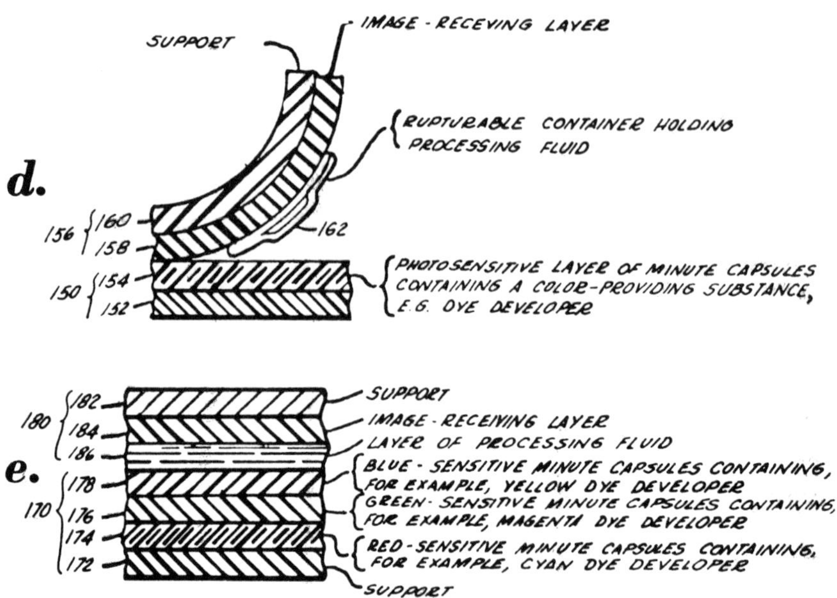

(a) Side view of apparatus for thermal evaporation process for coating capsule with metallic film
(b) Cross section along line **2–2** of Figure 8.7a
(c) Film unit for one step photographic process
(d) Photographic film unit for monochromatic images
(e) Photographic film unit for multicolor images

Source: U.S. Patent 4,137,194

A photographic film unit or assembly useful in carrying out a one-step photographic process for the formation of an image of an individual color is illustrated in Figure 8.7c. This makes use of a positive sheet material or image-receiving element **70** comprising an image-receiving layer of opaque or transparent material which is liquid-permeable and dyeable from alkaline solutions and which has been illustrated for the purposes of simplicity as a single sheet of paper. However, the positive element **70** may comprise a support upon which at least one liquid-permeable and dyeable layer is mounted.

The film unit also employs a negative sheet material or photosensitive element **72** comprising a support **74** of paper or film base material upon which there is mounted, in the order or sequence named, a layer **76** comprising a profusion of minute capsules in substantial continuity, the capsules containing a dye such as a dye developer and having the outer surfaces thereof provided with a thin, light-reflecting coating and a conventional photosensitive layer **78** of silver halide. The use of a reflecting layer behind a silver halide emulsion layer but in front of a dye layer makes available otherwise wasted light for absorption by the emulsion while minimizing the absorption by the dye of light needed for exposure.

The photosensitive element **72** and the image-receiving element **70**, for the purpose of positive image formation, are adapted to be placed in superposed relation and are arranged so that the photosensitive layer or stratum **78** is next to the image-receiving element **70**.

A rupturable container **80**, adapted to carry an alkaline solution or liquid processing composition, is shown positioned transversely of and adhered to the image-receiving element **70**. Container **80** is of a length approximating the width of the film unit and is constructed to carry sufficient liquid to effect negative image formation in an exposed image area of the photosensitive layer **78** and positive image formation in the corresponding image area of image-receiving element **70**. In use, the container **80** is adapted to be positioned between the image-receiving element and the photosensitive element so that it will be adjacent the edges of the corresponding image areas of these elements which are to be processed by the liquid contents of the container. When the film unit is of the roll film type, a plurality of containers are employed, one for each corresponding pair of successive image areas in the photosensitive and image-receiving elements.

The photosensitive silver halide layer used is provided by silver halide emulsions of the conventional character and is coated onto layer **76** after the latter has dried. Emulsions of suitable sensitivity range are chosen to meet the particular requirements of use to which the photosensitive element will be put. The silver halide is in all instances used in a water- and alkali-permeable carrier material such as gelatin, although other water- and alkali-permeable materials known to the art may be substituted.

The image-receiving material of the positive element **70** includes any material dyeable by the dyes employed, preferably from alkaline liquid. The positive element **70** may, as shown, comprise a single sheet of permeable material or it may comprise a support which carries a layer or a stratum of a permeable image-receiving material. An example of such is imbibition paper or baryta paper or conventional film base material upon which a permeable stratum is coated.

A photographic film unit or assembly useful in carrying out a one-step photographic process for the formation of an image of an individual color is illustrated in Figure 8.7d as comprising a photosensitive element **150**, a print-receiving element **156** and a rupturable container **162** for holding a liquid processing fluid or composition.

The photosensitive element **150** comprises a conventional paper or plastic film base or support **152** and a photosensitive layer **154** comprising, in substantial contiguity, a profusion of minute capsules of alkali-permeable film-forming polymeric material coated with silver halide appropriately sensitized, the capsules containing a color-providing substance such as a dye developer.

The photosensitive element **150** is shown in a spread-apart relationship with an image-receiving element **156** having mounted thereon a rupturable container **162** holding a processing composition. The image receiving element **156** comprises a dyeable material and may comprise a single image-receiving layer or, as shown, an image-receiving layer **158** carried by a support **160**.

After exposure, the image-receiving element **156** is brought into superposed relationship with the photosensitive element **150**, and the rupturable container **162** is ruptured by application of suitable pressure, e.g., by advancing between a pair of rollers (not shown); and a layer of the liquid processing composition is spread between the superposed elements. The processing composition permeates into the capsular photosensitized layer **154** to initiate development of the the latent image in the exposed silver halide regions.

In exposed silver halide areas, the dye developer, for example, carried by the capsules, will be reacted and become immobilized. In unexposed areas, the dye developer will be mobile and will diffuse to the superposed image-receiving element **156**. After a suitable imbibition period, the photosensitive element **150** and the image-receiving element **156** are separated to reveal the positive colored image.

Multicolor images may be obtained using dye developers in diffusion-transfer reversal processes by several techniques. One such process for obtaining multicolor transfer images utilizing dye developers employs an integral multilayer photosensitive element wherein at least two selectively sensitized photosensitive layers are superposed on a single support and are processed simultaneously and without separation, with a single common image-receiving layer.

A suitable arrangement of this type comprises a support carrying a red-sensitive silver halide layer, a green-sensitive silver halide layer and a blue-sensitive silver halide layer, the layers having associated therewith, respectively, a cyan dye developer, a magenta dye developer and a yellow dye developer. Each dye developer is encapsulated within minute capsules of alkali-permeable polymeric materials, the outermost walls of the capsules being suitably sensitized with silver halide. A multilayer photosensitive element of the type just described is illustrated in Figure 8.7e.

COMPANY INDEX

INVENTOR INDEX

U.S. PATENT NUMBER INDEX

NOTICE

Nothing contained in this Review shall be construed to constitute a permission or recommendation to practice any invention covered by any patent without a license from the patent owners. Further, neither the author nor the publisher assumes any liability with respect to the use of, or for damages resulting from the use of, any information, apparatus, method or process described in this Review.